Small Animal Microbiomes and Nutrition

# Small Animal Microbiomes and Nutrition

*Robin Saar*
RAS4Pets
Lethbridge
AB, Canada

*Sarah Dodd*
University of Guelph
Garafraxa
ON, Canada

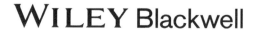

*Library of Congress Cataloging-in-Publication Data*
Names: Saar, Robin, author. | Dodd, Sarah (Veterinary nutritionist) author.
Title: Small animal microbiomes and nutrition / Robin Saar, Dr. Sarah Dodd.
Description: Hoboken, NJ : Wiley-Blackwell, 2024. | Includes bibliographical references and index.
Identifiers: LCCN 2023002572 (print) | LCCN 2023002573 (ebook) | ISBN 9781119862604 (paperback) | ISBN 9781119862635 (adobe pdf) | ISBN 9781119862628 (epub) | ISBN 9781119862611 (obook)
Subjects: MESH: Animal Nutritional Physiological Phenomena | Pets–physiology | Microbiota
Classification: LCC SF414 (print) | LCC SF414 (ebook) | NLM SF 414 | DDC 636.089/32–dc23/eng/20230523
LC record available at https://lccn.loc.gov/2023002572
LC ebook record available at https://lccn.loc.gov/2023002573

Cover Design: Wiley
Cover Images: Courtesy of Robin Saar

Set in 9.5/12.5pt STIXTwoText by Straive, Pondicherry, India
SKY10052543_080723

# Contents

# Preface

Microorganisms coexist in communities everywhere, soil, plants, oceans, and as a part of animals' physiological systems. What is interesting is the essential and intrinsic roles the microbiota in these communities play in the health and function of the environment in which they reside. Researchers in the field now recognize the gut microbiome as a super organ in the body as it completes or assists in multiple normal physiological and metabolic processes. This super organ influences and co-functions within the body of animals, and we are just starting to peel away the layers of how the microbiota influence animal health.

Nutrition has historically taken a back seat in veterinary education and client conversations. Recently, pressure from pet parents to receive our recommendations and guidance on the best nutrition for their pets has invigorated the nutrition education sector. Nutrition goes hand in hand with the gut microbiome; nutrients not absorbed in the small intestine continue to the large intestine and undergo microbial fermentation. The results of these interactions influence both microbial and host health. Currently, we design diets to meet the pet's nutritional needs and rarely consider the health of the gut microbes or the resulting influence when formulating a diet. Nutritional knowledge, diet varieties, and pet parent willingness to participate in their pet's health has also increased in the last decade, evoking the need for veterinary professionals to evolve how they practice nutritional medicine and engage with pet parents.

This textbook's final chapters review basic nutritional math equations, practical tips, and best practices when communicating with pet parents. In my experience, communication with pet parents is the most substantial skill a veterinary professional must master to be successful.

While there is a growing aggregate of research papers in this field of study, a textbook providing an all-encompassing practical guide for all veterinary professionals did not exist, until now. Microbiome medicine is not part of veterinary or veterinary technology curricula to the extent that it should be. I wanted to provide a practical guide that would review the normal physiological processes in such a manner that anyone with a basic understanding of animal physiology could comprehend and create a practical application within a veterinary practice. While we need further research in this vast field, and I acknowledge that a few of these concepts require a deeper dive, I feel that this format will provide an introductory learning platform about microbiomes in dogs and cats. This topic is in its infancy, and I am excited to provide vet professionals with an introductory textbook on small animal microbiomes and nutrition.

Finally, I acknowledge Dr. Holly Ganz, Dr. Dawn Kinsbury who wrote chapters 5 and 6 and Nicole Stevens and Andrew Abernathy who added figures and tables.

# About the Companion Website

This book is accompanied by a companion website.

**www.wiley.com/go/saar/1e**

This website includes chapter 26.

# Section I

# Understanding a Microbiome

# 1

# Common Definitions

## 1.1 Microbiome

There are multiple functional definitions of the term "microbiome." According to the Human Microbiome Consortium, the microbiome is considered as the community of all microbes recovered from a particular habitat or ecosystem [1]. These microscopic communities, including bacteria, fungi, and viruses, can be found in all living things, including plants, and are found in every different imaginable habitat, from life-forms to soils and bodies of water [2, 3]. Microbiomes can be found on outer surfaces, particularly as biofilms, and within several body systems of animals including the respiratory tract, reproductive organs, integumentary, oral cavity, urinary tract, neurological pathways via the brain-gut axis, and the gastrointestinal (GI) tract. Over 30 trillion microbes may reside within the GI system alone [4, 5]. This list is not exhaustive, as this area of knowledge is relatively novel, and innovations allow us to discover microbiomes in organs and systems once thought to be sterile. The total cumulative microbiomes in a human host may weigh as much as 1–3% body mass [4].

While some common trends are being observed in current research, microbiomes are unique for each individual with their diversity and density affected by several intrinsic (genetics, age, sex) and extrinsic (environment, physiological state, antibiotic therapy, health and nutrition) factors [6]. These incredibly diverse communities shape the health of the host and influence its physiology, through multiple complex

*Small Animal Microbiomes and Nutrition*, First Edition. Robin Saar and Sarah Dodd.
© 2024 John Wiley & Sons, Inc. Published 2024 by John Wiley & Sons, Inc.
Companion website: www.wiley.com/go/saar/1e

pathways, including influencing remote organ and immune responses. A main focus of research is on the microbiomes of the GI tract, and how perturbations of these complex communities are associated with multiple health conditions in humans: depression, autism spectrum disorder, oral health, chronic obstructive pulmonary disease (COPD), asthma, pneumonia, dermatological, obesity, cardiovascular, diabetes, rheumatoid arthritis, hepatic associated disorders, cancer, inflammatory bowel disease (IBD), and infection due to bacterial translocation [4–7]. Microbiome communities affect the status of, and rely on, each other for daily functions, communicating through the release of metabolites – products of microbial fermentation [8]. One recognized influence is the cumulative genetic material, the metagenome, of all the microbes in one animal's singular microbiome. A metagenome may contain over 200 times the number of genes in a host's genome; therefore, the level of influence these genes have over host gene expression is one explanation for the microbiota influence on the host's physiological systems [8].

The development of new innovative research tools allows us to see, understand, and evaluate previously unidentifiable concepts regarding the body's microbiomes. Some obstacles that remain with identifying and determining the effects of microbiomes are reproducing their environment, including food sources, to enhance growth and preventing the death of the microbes when sampling. Research is also limited at this time, with many research projects utilizing small study groups, which are not always representative of the wider population, or reproducible in future projects. This is a common limitation for quantitative research [9].

## 1.2 Microbiota

The microbiota may be defined as the individual bacteria, fungi, viruses, and protozoa that can be found in a microbiome community. Microbes pre-date the Earth's eukaryotic biodiversity and are numerous, diverse, and ubiquitous. They have adapted to live in extreme environments such as the high pressure, as in the deep ocean, extreme heat, or chemical exposure. Different types of bacteria survive in both aerobic and/or anaerobic environments. Environmental differences are one reason that it has been difficult to identify microbiota in discovered and undiscovered communities [8]. Those that live in an anaerobic environment may have a shorter survival rate when removed, for example in biopsy samples, and then brought into an aerobic environment. It is estimated that only 20–30% of organisms are culturable, which leaves a large group of microbiota that are unidentified through routine culture [10]. The main phyla composing the gut microbiome vary from species to species, but *Fusobacteria, Bacteroidetes,* and *Firmicutes,* as well as, to a lesser extent, *Proteobacteria* and *Actinobacteria,* are typically prevalent in dogs and cats [3, 11].

Communication occurs between the microbes within their microbiome and with host body systems, which in turn can change or influence the physiology of the host. The host relies on the microbiota to complete functions that may not be encoded in their genes to complete [5]. The roles of microbiota are complex and may change as resource availabilities change [8]. Currently, we understand that microbiota plays roles in the production of vitamins, mineral absorption, structural integrity of barriers, metabolism of nondigestible products and provision of energy sources (short-chain fatty acids – SCFAs), interactions with or involved in the production of chemical and neurotransmitter metabolites affecting other organs of the body (bidirectional axis), host genomic expression, inflammatory processes, intestinal permeability, immune function, and food intake and energy expenditure [4, 6, 8, 11–16].

## 1.3 Pathogens

Pathogens are defined as a biological agent that causes disease or illness to its host. Although in the minority, these microbes are generally known to cause illness, at least in certain circumstances. Pathogens can be divided into five groups: viruses, bacteria, fungi, protozoa, and helminths [17]. Characteristics of pathogens are the mode of transmission, mechanism of replication, pathogenesis (how it causes diseases), and ability to elicit a response. Depending on the pathogen, replication may occur in the intracellular and/or extracellular compartments, while host defense mechanisms work to destroy the pathogen and stop its growth. Common canine and feline pathogens are summarized by group in Table 1.1.

Pathobionts are commensal microbes that can be present at low levels in healthy microbiomes without causing harm to the host but can be pathogenic under certain circumstances [10]. While a general previous

**Table 1.1** Common canine and feline pathogens.

| Common causes of disease in dogs and cats | | | |
| --- | --- | --- | --- |
| Viruses | DNA viruses | Adenoviruses | Canine adenoviruses |
| | | Herpesviruses | Canine herpesvirus |
| | | | Feline herpesvirus |
| | | Parvoviruses | Canine parvovirus |
| | | | Feline panleukopenia virus |
| | RNA viruses | Orthomyxoviruses | Canine influenza |
| | | Paramyxoviruses | Canine distemper virus |
| | | | Canine parainfluenza virus |
| | | Coronaviruses | Canine respiratory coronavirus |
| | | | Feline enteric coronavirus |
| | | Picornaviruses | Feline calicivirus |
| | | Rhabdoviruses | Rabies |
| | | Retroviruses | Feline leukemia virus |
| | | | Feline immunodeficiency virus |
| Bacteria | Gram +ve cocci | Staphylococci | *Staphylococcus* spp. |
| | | Streptococci | *Streptococcus* spp. |
| | Gram −ve cocci | | *Bartonella henselae* |
| | Gram +ve bacilli | | *Corynebacteria* |
| | | | *Bacillus anthracis* |
| | | | *Listeria monocytogenes* |
| | Gram −ve bacilli | | *Bordetella bronchiseptica* |
| | | | *Yersinia pestis* |
| | Anaerobes | Clostridia | *Clostridia* spp. |
| | Spirochetes | | *Borrelia burgdorferi* |
| | | | *Leptospira interrogans* |
| | Rickettsials | | *Ehrlichia canis* |
| | | | *Anaplasma* spp. |

**Table 1.1** (Continued)

**Common causes of disease in dogs and cats**

| | | |
|---|---|---|
| | Chlamydias | *Chlamydophila felis* |
| | Mycoplasmas | *Mycoplasma haemocanis* |
| | | *Mycoplasma felis* |
| Fungi | | *Candida albicans* |
| | | *Cryptococcus neoformans* |
| | | *Aspergillus* |
| | | *Histoplasma capsulatum* |
| | | *Coccidioides immitis* |
| Protozoa | | *Giardia* spp. |
| | | *Leishmania* |
| | | *Babesia* spp. |
| | | *Hepatozoon canis* |
| | | *Cystoisospra* |
| | | *Cryptosporidium* |
| | | *Toxoplasma gondii* |
| Helminths (worms) | Nematodes (roundworms) | *Dirofilaria immitis* |
| | | *Toxocara* spp. |
| | | *Toxascaris leonina* |
| | | *Uncinaria stenocephala* |
| | | *Trichuris vulpis* |
| | | *Ancylostoma* spp. |
| | | *Capillaria* spp. |
| | Cestodes (tapeworms) | *Taenia* spp. |
| | | *Echinococcus* spp. |
| | | *Sarcocystis* |

*Source:* Adapted from Alexander et al. [18], Inpankaew et al. [19], Day et al. [20], Riley et al. [21], Millán and Rodriíguez [22], Biek et al. [23] and Villeneuve et al. [24].

concept was a simple overgrowth of a pathogenic bacteria was the cause of dysbiosis, new information shows that a barrier dysfunction plays a larger role in pathogenic bacteria being allowed to either colonize or translocate (cross the surface of an epithelial barrier) causing illness in the host [10, 17]. In some circumstances, it may be a combination of genetics along with the presence of specific microbiota or metabolites that lead to disease or illness in the host. The immune response cannot eliminate most pathogens, and most pathogens are not universally lethal as this would affect the long-term survival of that pathogen [17]. However, some pathogens may cause an attack on the immune response that can affect other microbiomes in the body and may be detrimental for the host [25, 26].

## 1.4 Symbiosis

Symbiosis describes a relationship or interaction between two organisms of different types, and the specific classification of symbiosis depends on whether either or both organisms benefit from the relationship [27]. These different species inhabit the same spaces and share or compete for the same resources. They interact in a variety of ways, known collectively as symbiosis. There are five main symbiotic relationships: mutualism, commensalism, predation, parasitism, and competition. Table 1.2 shows examples of each.

1) Mutualism – All species benefit from positive effects focusing on pro-tection from pathogens and/or the provision of nutrients [28]. An example of mutualism is the dependence of symbionts (microbiotas) on resources (cellulose) that are not utilized by the host. Another example is *Bifidobacterium longum* (subspecies *infantis – B. infantis*), which is found in human breast milk. This breast milk contains 30% of calories coming from oligosaccharides that cannot be digested by the infant and are instead digested by *B. infantis* in the GI tract. *Bifidobacterium* and *Lactobacillus* are generally regarded as beneficial microbes because of their ability to exclude harmful bacteria by pro-ducing various antimicrobial agents [26].
2) Predation – One species benefits from consuming another species. When looking for means to precisely modulate microbiomes, predation

**Table 1.2**  Examples of symbiotic relationships.

| | | |
|---|---|---|
| Strongly positive | Obligate mutualism | Lichen |
| | Strong mutualism | Most vertically transmitted gut mutualists and their host |
| | Moderate mutualism | Clownfish and anemones |
| | Marginal mutualism | Ants and aphids |
| Neutral | Commensalism | Clown fish and anemones |
| | Benign parasitism | *Dipylidium caninum* and canids |
| | Conspicuous parasitism | Many GI nematodes and their host |
| | Severe parasitism | Parvovirus and their host |
| Strongly negative | Lethal parasitism | *Dirofilaria immitis* and their host |

*Source:* Adapted from Swain Ewald and Ewald [28].

is being researched as a promising approach [29]. Bacteriophages (phages) are viruses that prey on bacteria [30]. Phages can enter a bacterium and rapidly multiply producing hundreds of new viruses. Benefits of using predation as an approach in modulating microbiomes are the ability to (i) deliberately perturb specific bacteria, (ii) develop a deeper understanding of interbacterial and bacterial-mammalian host interactions, and (iii) be able to plan and create reproducible approaches to remodel microbiota for therapeutic purposes [29].

3) Parasitism – One species benefits from living with, on, or in a host species at the expense of the host. Some negative effects of parasitism are vitamin deficiency, immunopathy, tissue damage, and mortality [28]. While parasitism is generally thought of to have a negative effect, there are some instances where utilization of select organisms may induce a more positive effect on the host, particularly in chronic infections. In mice, chronic intestinal helminth infection has been documented to increase susceptibility to co-infection, and lower the efficacy of vaccination, while also downregulating allergic immune responses to harmless antigens creating protection against allergic diseases [29, 31].

4) Competition – Different species benefit from limited resources in the same ecosystem at the expense of each other. Competition exclusion is

a common trait of some probiotics. These nonpathogenic bacterial cultures are used to reduce colonization or decrease populations of pathogenic bacteria [32]. Competitive exclusion for intestinal bacteria is the bacteria to bacteria competition for available nutrients and mucosal adhesion sites [33]. They can also change the environment to make it less suitable for their competitors. Bacteria may also displace pathogens by taking up space in the biofilm or mucosa, inhibit the adhesion of pathogens, and decrease the competitor's ability to attach to receptor sites. The level of effectiveness of a bacterium using this relationship depends on the strain, species, and genus to receive reproducible results. Another form of competition exclusion is the production of debilitating metabolites by beneficial bacteria. Bacteriocins are one example of antimicrobial metabolites, which affect the pathogens but not the bacteriocins themselves. There are three main classes of bacteriocins based on their structure and function [34]:

   i) Class I – small peptides possessing lanthionine residues

   ii) Class II – which is heat-stable and does not contain lanthionine residues

   iii) Class III referred to as bacteriolysins – which are large, heat-labile murein hydrolases

5) Commensalism – One species benefits with no net positive or negative effect to the other [35]. Many discussions about the microbiota in microbiomes regard the relationship between the host and the microbiota to be commensal. This term when used in a simplistic definition does not consider the complexity of these relationships. One paper describes commensalism as the dividing line between parasitic and mutualistic associations, with the overall effects of this relationship as being positive or negative, difficult to accurately assess [28]. Additionally, because these effects are not able to be precisely measured, it is difficult to always place microbiota appropriately on this continuum of mutualistic to commensal to parasitic. This group of microorganisms is called indeterminate symbionts. There are situations where some bacteria can move from being mutualistic to parasitic in different circumstances. These ambisymbionts can be identified as either mutualistic or parasitic, whereas indeterminate symbionts have an uncertain net effect.

Positive "commensal relationships" are providing the host with essential nutrients, metabolism of indigestible compounds, protection against colonization of

| Box 1.1 Positive Effects of Host–Symbiote Relationship |
|---|
| • Providing the host with essential nutrients<br>• Metabolism of indigestible compounds<br>• Protection against colonization of opportunistic pathogens<br>• Contribution to the development of the intestinal architecture<br>• Stimulation of the immune system |

opportunistic pathogens, contribution to the development of the intestinal architecture, and stimulation of the immune system [36] (Box 1.1).

## 1.5 Dysbiosis

If there is a microbial shift, brought on by genetics of the host, infectious illnesses, diets, or the prolonged use of antibiotics or other bacteria-destroying medications, these perturbations to the structure of the community is referred to as dysbiosis [10, 37]. When this occurs, normal interactions stop, resulting in the host body being more susceptible to disease [10]. Perturbation of normal host microbiota has been associated with several pathologies in dogs and cats, including chronic enteropathies, idiopathic IBD, acute hemorrhagic diarrhea syndrome, small bowel strictures or adhesions, neoplasia, chronic intussusception, hypothyroidism, diabetic autonomic neuropathy, scleroderma, abnormal migrating motor complexes, atrophic gastritis, and exocrine pancreatic insufficiency [3]. Table 1.3 lists some dysbiotic conditions recognized in humans.

Three types of dysbiosis can occur concurrently [10]:

1) Loss of beneficial microbial organisms – There are several mechanisms where commensal bacteria can positively influence host biology to prevent disease. Beneficial microbiota influences the host immune response with the tolerance of resident commensals being governed in part by T regulatory (Treg) cells, which are a specialized subset of T lymphocytes. When beneficial microbiota ferments dietary products, they can produce SCFAs, which have been shown to regulate the Treg pool to protect the body from inflammation and disease states such as colitis. Beneficial bacteria may also directly reduce

**Table 1.3** Dysbiosis-associated conditions in humans.

| |
|---|
| Periodontal disease |
| Neurological diseases – depression/anxiety |
| Respiratory diseases |
| Dermatological diseases |
| Obesity |
| Diabetes |
| Arthritis and joint diseases |
| Inflammatory bowel diseases |
| Allergic diseases |
| Autism |

*Source:* Adapted from DeGruttola et al. [38] and Sudhakara et al. [39].

inflammation by targeting cytokines and play a role in regulating invariant Natural Killer T cells (NKT) cells, which influence lipid antigens along with innate and adaptive inflammation.

2) Expansion of pathobionts – Pathobionts may create harmful effects when given the opportunity to expand. Multiple studies have demonstrated how pathobionts can increase their numbers by taking advantage of an inflamed environment. For example, when animals are treated with antibiotics, then have colitis induced using dioctyl sodium sulfosuccinate, a multi-drug-resistant stain of *Escherichia coli,* increases in numbers and can penetrate the intestinal mucosal barrier and translocate causing sepsis.

3) Loss of diversity – With multiple varieties of microbiota eliciting health benefits to the host, having a more diverse and complex pool of organisms has been shown to provide maximum benefits. Some studies have observed a difference in disease processes later in life associated with lower microbial diversity at a crucial development stage.

## 1.6  Probiotics

The Food and Agriculture Organization of the United Nations and the World Health Organization defined a probiotic as "live microorganisms, which when administered in adequate amounts, confer a health benefit upon the host" [40, 41]. Probiotics in the form of cultured and fermented food sources (examples: yogurt, sauerkraut) have been anecdotally known to have health benefits, with research now looking at specific microbiota strains, species, and subspecies of bacteria, correlating them with direct benefits via commensal interactions with the GI tract resident microbiota [42]. Probiotics may be utilized to manage GI dysbiosis and have been shown in some cases to strengthen the immune response. Some probiotics can stimulate the production of anti-inflammatory substances and may participate in communication with other organs via bidirectional communication [42] (Figure 1.1).

There are characteristics of probiotics that allow them to be beneficial:

1) The microbiota in the probiotic must be alive and viable at the time of consumption [40, 43].
2) It must be able to survive varying environments through GI transit including gastric acid and be resistant to digestion by intestinal enzymes [40, 43].
3) The probiotic being used should be considered safe [40, 43].
4) Probiotics must either enhance the commensal bacteria or suppress the growth or colonization of pathogenic bacteria. There are three main actions through competition and exclusion that probiotics protect the host from pathogenic bacteria:
    i) Bacteria to bacteria competition for available nutrients [32]
    ii) Competition for space and acting as a physical barrier prevent pathogens from attaching to the gut surface [33, 43] – the action

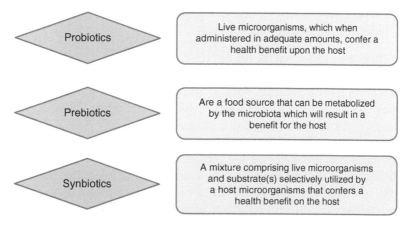

Figure 1.1 Definitions of probiotics, prebiotics, and synbiotics.

of the probiotic bacteria may be to adhere to the intestinal epithelia or receptors of the GI tract preventing the colonization of pathogenic bacteria

iii) Secretion of antimicrobial metabolites or mediators such as bacteriocins [34, 43]

5) The result of giving a probiotic should enhance the overall health of the pet. One example of positive action is the fermentation of undigested nutrients resulting in the production of SCFAs [44, 45]. SCFAs nourish enterocytes, increasing the health of the intestinal wall. SCFAs when produced in larger volumes can lower intestinal pH inhibiting the growth of pathogenic bacteria that prefer a more alkaline environment.

The main uses of probiotics are to:

1) Promote a positive change in a GI microbiome – utilizing the actions listed above the probiotic microbiota may elicit a change back to the host's normal diversity and density of microbiota [45].
2) Stimulate or enhance an immune response, without being proinflammatory – the modulation of the host GI immune system both locally and systemically via their interaction with the resident microbiota, GI epithelia, and gut immune cells [43, 46].
3) Increase or stimulate the production of neurochemicals and interaction with the gut-brain axis [47]. Probiotics that act as psychobiotics are utilized to affect many neurochemical disorders such as anxiety in pets.
4) Modulation of the immune system, help in stress management, protection from infection, improve growth and development, control allergies, and manage obesity [44].

There are times when the use of probiotics is possibly contraindicated. In an instance where a pet has a compromised GI barrier (barrier dysfunction), it is not recommended to take oral dosages of probiotics (live bacteria) as there is a rare, yet severe risk of bacterial translocation and sepsis, particularly in unregulated products [48].

In North America, as long as the probiotic label does not indicate any health claims, probiotics are not considered to be pharmaceuticals, and the classes of nutraceuticals or supplements are not recognized for animals and therefore do not have the same regulations placed upon them as pharmaceuticals, with regards to viability studies, dosing, and expiry of products. This lack of regulation could result in inconsistencies in the product contents with concerns that:

1) The product is not what is indicated on the label [49].
2) The bacteria may not be viable or in an carrier promoting survival to the target location [44].
3) The product may not provide benefits and may be pathogenic [37, 44, 49].
4) The bacteria are not listed at the subspecies level and may not result in the same or any benefits for the host [37].
5) The product may not contain sufficient bacteria to elicit a change [50]
6) The product may not be tested to identify the specific genus and dosage, nor have been tested for safety, stability, and consistent positive results [37, 50].
7) The strain used may release harmful metabolites [43].
8) The strain may be prone to transmit antibiotic resistance [44, 51].
9) Bacterial translocation may result in infection [44, 48].

## 1.7 Prebiotics

As opposed to probiotics, which consist of viable organisms, prebiotics are nutrients predominantly undigestible by the host animal that serve as a food source to be metabolized by the microbiota, resulting in benefit to the host [40, 45, 52]. These food sources consist of nutrients that can be fermented by the microbiota, which increases the survivability of beneficial microbes. Each species of microbiota has preferential food sources. Sources of indigestible nutrients are mainly from carbohydrates, with psyllium husk and/or yeast cell walls being a common ingredient used in commercial prebiotics at this time. As microbiota ferment cellulose, they may create the metabolites butyrate and acetate, SCFAs that are energy sources for colonocytes, and provide multiple other beneficial effects [44, 45].

To be classified as a prebiotic, the substrate must meet certain criteria [53]:

1) Resistant to digestion – does not break down in the acidic pH of the stomach, cannot be hydrolyzed by digestive enzymes, and is not absorbed in the upper GI tract.
2) Fermentable – it is fermentable by intestinal microbiota.

3) Produces a positive result – there is selective growth and/or activity of the intestinal microbiota that conveys a health benefit to the host.

There are different types of prebiotics: oligosaccharides like fructo-oligosaccharide (FOS), oligofructose, mannose-oligosaccharide (MOS), galacto-oligosaccharide (GOS), pectic oligosaccharide (POS), inulin, and glucan and noncarbohydrate compounds such as flavanols. Fructans, pectins, inulin, and flavanols are predominantly derived from vegetation like fruits and vegetables, GOS can be derived from lactose or synthetic lactulose, and resistant starches and glucan may be derived from plants and yeast cells [53].

## 1.8 Synbiotics

Compounds comprising of a mixture of both live microorganisms (probiotics) and a substrate selectively utilized by beneficial microorganisms that confer a health benefit to the host (prebiotic) are termed synbiotics [54]. The International Scientific Association for Probiotics and Prebiotics (ISAPP) has created another class of synbiotics called synergistic synbiotics, defined as "a synbiotic for which the substrate is designed to be selectively utilized by the co-administered microorganisms" [54]. These terms should be reserved for products where the prebiotic will selectively favor the specific probiotic organisms.

Reasons to feed a specific prebiotic with the probiotic are to [53]:

1) Selectively support the growth of the preferred microbiota once in the desired location (GI tract)
2) Aid in the metabolism of one or more health-promoting bacteria

## 1.9 Biological Markers (Biomarkers) and Their Measurement

Biomarkers are cellular, biochemical, or molecular indicators detectable in biological media that suggest changes to normal or pathological processes, as well as responses to a therapeutic intervention [55]. When assessing a healthy patient or a patient experiencing a disease state, biomarkers as a tool can aid in the prediction, cause, diagnosis, progression, regression, or outcome of treatment. Biomarkers can be divided into Exposure, where the level of risk is predicted, and Disease, where screening, diagnosis, and progression are monitored (Chart slide 13). The methods of detection and measurement of biomarkers can also be divided into targeted or untargeted, depending on the aim of the study [56]. When relationships between specific biomarkers and outcomes are known, they are typically measured by targeted processes, meaning quantitative measurements of specific metabolites are made. Alternatively, untargeted approaches allow for a more discovery-based approach, where a potentially vast number of individual or classes of biomarkers may be measured.

### 1.9.1 Genes, the Genome, and Genomics

The genome is the complete set of deoxyribonucleic acid (DNA) bearing all the genetic information of an organism [57]. The genes encoded in the DNA provide instructions to the cell on how to make each specific protein, which is then utilized to carry out functions in the body.

Proteins are synthesized through two processes:

1) Transcription – the synthesis of DNA into functional forms of ribonucleic acid (RNA), including mRNA, tRNA, rRNA, and noncoding RNA, which are used in the translation process.
2) Translation – the synthesis of mRNA into an amino acid sequence. The final polypeptide chain can then further undergo post-translation modifications along with subsequent enzymatic and nonenzymatic alterations to increase the number of protein species.

Genomes are complex and can be influenced by environmental factors. The microbiome and their respective genome have been shown to play a major role in human health and disease.

Genome-wide association studies (GWAS) is a scientific collaboration to create a large database to look for similar variants across the human genome, intending to determine links between genotypic and phenotypic variabilities [58]. Microbiome genome-wide association studies (mGWAS) explain the interaction of host genetic variation with the microbiome.

Genomics refers to the study of an organism's genome, the entire complement of genes, including interactions between genes with both each other and the organism's environment [59, 60]. This may include analysis of all nucleotide sequences in the genome, and the structure, function, evolution, and mapping of the genome, in order to understand the entire genetic information of the organism. Next-generation sequencing technology enables the investigation of the complex interaction between host genetics and microbial communities [58].

In comparison to genomics that study the genome of a singular organism, metagenomics is the study of a collection of genomes from a community of organisms [61]. This platform may be used to examine all DNA sequences across multiple organisms, particularly useful when culture or separation of microbes is not feasible or required.

Lastly, epigenetics refers to the study of how internal and external factors can influence the expression of genes [62–64]. Epigenetic changes are reversible and do not alter the sequence of DNA, or genotype, but instead affect the way the encoding of the DNA is interpreted – the phenotype.

Three ways epigenetics can affect gene expression are:

1) DNA methylation – a chemical group is added to a specific place on the DNA where it "blocks" the proteins "read" the gene [63, 64]. The chemical group can then be removed by a process called demethylation. To "silence" or turn genes "off," methylation is used while demethylation turns genes "on."

2) Histone (chromatin) modification – histones are proteins that allow or stop DNA from being "read" depending on how tightly the DNA is wrapped around it [64]. Chromatin is the complex of histones and DNA combined. Chemical groups are added or removed from histones to alter the wrap. A wrapped gene is considered "off," while an unwrapped gene is considered "on" or able to be "read."

3) Noncoding RNA – while coding RNA is used to make proteins, noncoding RNA helps control gene expression by attaching to and breaking down coding RNA so it cannot be used to make proteins [63]. Noncoding RNA can also modify histones with the use of other proteins to influence whether the gene is "on" or "off."

Epigenetics can change as part of growth and development, with some changes being reversible. These changes can affect an organism's health by affecting the immune system, developing neoplasia due to mutations, and affecting fetal epigenetics based on the maternal environment and behavior during pregnancy [64]. Known associated illnesses include cognitive dysfunction, respiratory, cardiovascular, reproductive, autoimmune, neurobehavioral illnesses along with a wide variety of behaviors and cancers. Epigenetic modifications can be induced by several drivers, including exposure to toxins, nutrition during pregnancy and early development, and behavioral influences such as maternal-neonatal care, mental health, and the aging process.

### 1.9.2 Metabolites, the Metabolome, and Metabolomics

Microbial metabolism and fermentation results in production of small molecular substrates, intermediates, and products, collectively termed metabolites [65]. The vast diversity of metabolites are produced by microbiota from the metabolism or fermentation of macronutrients and micronutrients, which then can interact with multiple body systems. The effect of specific microbiota-derived metabolites depends on multiple factors including the strain of microbiota, the food source provided, the volume of metabolites produced, and the health status of the host (Figure 1.2).

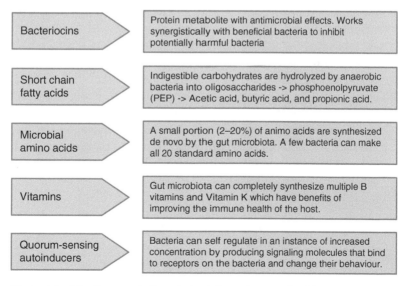

| Bacteriocins | Protein metabolite with antimicrobial effects. Works synergistically with beneficial bacteria to inhibit potentially harmful bacteria |
| Short chain fatty acids | Indigestible carbohydrates are hydrolyzed by anaerobic bacteria into oligosaccharides -> phosphoenolpyruvate (PEP) -> Acetic acid, butyric acid, and propionic acid. |
| Microbial amino acids | A small portion (2–20%) of animo acids are synthesized de novo by the gut microbiota. A few bacteria can make all 20 standard amino acids. |
| Vitamins | Gut microbiota can completely synthesize multiple B vitamins and Vitamin K which have benefits of improving the immune health of the host. |
| Quorum-sensing autoinducers | Bacteria can self regulate in an instance of increased concentration by producing signaling molecules that bind to receptors on the bacteria and change their behaviour. |

**Figure 1.2** The five metabolites derived from the gut microbiota and their main function.

There are currently 5 gut microbiota-derived metabolites identified:

1) Bacteriocins – A protein metabolite that has antimicrobial effects and works synergistically with beneficial bacteria to inhibit potentially harmful bacteria. The synergy of bacteriocins and antibiotics may help address the problem of antimicrobial resistance as a future approach in the treatment of infectious diseases [34].

2) Short-chain fatty acids – Indigestible carbohydrates such as some fiber sources are hydrolyzed by anaerobic bacteria into oligosaccharides that are then converted into phosphoenolpyruvate (PEP) and finally into acetic acid, butyric acid, and propionic acid depending on the bacteria of origin [66]. These metabolites in particular have been highly studied for their effect on the host [45].

3) Microbial amino acids – While most amino acids in the intestines originate from the consumption of nitrogenous ingredients (animal and plant sources along with from the host muscle tissue), a small portion is synthesized *de novo* by the gut microbiota. A few bacteria can make all 20 of the standard amino acids, contributing to the host's amino acid homeostasis [66]. Microbial synthesized lysine, in particular, has been shown to contribute 2–20% of the total circulating volume in a study in humans, pigs, and rats.

4) Vitamins – Some vitamins can be completely synthesized by the gut microbiota including multiple B vitamins and vitamin K, which have benefits at improving immune health for the host – though sites of production and absorption must be considered [67].

5) Quorum-sensing autoinducers – Over time there is a gradual and accumulative increase in bacteria concentrations in a certain area. The bacteria will self-regulate by producing and releasing signaling molecules to detect the bacterial concentration. The signaling molecules will bind to receptors on the bacteria and ultimately change the behavior of the bacteria [66].

Metabolites have a variety of functions:

1) Key factors in a variety of host to microbiota and cell to cell communication [65]

2) Metabolite signaling through a series of innate immune receptors affecting host immunity [65, 68], along with regulation of the adaptive immune cell development (T lymphocytes) [66]

3) Drive changes in the composition and function of the microbiota through signaling (quorum sensing) [66, 68]
4) Production of SCFAs, which provide multiple benefits to the host [45, 68]
5) Participate in various physiological processes, including energy metabolism [65]
6) Represent potential biomarkers for early diagnosis of multiple disorders [65]
7) Directly kill pathogens by:
    i) disrupting bacterial cell structures.
    ii) interfering with bacterial DNA, RNA, and protein metabolism.
    iii) resource competition between commensal bacteria and pathogens.
    iv) affect cell adhesion and biofilm formation.
    v) regulation of the immune system by activating innate immunity [66]
8) Production of vitamins and metabolism of some minerals [67]

The phrase "metabolome" refers to the biochemical environment derived from the symbiosis of nutrient-rich milieu provided by the host and the products and metabolites produced by the microbiota [69]. It provides a functional interpretation of cellular activity and physiological status.

The metabolome includes simple amino acids and related amines, lipids, sugars, nucleotides, vitamins, and other intermediary metabolites. The molecules in a metabolome will change depending on the organism being studied and what chemical reactions are occurring in the cell. Metabolomics analyses include sensitive chromatographic methods coupled with mass spectrometry – gas chromatography-mass spectrometry (GC-MS) and liquid chromatography-mass spectrometry (LC-MS) – as well as nuclear magnetic resonance to identify and quantify compounds in the metabolome [59].

The study of the metabolome is termed metabolomics. This platform includes analytical profiling, quantification, and comparison of metabolites present in biological samples [56, 65].

Metabolomics offers a window into metabolic mechanisms through the use of analytical chemistry and multivariate data analysis [59]. Examples of metabolomics in disease research include certain types of neoplasia with dogs and the use of dogs as a translation model for humans, with the data possibly being bidirectionally beneficial [70, 71]. Due to the complexity of the metabolome, there are two main types of analytic platforms used in metabolomics [56, 59, 71–73]:

1) Mass spectrometry – achieves a high sensitivity in the analysis. Mass spectrometry may require extensive sample preparation, which can result in the loss of certain compounds. This technique can be limited with respect to the range of metabolite detection per sample and require different preparations of multiple samples to detect maximum number of metabolites. Types of mass spectrometry include:
    i) Gas chromatography-mass spectrometry (GC-MS) – oldest tool for qualitative metabolic profiling while providing high chromatographic resolution
    ii) Liquid chromatography-mass spectrometry (LC-MS) – high sensitivity and provides information regarding metabolite structure.
    iii) Capillary electrophoresis-mass spectrometry (CE-MS) – high efficiency allowing separation of chemically diverse metabolites in smaller sample volumes with little to no pretreatment required.
2) Nuclear magnetic resonance (NMR) – quantitative, highly reproducible nondestructive technique. Requires comparatively large sample volumes, but little to no pretreatment of samples, and a range of metabolites can be analyzed in a single sample. Specificity is limited as metabolite resonances may overlap.

These technological advances allow for large quantities of data to be obtained at multiple levels – organelle, cell, tissue/fluid, organ, and entire organism, which provide information on biomolecular functions. Databases for metabolomes and metabolic analyses are available through online platforms:

1) The Human Metabolome Database – https://hmdb.ca/ [74]
2) The Livestock Metabolome Database – https://lmdb.ca/ [75]
3) The Bovine Metabolome Database – https://bovinedb.ca/ [76]
4) Metaboanalyst – https://www.metaboanalyst.ca [77]

### 1.9.2.1 Metabonomics

A specific branch of metabolomics, termed metabonomics, is dedicated to the study of how the metabolic profile of biological systems change in response to alterations, such as environmental exposures, pathophysiologic events, and nutrition [56, 71, 78]. Thus, this profile is determined by both host genetics and exogenous factors. The term is not always used; however, often the term metabolomics is used to include what could be more strictly defined as metabonomics.

### 1.9.3 The Proteome and Proteomics

The proteome is the complete set of proteins expressed by an organism [79]. It represents the expression of an organism's genome and actively changes in response to various factors, including the organism's developmental stage, and other internal and external conditions.

"a large-scale study of protein properties produced by the cell. This includes the expression level, post-transcriptional modification, and protein interaction, in order to obtain a global view of disease processes or cellular processes at the protein level." Proteomics aims to catalog the entire protein products of the human genome. Other specific "omics" studies exist, such as lipidomics, which is the study of biological lipids [56].

There are three main strategies of proteomics showing to have an impact:

1) Protein–protein linkage maps
2) Genomic DNA sequences of peptide sequences from mass spectrometry
3) Quantitative protein expression 42.2

## Glossary

**Biological marker (biomarker)** – cellular, biochemical, or molecular alterations that are measurable in biological media such as tissues, cells, or fluids; include biological characteristics that can be objectively measured and evaluated as an indicator of normal biological processes, pathogenic processes, or pharmacological responses to a therapeutic intervention

**Commensalism** – a form of symbiosis where one species lives with, on, or in a host and provides no benefit or detriment to the host

**Competition** – different species using similarly limited resources in the same ecosystem

**Dysbiosis** – a change to the composition of resident commensal communities relative to the community found in healthy individuals

**Genome** – the complete set of DNA (genetic information) in an organism; contains all the information needed to build and maintain that organism throughout its life

**Genomics** – the study of an organism's genome (genes), including interactions of those genes with each other and the organism's environment

**Epigenetics** – the study of how behaviors and environment can cause changes that affect the way genes work

**Metabolites** – small molecular substrates, intermediates, and products of metabolism

**Metabolome** – the collection of small compound metabolites in an organism

**Metabolomics** – an analytical profiling technique for measuring and comparing large numbers of metabolites present in biological samples

**Metabonomics** – the quantitative study of how the metabolic profile of biologic systems change in response to alterations caused by pathophysiologic stimuli, toxic exposures, or dietary changes

**Metagenomic** – the study of a collection of genetic material (genomes) from a mixed community of organisms

**Microbiome** – the microbiome is the genetic material of all the microbes – bacteria, fungi, protozoa, and viruses – that live in a particular ecosystem. These microscopic communities can be found in all biological systems, including inside humans and other animals, along with residing in plants, soils, and oceans

**Microbiota** – the individual bacteria, fungi, virus, and protozoa that make up the microbiome community

**Mutualism** – both (or all) species benefit in a mutualistic symbiotic relationship

**Parasitism** – a symbiotic relationship in which one species lives with, on, or in a host species at the expense of the host

**Pathogens** – a biological agent that causes disease or illness to its host

**Prebiotics** – food sources that can be utilized by the microbiota and in turn result in a benefit for the host; typically indigestible to the host but rapidly fermented by the host's microbiota

**Predation** – a symbiotic relationship in which one species hunts, kills, and consumes (an)other species

**Probiotics** – viable microbes intended to be beneficial to the commensal microbiota

**Proteome** – the complement of proteins produced by a cell

**Proteomics** – large-scale study of proteins produced by a cell; includes the expression level, post-transcriptional modification, and protein interaction in order to obtain a global view of disease processes or cellular processes at the protein level

**Short-chain fatty acids (SCFAs)** – metabolites of microbial fermentation – predominantly acetic acid, butyric acid, and propionic acid

**Symbiosis** – any relationship or interaction between two dissimilar organisms, with the specific kind of symbiosis depending on whether either or both organisms benefit from the relationship

**Symbiotic** – a product consisting of a probiotic and prebiotic in combination

# References

1 Consorium, T.H.M.P. (2012). Structure, function and diversity of the healthy human microbiome. *Nature* 486 (7402): 207–214.

2 Marchesi, J. (2017). What is a microbiome? https://microbiologysociety. org/blog/what-is-a-microbiome.html (accessed 11 May 2021).

3 Suchodolski, J. (2016). Diagnosis and interpretation of intestinal dysbiosis in dogs and cats. *The Veterinary Journal* 215: 30–37.

4 Ruan, W., Engecik, M., Spinler, J., and Versalovic, J. (2020). Healthy human gastrointestinal microbiome: composition and function after a decade of exploration. *Digestive Diseases and Sciences* 65: 695–705.

5 Shahab, M. and Shahab, N. (2022). Coevolution of the human host and gut microbiome: metagenomics of microbiota. *Cureus* 14 (6): e26310.

6 Tengeler, A., Kozicz, T., and Kiliaan, A. (2018). Relationship between diet, the gut microbiota, and brain function. *Nutrition Reviews* 76 (8): 603–617.

7 Murtaza, N., Cuív, P., and Morrison, M. (2017). Diet and the microbiome. *Gastroenterology Clinics of North America* 46: 49–60.

8 Rowland, I., Gibson, G., Heinken, A. et al. (2018). Gut microbiota functions: metabolism of nutrients and other food components. *European Journal of Nutrition* 57.

9 Queirós, A., Faria, D., and Almeida, F. (2017). Strengths and limitations of qualitative and quantitative research methods. *European Journal of Education Studies* 3 (9): 369–387.

**10** Petersen, C. and Round, J. (2014). Defining dysbiosis and its influence on host immunity and disease. *Cellular Microbiology* 16 (7): 1024–1033.

**11** Alessandri, G., Argentini, C., Milani, C. et al. (2020). Catching a glimpse of the bacterial gut community of companion animals: a canine and feline perspective. *Microbial Biotechnology* 13 (6): 1708–1732.

**12** Benyacoub, J., Czarnecki-Maulden, G., Cavadini, C. et al. (2003). Supplementation of food with enterococcus faecium (sf68) stimulates immune functions in young dogs. *Journal of Nutrition* 133 (4): 1158–1162.

**13** Sauter, S., Benyacoub, J., Allenspach, K. et al. (2006). Effects of probiotic bacteria in dogs with food responsive diarrhoea treated with an elimination diet. *Journal of Animal Physiology and Animal Nutrition* 90: 269–277.

**14** Bybee, S., Scorza, A., and Lappin, M. (2011). Effect of the probiotic enterococcus faecium sf68 on presence of diarrhea in cats and dogs housed in an animal shelter. *Journal of Veterinary Internal Medicine* 25 (4): 856–860.

**15** Lappin, M., Satyaraj, E., and Czarnecki-Maulden, G. (2009). Pilot study to evaluate the effect of oral supplementation of enterococcus faecium sf68 on cats with latent feline herpesvirus 1. *Journal of Feline Medicine and Surgery* 11: 650–654.

**16** Veir, J., Knorr, R., Cavadini, C. et al. (2007). Effect of supplementation with enterococcus faecium (sf68) on immune functions in cats. *Veterinary Therapeutics* 8 (4): 229–238.

**17** Janeway, C. Jr., Travers, P., Walport, M., and Shlomchik, M. (2001). Infectious agents and how they cause disease. In: *Immunology: The Immune System in Health and Disease*. New York: Garland Science. https://www.ncbi.nlm.nih.gov/books/NBK27114/.

**18** Alexander, K., Kat, P., Wayne, R., and Fuller, T. (1994). Serologic survey of selected canine pathogens among free-ranging jackals in kenya. *Journal of Wildlife Diseases* 30 (4): 486–491.

**19** Inpankaew, T., Hii, S., Chimnoi, W., and Traub, R. (2016). Canine vector-borne pathogens in semi- domesticated dogs residing in northern cambodia. *Parasites & Vectors* 9 (253).

**20** Day, M., Carey, S., Clercx, C. et al. (2020). Aetiology of canine infectious respiratory disease complex and prevalence of its pathogens in europe. *Journal of Comparative Pathology* 176: 86–108.

**21** Riley, S., Foley, J., and Chomel, B. (2004). Exposure to feline and canine pathogens in bobcats and gray foxes in urban and rural zones of a national park in california. *Journal of Wildlife Diseases* 40 (1): 11–22.

**22** Millán, J. and Rodriíguez, A. (2009). A serological survey of common feline pathogens in free-living european wildcats (*Felis silvestris*) in central spain. *European Journal of Wildlife Research* 55: 285–291.

**23** Biek, R., Ruth, T., Murphy, K. et al. (2006). Factors associated with pathogen seroprevalence and infection in rocky mountain cougars. *Journal of Wildlife Diseases* 42 (3): 606–615.

**24** Villeneuve, A., Polley, L., Jenkins, E. et al. (2015). Parasite prevalence in fecal samples from shelter dogs and cats across the canadian provinces. *Parasites & Vectors* 8: 281.

**25** Weese, S., Nichols, J., Jalali, M., and Litster, A. (2015). The oral and conjunctival microbiotas in cats with and without feline immunodeficiency virus infection. *Veterinary Research* 46 (21): https://doi.org/10.1186/s13567-014-0140-5.

**26** Lubbs, D., Vester, B., Fastinger, N., and Swanson, K. (2009). Dietary protein concentration affects intestinal microbiota of adult cats: a study using dgge and qpcr to evaluate differencesin microbial populations in the feline gastrointestinal tract. *Journal of Animal Physiology and Animal Nutrition* 93: 113–121.

**27** Hirsch, A. (2004). Plant-microbe symbioses: a continuum from commensalism to parasitism. *Symbiosis* 37 (1–3): 345–363.

**28** Swain Ewald, H. and Ewald, P. (2018). Natural selection, the microbiome, and public health. *Yale Journal of Biology and Medicine* 91: 445–455.

**29** Hsu, B., Gibson, T., Yeliseyev, V. et al. (2019). Dynamic modulation of the gut microbiota and metabolome by bacteriophages in a mouse model. *Cell Host & Microbe* 25: 803–814.

**30** De Paepe, M. and Petit, M.-A. (2014). Killing the killers. *eLife* 3: e04168.

**31** Smits, H. and Yazdanbakhsh, M. (2007). Chronic helminth infections modulate allergen-specific immune responses: protection against development of allergic disorders? *Annals of Medicine* 39 (6): 428–439.

**32** Callaway, T., Anderson, R., Edrington, T. et al. (2013). Novel methods for pathogen control in livestock pre-harvest: an update. In: *Advances in Microbial Food Safety* (ed. J. Sofos), 275–304. Woodhead Publishing Series in Food Science, Technology and Nutrition.

**33** Collado, M., Gueimonde, M., and Salminen, S. (2010). Probiotics in adhesion of pathogens: mechanisms of action. In: *Bioactive Foods in promoting health* (ed. R. Watson and V. Preedy), 353–370. Cambridge, MA: Academic Press.

**34** Eijsink, V., Axelsson, L., Diep, D. et al. (2022). Production of class ii bacteriocins by lactic acid bacteria; an example of biological warfare and communication. *Probiotics and Antimicrobial Proteins* 8 (4): 177–182.

**35** Mathis, K. and Bronstein, J. (2020). Our current understanding of commensalism. *Annual Review of Ecology, Evolution, and Systematics* 51: 167–189.

**36** Martín, R., Miquel, S., Ulmer, J. et al. (2013). Role of commensal and probiotic bacteria in human health: a focus on inflammatory bowel disease. *Microbial Cell Factories* 12 (71): https://doi.org/10.1186/1475-2859-12-71.

**37** Perez-Carrasco, V., Soriano-Lerma, A., Soriano, M. et al. (2021). Urinary microbiome: yin and yang of the urinary tract. *Frontiers in Cellular and Infection Microbiology* 11.

**38** DeGruttola, A., Low, D., Mizoguchi, A., and Mizoguchi, E. (2016). Current understanding of dysbiosis in disease in human and animal models. *Inflammatory Bowel Diseases* 22 (5): 1137–1150.

**39** Sudhakara, P., Gupta, A., Bhardwaj, A., and Wilson, A. (2018). Oral dysbiotic communities and their implications in systemic diseases. *Dentistry Journal* 6 (10).

**40** Hill, C., Guarner, F., Reid, G. et al. (2015). The international scientific association for probiotics and prebiotics consensus statement on the scope and appropriate use of the term probiotic. *Nature* 11: 506–514.

**41** Food and Agricultural Organization of the United Nations and World Health Organization (2001). Health and nutritional properties of probiotics in food including powder milk with live lactic acid bacteria. www.who.int/foodsafety/publications/fs_management/en/probiotics.pdf (accessed 11 November 2022).

**42** Johnson, B. and Klaenhammer, T. (2014). Impact of genomics on the field of probiotic research: historical perspectives to modern paradigms. *Antonie Van Leeuwenhoek* 106: 141–156.

**43** Saarela, M., Mogensen, G., Fondén, R. et al. (2000). Probiotic bacteria: safety, functional and technological properties. *Journal of Biotechnology* 84: 197–215.

**44** Grześkowiak, L., Endo, A., Beasley, S., and Salminen, S. (2015). Microbiota and probiotics in canine and feline welfare. *Anaerobe* 34: 14–23.

**45** Gagné, J., Wakshlag, J., Simpson, K. et al. (2013). Effects of a synbiotic on fecal quality, short-chain fatty acid concentrations, and the microbiome of healthy sled dogs. *BMC Veterinary Research* 9 (246): https://doi.org/10.1186/1746-6148-9-246.

**46** Lee, D., Goh, T., Kang, M. et al. (2022). Perspectives and advances in probiotics and the gut microbiome in companion animals. *Journal of Animal Science and Technology* 64 (2): 197–217.

**47** Bercik, P., Park, A., Sinclair, D. et al. (2011). The anxiolytic effect of bifidobacterium longum ncc3001 involves vagal pathways for gut–brain communication. *Neurogastroenterology and Motility* 23 (12): 1132–1139.

**48** Liong, M. (2008). Safety of probiotics: translocation and infection. *Nutrition Reviews* 66 (4): 192–202.

**49** Siddiqi, R. and Moghadasian, M. (2020). Nutraceuticals and nutrition supplements: challenges and opportunities. *Nutrients* 12: https://doi. org/10.3390/nu12061593.

**50** Weese, J. and Martin, H. (2011). Assessment of commercial probiotic bacterial contents and label accuracy. *Canadian Veterinary Journal* 52: 43–46.

**51** Fatahi-Bafghi, M., Naseri, S., and Alizehi, A. (2022). Genome analysis of probiotic bacteria for antibiotic resistance genes. *Antonie Van Leeuwenhoek* 115: 375–389.

**52** Strompfová, V., Lauková, A., and Cilik, D. (2013). Synbiotic administration of canine-derived strain lactobacillus fermentum ccm 7421 and inulin to healthy dogs. *Canadian Journal of Microbiology* 59 (5): 347–352.

**53** Pandey, K., Naik, S., and Vakil, B. (2015). Probiotics, prebiotics and synbiotics – a review. *Journal of Food Science and Technology* 52 (12): 7577–7587.

**54** Swanson, K., Gibson, G., Hutkins, R. et al. (2020). The international scientific association for probiotics and prebiotics (isapp) consensus statement on the definition and scope of synbiotics. *Nature* 17: 687–701.

**55** Mayeux, R. (2004). Biomarkers: potential uses and limitation. *NeuroRx* 1: 182–188.

**56** Rezzi, S., Ramadan, Z., Fay, L., and Kochhar, S. (2007). Nutritional metabonomics: applications and perspectives. *Journal of Proteome Research* 6: 513–525.

**57** Goldman, A. and Landweber, L. (2016). What is a genome? *PLoS Genetics* 12 (7): https://doi.org/10.1371/journal.pgen.1006181.

**58** Awany, D., Allall, I., Dalvie, S. et al. (2019). Host and microbiome genome-wide association studies: current state and challenges. *Frontiers in Genetics* 9: 637.

**59** Zhang, X., You, L., Wang, W., and Xiao, K. (2015). Novel omics technologies in food nutrition. In: *Genomics, Proteomics and Metabolomics in Nutraceuticals and Functional Foods* (ed. D. Bagchi, A. Swaroop, and M. Bagchi), 46–65. Chichester: Wiley.

**60** Mellersh, C. (2008). Give a dog a genome. *The Veterinary Journal* 178: 46–52.

**61** Chiu, C. and Miller, S. (2019). Clinical metagenomics. *Nature Reviews* 20: 341–355.

**62** Jablonka, E. and Lamb, M. (2002). The changing concept of epigenetics. *Annals of the New York Academy of Sciences* 981: 82–96.

**63** Berger, S., Kouzarides, T., Shiekehattar, R., and Shilatifard, A. (2009). An operational definition of epigenetics. *Genes & Development* 23: 781–783.

**64** Weinhold, B. (2006). Epigenetics: the science of change. *Environmental Health Perspectives* 114 (3): A160–A167.

**65** Agus, A., Clément, K., and Sokol, H. (2020). Gut microbiota-derived metabolites as central regulators in metabolic disorders. *Gut* 70: 1174–1182.

**66** Li, Z., Quan, G., Jiang, X. et al. (2018). Effects of metabolites derived from gut microbiota and hosts on pathogens. *Fronteirs in Cellular and Infection Microbiology* 8: 314.

**67** Guetterman, H., Huey, S.L., Knight, R. et al. (2021). Vitamin b-12 and the gastrointestinal microbiome: a systematic review. *Advances in Nutrition* 13 (2): 530–558.

**68** Levy, M., Thaiss, C., and Elinav, E. (2016). Metabolites: messengers between the microbiota and the immune system. *Genes & Development* 30: 1589–1597.

**69** Honneffer, J., Steiner, J., Lidbury, J., and Suchodolski, J. (2017). Variation of the microbiota and metabolome along the canine gastrointestinal tract. *Metabolomics* 13 (26): https://doi.org/10.1007/s11306-017-1165-3.

**70** Zhang, J., Wei, S., Liu, L. et al. (2012). Nmr-based metabolomics study of canine bladder cancer. *Biochimicha et Biophysica Acta* 1822: 1807–1814.

**71** Carlos, G., dos Santos, F., and Fröehlich, P. (2020). Canine metabolomics advances. *Metabolomics* 16.

**72** Gika, H., Theodoridis, G., Plumb, R., and Wilson, I. (2014). Current practice of liquid chromatography–mass spectrometry in metabolomics and metabonomics. *Journal of Pharmaceutical and Biomedical Analysis* 87: 12–25.

**73** García-Pérez, I., Whitfield, P., Bartlett, A. et al. (2008). Metabolic fingerprinting of schistosoma mansoni infection in mice urine with capillary electrophoresis. *Electrophoresis* 29: 3201–3206.

**74** Centre, T.M.I. (2022). The human metabolome database. https://hmdb.ca (accessed 27 July 2022).

**75** Centre, T.M.I. (2022). Livestock metabolome database. https://lmdb.ca (accessed 27 July 2022).

**76** Centre, T.M.I. (2022). Bovine metabolome databse. https://bovinedb.ca (accessed 27 July 2022).

**77** MetaboAnalyst (2022). Metaboanalyst 5.0. https://www.metaboanalyst.ca (accessed 27 July 2022).

**78** Antcliffe, D. and Gordon, A. (2016). Metabonomics and intensive care. *Critical Care* 20: 68.

**79** Westergren-Thorsson, G., Marko-Vagra, G., Malmsröm, J., and Larsen, K. (2006). Proteome. In: *Encyclopedia of Respiratory Medicine* (ed. G. Laurent and S. Shapiro), 527–532. Cambridge, MA: Academic Press.

# 2

# Functions of the Gastrointestinal Microbiome

## 2.1 What Is the Gastrointestinal Microbiome?

The microbiome is the community of all microbiota within a particular habitat or ecosystem [1]. Within the context of this text, this refers to the microbial population within the gastrointestinal (GI) tract of dogs and cats. The microbiome has multiple known functions and effects that impact physiological functions of the host. Many of the actions of microbiota are multifunctional and can result in widespread impacts or elicit a change across a variety of areas within the host body. While many of these functions will be discussed in greater detail in the corresponding chapters, this chapter will provide a brief overview of some ways the GI microbiome plays a role in metabolic functions, how it provides benefit to the host in protection from non-beneficial or pathobiont bacteria, and how it maintains the structure of some organs and cells and participates in bidirectional communications.

## 2.2 Metabolic Functions

The microbiota in the GI can exert local metabolic functions specific to ingested nutrients within the fed intestine, including modulating digestion, extraction, and absorption of nutrients, excretion of byproducts, alterations in intestinal permeability and motility, and secretion of hormones [2–4]. Furthermore, effects on the host's extra-GI physiology and

*Small Animal Microbiomes and Nutrition*, First Edition. Robin Saar and Sarah Dodd.
© 2024 John Wiley & Sons, Inc. Published 2024 by John Wiley & Sons, Inc.
Companion website: www.wiley.com/go/saar/1e

metabolic state may be induced through microbially produced metabolites and the wider metabolomes. For example, metabolites produced within the GI tract may be absorbed into the circulatory system via the portal vein, which travels to the liver [2]. The liver's role is to act as a second protector against, or filter for, harmful substances that may have been absorbed in the intestine. While many metabolites are altered or degraded in the liver, some are converted into biologically active metabolites by hepatic enzymes. In this way, microbially derived metabolites may contribute to active metabolites affecting the host in locations distant from the GI tract.

There is a vast diversity of known metabolites that can be produced by a variety of microbiota metabolizing or fermenting macronutrients and micronutrients ingested by the host [5]. These metabolites can then interact with multiple body systems. Metabolites may participate in various physiological processes, essential to the normal function of the host system. The effect of specific microbiota-derived metabolites depends on multiple factors, including the specific microbe, the food source provided, the volume of metabolites produced, and the health status of the host.

### 2.2.1 Short-Chain Fatty Acids

Carbohydrates indigestible by the host, such as some fiber sources, can be hydrolyzed by anaerobic bacteria into oligosaccharides, which are then converted into phosphoenolpyruvate, and finally into short-chain fatty acids (SCFA): acetic, butyric, and propionic, depending on the nutrient and bacteria of origin [2, 6–8] (Table 2.1).

1) Butyric acid (butyrate) is a primary source of energy for colonocytes and has potential for anti-inflammatory and anticancer activity [6, 9–11]. Additionally, there is evidence that butyrate can activate intestinal gluconeogenesis helping to regulate glucose and energy homeostasis. Predominant producers of butyrate in the canine microbiome include *Faecalibacterium*, *Firmicutes*, *Fusobacteriaceae* and *Lachnospiraceae* [5], while in carnivores, like cats, and omnivorous dogs consuming low carbohydrate diets, butyrate synthesis is predominantly from fermentation of proteins, associated with *Clostridiaceae* and *Fusobacterium* [12–16].

**Table 2.1** Short chain fatty acids (SCFA), their main roles in the body, and related bacteria.

| | Short chain fatty acids | |
| --- | --- | --- |
| **Butyric acid (butyrate)** | **Propionic acid (propionate)** | **Acetic acid (acetate)** |
| • Primary source of energy for colonocytes <br> • Potent anti-cancer activity | • Additional energy source for epithelial cells <br> • Reduces hepatic glucose production | • Most abundant SCFA <br> • Provides energy for peripheral tissues <br> • Aids in metabolism of cholesterol and lipogenesis |
| Produced by *Firmicutes* *Lachnospiraceae* and *Faecalibacterium prausnitzii* | Produced by *Bacteroides species,* *Negativicutes* *Clostridium species* | Produced by many bacteria <br> Is required for growth of *Faecalibacterium prausnitzii* |

2) Propionic acid (propionate) is an additional energy source for epithelial cells. Once converted to glucose in the intestine, it is transferred to the liver where it reduces hepatic glucose production. In dogs and cats, propionate appears to largely be produced by *Bacteroidetes* and *Clostrdidiaceae* [11, 17].

3) Acetic acid (acetate) is the most abundant SCFA though specific roles are still under investigation. Acetate may be used as energy for peripheral tissues and, at least in some species, it may play a role in the metabolism of cholesterol and lipogenesis and aid in appetite regulation [18, 19]. Furthermore, it is a co-factor and metabolite for other bacteria, and can be required for the growth of some bacteria species.

Fermentation of protein derivatives and amino acids can also result in the production of some SCFA. Aspartate, alanine, threonine, and methionine are the main sources of propionate, while glutamate, lysine, histidine, cysteine, serine, and methionine fermentation predominantly result in the production of butyrate [8].

## 2.2.2 Gases

Gas is a product of anaerobic microbial fermentation in particular, with the majority of bacterial-generated gases comprised of hydrogen, carbon dioxide, methane, and nitrogen. The characteristic odor attributable to fermentative gases arise from odiferous particularly from protein putrefaction, such as ammonia, sulfides, indoles, phenols, and volatile amines [20, 21]. While some of these gases can be used as energy, others may have pathological consequences for the host. Putrefactive compounds have been suggested to promote development of colonic cancer and may exacerbate underlying health conditions such as ulcerative colitis [21].

## 2.2.3 Amino Acids

While most amino acids in the intestines originate from the consumption of protein-containing foods (animal and plant sources along with some digestion of microbes and sloughed host tissue), a small portion is synthesized de novo by the gut microbiota. Some gut microbes are capable of synthesizing all 20 protein-building amino acids, which in turn may contribute to the host's amino acid homeostasis [22]. The contribution of microbial amino acids to host amino acid status is variable depending on species. In ruminants, microbial protein and essential amino acid synthesis is critical and can entirely meet the animal's needs under some circumstances [23]. In nonruminants, dietary protein has long been more of a focus, with microbial synthesis of amino acids largely disregarded. However, microbially synthesized lysine has been shown to contribute between 2 and 20% of the total circulating lysine volume in humans, pigs, and rats, indicating a potential significant source of essential amino acids even in monogastrics [24] (Figure 2.1).

The concentration of individual amino acids can also play a role on overall amino acid utilization. For example, L-glutamine can regulate the bacterial metabolism of arginine, serine, and aspartate and reduce the catabolism of essential and nonessential amino acids [8]. Butyrate and propionate also play a role in the creation of some amino acids and peptides.

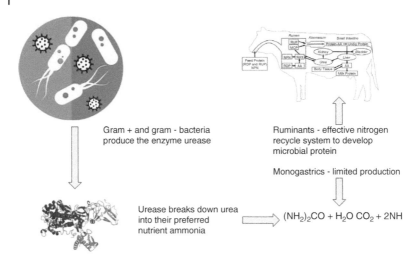

Gram + and gram - bacteria produce the enzyme urease

Ruminants - effective nitrogen recycle system to develop microbial protein

Monogastrics - limited production

Urease breaks down urea into their preferred nutrient ammonia

$(NH_2)_2CO + H_2O\ CO_2 + 2NH$

**Figure 2.1** Contribution of microbiota to amino acid synthesis. While most amino acids in the intestines originate from the consumption of nitrogenous ingredients (animal and plant sources along with the host muscle tissue), a small portion are synthesized de novo by the gut microbiota.

### 2.2.4 Vitamins and Minerals

Many microbes in the small animal GI microbiome are capable of synthesizing vitamins, particularly menaquinones and phylloquinones (forms of vitamin K) and B vitamins, including biotin, cobalamin ($B_{12}$), folate ($B_9$), pyridoxine ($B_6$), riboflavin ($B_2$), and thiamin ($B_1$) [25]. Others may not be able to synthesize vitamins *de novo*, but may absorb and transform vitamins using co-factors produced by other organisms [26]. In addition to their wider functions, some vitamins may play a role in local applications, such as gut barrier function, or assist with the uptake of nutrients by the GI epithelial cells [27]. For example, $B_{12}$ has been demonstrated to influence the composition of the GI microbiome [28]. An analysis of 22 studies from a variety of subjects (*in vitro*, animals, and humans) found that a majority reported $B_{12}$ was associated with alterations in both alpha-diversity and beta-diversity, the relative abundance of bacteria in the colon, and SCFA production [29]. Vitamins A, $B_2$, D, and E may increase commensal abundance, while vitamins A, $B_2$, $B_3$, C, and K may increase or maintain microbial diversity in the GI microbiome [26]. Vitamin D can alter the number of species (diversity or richness), and vitamin C, the production of SCFAs. Vitamins $B_2$ and E may increase the species that produce SCFAs.

Though microbes are incapable of synthesizing minerals, as minerals are inorganic substances, they may influence host absorption and utilization of ingested minerals [30]. Additionally, dietary mineral content may in turn modulate the gut microbiome [31].

## 2.3  Structural Functions

### 2.3.1  Tight Junctions and Intestinal Permeability

The epithelial cells of the intestine are joined together in junctional complexes: tight junctions, adherent junctions, and desmosomes [32]. These junctional complexes mechanically seal the cells together to create the intestinal epithelial barrier though each complex has differing permeability and ability to allow passage of water and small molecules. The tight junctions are narrow adhesions consisting of specific proteins connected to the cytoskeleton that connect or create fusion points between adjacent epithelial cells. They have fluctuating permeability as they respond to both external and internal cellular stimuli. Some functions are to maintain cellular polarity by passively regulating transepithelial movement of molecules including macronutrients, micronutrients, and cellular communication molecules. In disease states, dysfunction of the tight junctions can result in increased permeability, attributable to and/or modifiable in some cases by bacterial toxins, cytokines, hormones, and drugs [33].

Between the GI epithelial cells and the contents of the gut lumen, including the microbiome, lays a 2-tiered mucus layer [34]. This layer keeps some luminal microbes from directly contacting the epithelial cells. Intestinal goblet cells secrete mucin glycoproteins to create an inner layer that is denser and free of microorganisms and an outer layer that provides glycans as a source of nutrition for resident microbiota. In part of maintaining the structure of the GI tract, microbes have multiple functions in activating receptors, resulting in signaling of several pathways essential for promoting mucosal barrier function [35]. These include:

1) Maintenance of desmosomes at the epithelial villus by inducing protein expression
2) Stimulation of tight junctions via interaction with peptidoglycans in microbial cell wall
3) Cytokine-induced apoptosis (cell death) of the intestinal epithelial cells

4) Increase synthesis of endocannabinoids that decrease metabolic endotoxemia
5) Development of intestinal microvasculature by transcription factor induction
6) Maintenance of mucosal glycosylation patterns on cell surfaces and subcellular levels
7) Synthesis of antimicrobial proteins

## 2.4 Protective Functions

### 2.4.1 Bacteriocins

Bacteriocins are protein metabolites that have antimicrobial effects and work synergistically with beneficial bacteria to inhibit potential pathogens [36]. The synergy of bacteriocins and antibiotics may help address the problem of antimicrobial resistance as a future approach in the treatment of infectious diseases [22] (Figure 2.2).

Bacteriocins directly kill pathogens by [35, 36]:

1) Disrupting bacterial cell structures
2) Interfering with bacterial DNA, RNA, and protein metabolism
3) Compete for resources between commensal bacteria and pathogens
4) Affecting cell adhesion and biofilm formation
5) Regulating the immune system by activating innate immunity

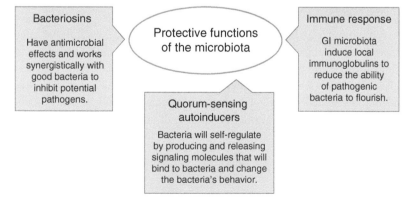

Figure 2.2   The protective functions of microbiota.

### 2.4.2 Quorum-Sensing

Over time if there is a gradual, and accumulative increase in bacteria concentrations in a certain area, certain microbes will self-regulate by producing and releasing signaling molecules to detect and control the bacterial concentration [37]. The signaling molecules will bind to receptors on the bacteria and ultimately change the behavior of the bacteria.

### 2.4.3 Immune Response

GI commensal microbiota also maintains the intestinal barrier by inducing local immunoglobulins to reduce the ability of pathogenic bacteria to flourish. For example Gram-negative microbiota (for example *Bacteroides*) can activate intestinal dendritic cells, resulting in the expression of mucosal IgA [35]. Additionally, they can use mechanisms to restrict bacterial translocation.

## 2.5 Participation in Bidirectional Axis Communication

Communication between different physiological systems can occur through metabolites and, more accurately, the metabolome [19]. Metabolites created from a variety of microbiota can travel across the epithelium and enter into the hepatic portal circulation. Some metabolites, such as SCFA, can cross the blood–brain barrier to influence a change on neurological systems [38]. Additionally, alternative systems such as the hepatic, renal, and subsequently urinary systems are affected by metabolites. For example, excessive uremic toxin production in the GI tract has been implicated in the development of renal diseases [39].

## 2.6 Chapter Summary

- The gastrointestinal microbiome is a diverse community of microbes that interact with the host animal in a plethora of ways
- Microbes in the gut metabolize or otherwise alter some ingested nutrients and can synthesize nutrients de novo for host animal absorption

- Short-chain fatty acids are synthesized by microbes in the colon and are of key importance for colonocyte health
- Gut microbes stimulate physical and immunological changes in the gut wall to maintain a barrier permeable to essential substances like nutrients but impermeable to pathogens
- The gastrointestinal microbiome is not static, it is constantly shifting and adapting.

## References

1 Marchesi, J. (2017). What is a microbiome? https://microbiologysociety.org/blog/what-is-a-microbiome.html (accessed 11 May 2022).

2 Olofsson, L. and Bäckhed, F. (2022). The metabolic role and therapeutic potential of the microbiome. *Endocrine Reviews* 43: 907–926.

3 Costa, M. and Weese, J. (2018). Understanding the intestinal microbiome in health and disease. *Veterinary Clinics of North America: Equine* 34: 1–12.

4 Lee, D., Goh, T., Kang, M. et al. (2022). Perspectives and advances in probiotics and the gut microbiome in companion animals. *Journal of Animal Science and Technology* 64 (2): 197–217.

5 Pilla, R. and Suchodolski, J. (2021). The gut microbiome of dogs and cats, and the influence of diet. *Veterinary Clinics of North America: Small Animal Practice* 51: 605–621.

6 Swanson, K., Grieshop, C., Flickinger, E. et al. (2002). Fructooligosaccharides and lactobacillus acidophilus modify gut microbial populations, total tract nutrient digestibilities and fecal protein catabolite concentrations in healthy adult dogs. *Journal of Nutrition* 132: 3721–3731.

7 Gagné, J., Wakshlag, J., Simpson, K. et al. (2013). Effects of a synbiotic on fecal quality, short-chain fatty acid concentrations, and the microbiome of healthy sled dogs. *BMC Veterinary Research* 9: 246.

8 Rowland, I., Gibson, G., Heinken, A. et al. (2018). Gut microbiota functions: metabolism of nutrients and other food components. *European Journal of Nutrition* 57: 1–24.

9 Roediger, W. (1982). Utilization of nutrients by isolated epithelial cells of the rat colon. *Gastroenterology* 83 (2): 424–429.

10 Lazarova, D. and Brodonaro, M. (2017). P300 knockout promotes butyrate resistance. *Journal of Cancer* 8: 3405–3409.

**11** Tizard, I. and Jones, S. (2018). The microbiota regulates immunity and immunologic diseases in dogs and cats. *Veterinary Clinics of North America: Small Animal Practice* 48: 307–322.

**12** Potrykus, J., White, R., and Bearne, S. (2008). Proteomic investigation of amino acid catabolismin the indigenous gut anaerobe fusobacterium varium. *Proteomics* 8: 2691–2703.

**13** Bermingham, E., Young, W., Kittelmann, S. et al. (2013). Dietary format alters fecal bacterial populations in thedomestic cat (felis catus). *MicrobiologyOpen* 2 (1): 173–181.

**14** Bermingham, E., Young, W., Butowski, C.F. et al. (2018). The fecal microbiota in the domestic cat (felis catus) is influenced by interactions between age and diet; a five year longitudinal study. *Frontiers in Microbiology* 9: 1231.

**15** Bermingham, E., Maclean, P., Thomas, D. et al. (2017). Key bacterial families (clostridiaceae, erysipelotrichaceae and bacteroidaceae) are related to the digestion of protein and energy in dogs. *PeerJ* 5: e3019.

**16** Sandri, M., Dal Monego, S., Conte, G. et al. (2017). Raw meat based diet influences faecal microbiome and end products of fermentation in healthy dogs. *BMC Veterinary Research* 13: 65.

**17** Van den Abbeele, P., Moens, F., Pignataro, G. et al. (2020). Yeast-derived formulations are differentially fermented by the canine and feline microbiome as assessed in a novel in vitro colonic fermentation model. *Journal of Agricultural and Food Chemistry* 68: 13102–13110.

**18** Frost, G., Sleeth, M., Sahuri-Arisoylu, M. et al. (2014). The short-chain fatty acid acetate reduces appetite via a central homeostatic mechanism. *Nature Communications* 5: 3611.

**19** Perry, R., Peng, L., Barry, N. et al. (2016). Acetate mediates a microbiome-brain–β-cell axis to promote metabolic syndrome. *Nature* 534: 213–217.

**20** Pinna, C., Vecchiato, C., Cardenia, V. et al. (2017). An in vitro evaluation of the effects of a yucca schidigera extract and chestnut tannins on composition and metabolic profiles of canine and feline faecal microbiota. *Archives of Animal Nutrition* 71 (5): 395–412.

**21** Hussein, H., Flickinger, E., and Fahey, G. Jr. (1999). Petfood applications of inulin and oligofructose. *Journal of Nutrition* 129 (7): 1454S–1456S.

**22** Mousa, W., Chehadeh, F., and Husband, S. (2022). Recent advances in understanding the structure and function of the human microbiome. *Frontiers in Microbiology* 13: 825338.

**23** Wu, G., Bazer, F., Dai, Z. et al. (2014). Amino acid nutrition in animals: protein synthesis and beyond. *Annual Review of Animal Biosciences* 2: 387–417.

**24** Metges, C. (2000). Contribution of microbial amino acids to amino acid homeostasis of the host. *Journal of Nutrition* 130 (7): 1857S–1864S.

**25** Swanson, K., Dowd, S., Suchodolski, J. et al. (2011). Phylogenetic and gene-centric metagenomics of canine intestinal microbiome reveals similarities with humans and mice. *The ISME Journal* 5: 639–649.

**26** Pham, V., Dold, S., Rehman, A. et al. (2021). Vitamins, the gut microbiome and gastrointestinal health in humans. *Nutrition Research* 95: 35–53.

**27** Uebanso, T., Shimohata, T., Mawatari, K., and Takahashi, A. (2020). Functional roles of b-vitamins in the gut and gut microbiome. *Molecular Nutrition & Food Research* 64: e2000426.

**28** Xu, Y., Xiang, S., Ye, K. et al. (2018). Cobalamin (vitamin b12) induced a shift in microbial composition and metabolic activity in an in vitro colon simulation. *Frontiers in Microbiology* https://doi.org/10.3389/fmicb.2018.02780.

**29** Manúsdottir, S., Ravcheev, D., de Crécy-Lagard, V., and Thiele, I. (2015). Systematic genome assessment of b-vitamin biosynthesis suggests co-operation among gut microbes. *Frontiers in Genetics* https://doi.org/10.3389/fgene.2015.00148.

**30** Barone, M., D'Amico F, Brigidi P, Turroni S, Gut microbiome–micronutrient interaction: the key to controlling the bioavailability of minerals and vitamins? *BioFactors*, 2022. 48 (2): p. 307–314.

**31** Pereira, A., Pinna, C., Biagi, G. et al. (2020). Supplemental selenium source on gut health: insights on fecal microbiome and fermentation products of growing puppies. *FEMS Microbiology Ecology* 96: fiaa212.

**32** Jergens, A., Parvinroo, S., Kopper, J., and Wannemuehler, M. (2021). Rules of engagement: epithelial-microbe interactions and inflammatory bowel disease. *Frontiers in Medicine* 8: 669913.

**33** Gasbarrini, G. and Montalto, M. (1999). Structure and function of tight junctions. Role in intestinal barrier. *Italian Journal of Gastroenterology and Hepatology* 31 (6): 481–488.

**34** Kleessen, B. and Blaut, M. (2005). Modulation of gut mucosal biofilms. *British Journal of Nutrition* 93 (Suppl. 1): S35–S40.

**35** Jandhyala, S., Talukdar, R., Subramanyam, C. et al. (2015). Role of the normal gut microbiota. *World Journal of Gastroenterology* 21 (29): 8787–8803.

**36** Eijsink, V., Axelsson, L., Diep, D. et al. (2022). Production of class ii bacteriocins by lactic acid bacteria; an example of biological warfare and communication. *Probiotics and Antimicrobial Proteins* 8 (4): 177–182.

**37** Obst, U. (2007). Quorum sensing: bacterial chatting. *Analytical and Bioanalytical Chemistry* 387: 369–370.

**38** Cannas, S., Tonini, B., Belà, B. et al. (2021). Effect of a novel nutraceutical supplement (relaxigen pet dog) on the fecal microbiome and stress-related behaviors in dogs: a pilot study. *Journal of Veterinary Behavior* 42: 37–47.

**39** Chen, Y.-Y., Chen, D.-Q., Chen, L. et al. (2019). Microbiome–metabolome reveals the contribution of gut–kidney axis on kidney disease. *Journal of Translational Medicine* 17: 5.

# 3

# The Origin and Development of the Gastrointestinal Microbiome

## 3.1 In Utero

Initial colonization of the body's microbiomes is commonly considered to start during the birthing processes, with exposure to maternal microbiota [1, 2]. Historically, research suggested that there were no functional microbiomes *in utero*; however, more recent work has demonstrated microbial communities in the canine endometrium [3], as well as the uterus, placenta, amniotic fluid, meconium, and umbilical blood of healthy pregnancies [4]. It is thus possible that early colonization of the fetus may begin *in utero*, though development of the normal, healthy microbiome likely depends on colonization with maternal microbiota during parturition [4].

Microbiome research has utilized the study of xenobiosis, the creation of a "germ-free state," which has been experimentally achieved in birds, fish, insects, and mammals [5]. The term "germ-free" is used for animals that are completely devoid of all detectable microbes including bacteria, fungi, viruses, parasites, and protozoa [6]. The first germ-free animal was created in 1896 by Nuttall and Thierfelder. They utilized a guinea pig that survived for only 13 days due to a lack of appropriate knowledge about nutrition or provisions of adequate equipment. In 1946, the first rat and mice colonies were created. In 1981, Wostmann discovered that germ-free animals had smaller hearts, lungs, livers, and thinner intestinal walls with reduced gastrointestinal mobility [7]. Additionally, they had overall

*Small Animal Microbiomes and Nutrition*, First Edition. Robin Saar and Sarah Dodd.
© 2024 John Wiley & Sons, Inc. Published 2024 by John Wiley & Sons, Inc.
Companion website: www.wiley.com/go/saar/1e

stunted growth and required large quantities of nutrient-rich food, which did not alleviate these conditions. The introduction of intestinal microbiota from healthy animals induced a critical health benefit, demonstrating the role of gut microbes in maintenance of animal health. Today, researchers still utilize these animals to understand how the GI microbiota affects the host's physiology and metabolism [5, 6]. The term gnotobiotic refers to germ-free animals that are selectively colonized with one or more bacterial strains [5], though sometimes these words ("germ-free" and "gnotobiotic") are used synonymously. Different protocols have been developed to establish a germ-free state in different species. For example, some germ-free rodent models are born via cesarean section, with the concept that the fetus is sterile in the womb, though in this protocol the entire uterus with the fetus is removed and placed in a sterile isolator where the fetus(es) are removed and are raised in sterile conditions with a germ-free foster mother or fed a sterilized milk replacer [6]. These "sterile" rodents are then bred to produce generations of germ-free offspring.

Utilizing current technology and research, particularly with germ-free animal models, the womb is still generally recognized as being sterile, in the sense that it bears no functioning microbiome [2, 6]. However, there can be transient maternally-derived bacteria that come in contact with the fetus and developmental tissues (placenta, umbilical cord, etc.) through bacterial translocation. Transient microbiota from the mother's indigenous microbiomes plays a role in maturing the immune systems of the fetus through immunological and chemical exposure to this microbiota. Studies have identified a correlation in the type of bacteria identified in the meconium, or umbilical blood of fetuses with maternal microbiota, though some researchers feel more supporting evidence is required to claim the development of a functioning microbiome versus transient bacteria existing in the womb [2]. Another way bacteria may reach the fetus is by an adventitious infection – when an acute or chronic infection of the mother crosses the placenta, it can directly infect the fetus [8].

## 3.2 Factors Influencing the Initial Colonization of Microbiota

The exposure diversity may differ depending on a large number of intrinsic and extrinsic factors. The GI microbiome is considered to begin development at birth and proceeds to evolve and mature during

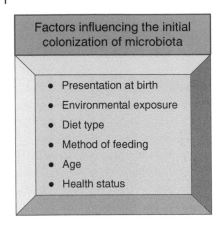

Figure 3.1 Factors influencing the initial colonization of microbiota.

the first weeks, months, and years of life, depending on the species [4, 9] (Figure 3.1).

### 3.2.1 Presentation at Birth

The first exposure of the fetus that allows for initial development of microbiomes begins during birth, with variations observed between neonates with vaginal exposure compared to those born via cesarean section [10, 11]. In animals like dogs and cats, the mothers will also lick the neonate, providing exposure to maternal oral microbes. Neonates born via vaginal delivery tend to have initial colonization with vaginal and fecal microbes. In puppies, *Staphylococcus, Enterobacter,* and *Escherichia coli* species were cultivable orally within days of birth, in comparison to caesarean-delivered puppies who lacked *Enterobacter* and *E. coli* but had cultivable *Streptococcus* and *Clostridium* species not present in the vaginally born pups [11]. This appears consistent with the reported vaginal and oral flora of dogs and fits with the birthing process of the dog, where some puppies may be born with intact amniotic membranes, separating the puppy from the vaginal flora, until the dam opens the membrane with her teeth, exposing the puppy to her oral microbes in the process [12].

To enhance the GI microbiomes of infants born by cesarean section, vaginal seeding has been proposed, where a vaginal swab is taken from the mother and rubbed over the neonate's skin, mouth, and nose post-delivery [13]. In humans, there is a positively related increase in the frequency of asthma, atopic disease, and immune disorders with the rate of cesarean delivery. By performing vaginal seeding, the theory is to allow for "normal" exposure and colonization of the fetal gut, reducing the subsequent risk of the associated diseases. However, research both in humans and companion animals have shown inconclusive results and at present there is insufficient evidence to either support or refute this practice [13, 14].

### 3.2.2 Environmental Exposure

The environment into which the neonate arrives also influences the type of pioneer microbiota to colonize. Newborn puppies and kittens are fairly immobile, with most of their microbial exposure coming from maternal interaction [12]. Physical contact with other individuals and even shared air are other environmental exposure influencers demonstrated in human infants [15]. For dogs and cats, these could include contact with the pet parent, other pets in the house, and the whelping box. Exposure to pathogenic sources during times of stress such as weaning also plays a role, as there is an increase in the risk of illness during this period [16].

### 3.2.3 Diet Type and Method of Feeding

Components of maternal milk shape the development of the neonatal microbiomes through a variety of components that may not be provided through milk from other species or commercial formulations. Maternal milk is initially high in colostrum, which provides a source of nutrients and immunoglobulins, and contributes to the maturation of the digestive tract [11]. In humans, breast-fed infants have microbiota enriched in *Lactobacillus, Staphylococcus, Bifidobacterium,* and *Bacteroides,* whereas formula-fed infants have predominantly facultative anaerobes (*Enterobacteriaceae*) and microbes that are associated with inflammation such as *Roseburia, Clostridium*, and *Anaerostipes* in their GI microbiomes [2, 9]. Formula-fed human infants have an increased maturation of their microbiome to match that of an adult composition [2]. Maternal milk contains beneficial components that are nutritional for both the infant and the GI microbiota including oligosaccharides that are considered to be prebiotics and provide antimicrobial and antiadhesive properties [2]. These milk oligosaccharides will enhance the density of specific bacterial populations such as *Bifidobacterium* genus in the GI microbiome [2]. Maternal milk contains GI and possibly oral microbes that have translocated in immune mediate cells to the mammary gland through an entero-mammary pathway [9]. These collections of bacteria can be identified in colostrum before the initial feeding of the neonatal. Bacteria from maternal milk is the second most significant bacterial exposure for a newborn after vaginal birth [9]. A recently published paper [12] found that none of the 12 colostrum/milk samples taken from canine dams postpartum were sterile [12]. Bacteria detected were *Staphylococci, Enterococci* along with *Escherichia coli* that were isolated in 50% of the colostrum samples and 17% of milk samples. *Proteus* spp. (*P. mirabilis*) was isolated in 50% of colostrum samples and 33.3% of milk samples. Five other bacteria species were detected, but they were only identified in one subject [8].

A dietary change during weaning can alter the density and diversity of microbiota in the GI microbiome [9]. In a small study following five litters of kittens from birth, differences in oral microbiomes were noted in neonates born by caesarian section versus those from vaginal delivery and those that ingested breast milk versus formula. The diversity of oral microbiomes was lowest at birth (week 0) and the highest at week 8. The composition of the microbiome became less variable once the kittens were all fed a commercial type of diet. The type of commercial diet itself has also been shown to reflect a difference in the populations of oral bacteria. Cats fed dry kibble have increased *Porphyromonas* spp. and *Treponema* spp., while wet canned diets show an increase in *Conchiformibius kuhniae* [6].

### 3.2.4 Age

Age does play a role in the establishment of microbiomes, with early colonization in the GI tract being crucial in establishing resistance to invading pathogens [9]. Gastrointestinal colonization occurs quickly and within 24 hours post-birth, with the number of bacteria being comparable to those of their dams [8]. Research consistently shows that GI microbiomes are frequently changing, along with fluctuating diversity and the density of these diverse groups during the first few weeks of life. In humans, differences between babies born vaginally and those by cesarean section cannot be separated based on the composition of their microbiota by only 1 month of age [9]. Examination of the fecal microbiota in puppies has demonstrated that initial colonization during the first 24 hours reflected similarities to the dam's samples, followed by an increase in microbial density and diversity during the first 21 days [12]. Fecal microbiota was significantly different from maternal samples by day 56, and it was noted that the overall change from day 1 to day 63 was an increase in the proportion of anaerobic bacteria in the distal portion of the colon [8]. Similarly, another study analyzing puppies' fecal microbiota over 2 months after birth and comparing it to a dam's fecal microbiota (*Bacteroidetes, Firmicutes, Fusobacteria, Actinobacteria,* and *Proteobacteria*) found a high variability within the major bacterial phyla *Firmicutes* in 2-day-old puppies, where dams experienced a lower variance of the same phyla. Once the puppies were 56 days old, the fecal microbiota was more similar to the dams (see Figure 3.2) [7]. In humans, the GI microbiome is considered to be stable by 3 years of age [8].

## 3.3 Dysbiosis During Microbiome Development

In comparison to the mature state, the juvenile microbiome has a low density of microbiota and is highly susceptible to instability, such as from exposure to antibiotic treatments or illness [15–19] (see Figure 3.3). Another common finding is the persistence of dysbiosis post antimicrobial treatment. In kittens treated with either amoxicillin/clavulanic acid or doxycyline, alterations to both serum and fecal metabolomic profiles, at least partially attributable to the antibiotics' effects on the microbiome, persisted for up to 10 months after treatment [17].

It is understood that GI microbiota are required for the normal maturation of the immune system from information gathered about "germ-free" mice; reduced development of gut-associated lymphoid tissue (GALT), decreased numbers of T cells, B cells, antimicrobial peptides, along with thinner mucous layer, and fewer Peyer's patches resulting in less immunotolerance and severe allergic responses to food antigens are some of the results of "germ-free mice" not a normal functioning GI microbiome [20, 21]. Another consideration is the association that autoimmune diseases

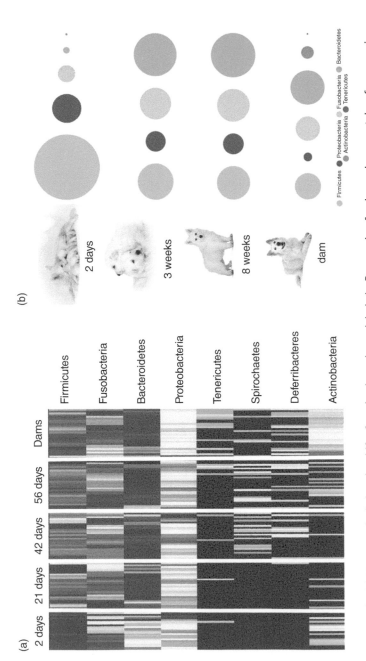

(a)

(b)

2 days    21 days    42 days    56 days    Dams

Firmicutes
Fusobacteria
Bacteroidetes
Proteobacteria
Tenericutes
Spirochaetes
Deferribacteres
Actinobacteria

2 days

3 weeks

8 weeks

dam

● Firmicutes ● Proteobacteria ● Fusobacteria ● Bacteroidetes
● Actinobacteria ● Tenericutes

**Figure 3.2** (a) Heatmap depicting the shift of predominant bacterial phyla. Preweaning fecal samples were taken from puppies and dams and tested for abundance of bacteria. Decrease in abundance is denoted by the green and blue bars, while increases in abundance is denoted by red and orange. (b) Bubble plot illustrating changing abundance of bacterial phylum in aging puppies. *Source:* Wostmann [7]. Creative Commons License: https://creativecommons.org/licenses/by/4.0/.

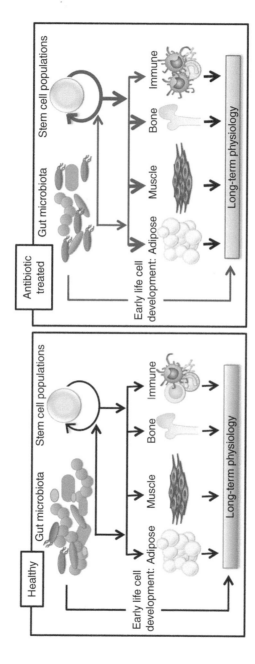

**Figure 3.3** Stem cell populations and long-term physiology are impacted by changes in the gut microbiota due to antibiotic use. *Source:* Del Carro et al. [12]. Creative Commons License: https://creativecommons.org/licenses/by/4.0/.

may be preceded by an increase in intestinal permeability [22]. There are dynamic changes in the commensal flora that occur during the first stages of life, and these developmental changes combined with an immature or weakened immune system can lead to a higher susceptibility to an infection or disease [23]. There is thus an importance in ensuring the integrity of the composition and proper maturation of the microbiomes early in life.

In humans, diseases suggested to be associated with dysbiosis during the development years of the microbiome and immune system include asthma (respiratory disease), allergies, obesity, diabetes, and inflammatory bowel disease [22]. The lack of specific or combination of microbiota species, lack of insufficient metabolite production due to the decreased density of specific microbiota, a change in host physiological function due to the reduction in specific microbiota or corresponding reduction in metabolite production, or the ability for a pathobiont to inhabit or colonize where it would have previously been excluded may all contribute to the etiopathogenesis of associated disease conditions. There is an association between low microbial richness with an increase of proinflammatory microbial species, insulin resistance, dyslipidemia, and a marked inflammatory phenotype [22]. With a juvenile microbiome, there is the consideration of an immature immune system, which may result in different outcomes compared to a pet with a functioning healthy mature immune system.

Genetics play a role in the risk of disease development, along with varying results between sexes. For example, one study in mice found that antibiotic treatment to "germ-free" mice early in life had an increased incidence of diabetes only in the male mice [24]. Another long-term study of over 12,000 human children found that in the first 6 years of life, there was a significant reduction of weight and height gain after neonatal antibiotic exposure in the boys only [25]. When a fecal transplant was completed from the neonatal antibiotic-treated boys and placed in "germ-free mice," the male but not female mice experienced significant growth impairment. Both boys and girls that received antibiotics before 6 years of age but after the neonatal period had a significantly higher body mass index. Those that had neonatal antibiotic treatment in the study had decreased fecal diversity and density of Bifidobacteria until 2 years of age.

# 3.4 Key Nutritional Factors

## 3.4.1 Maternal Colostrum and Maternal Milk

After exposure to the dam's own microbiome, maternal milk may be the second most influential source of microbes for the naive GI microbiome. Nutritionally, colostrum, while low in energy content, is a source of nutrients and most importantly maternal immunoglobulins, and it contributes to the maturation of the digestive tract. Canine colostrum contains 20–30 g/l, while feline colostrum contains 40–50 g/l of immunoglobulin G [26]. Both canine and feline neonates require the passive transfer of immunoglobulin G in the first 12–16 hours to stimulate immune protection. Immunoglobulin G decreases by 50% in colostrum after the first 24 hours or so, highlighting the critical nature of this early time period.

Milk is higher in energy content than colostrum and contains additional nutrients, such as milk glycans – oligosaccharides, glycoproteins, glycopeptides, and glycolipids. Interestingly, milk glycans require high energy to be produced by the mammary gland and yet are not intestinally digestible by the neonatal mammal. Milk glycans, particularly milk oligosaccharides, act like a prebiotic and function to protect and develop beneficial microbes, such as *Bifidobacteria* species, act as an antimicrobial by prophylactically binding bacteria, viruses, and toxins, promoting the immune system and enhancing intestinal epithelial barrier function [27, 28]. Furthermore, milk contains a large number of microbes, reportedly on the scale of 10-10 [5] in human milk, and these microbes contribute to early colonization of the neonatal gut, providing benefits such as defense against pathogens for the immunologically naïve system [29].

## 3.4.2 Prebiotics

With a high volume of indigestible oligosaccharides in maternal milk, a growth diet should ideally contain adequate levels of prebiotics. The use of prebiotics in the diet may assist with a smooth transition onto the new diet, along with continuing to support immune and gut health, including, though not limited to, the provision of microbially SCFAs. Indeed, in comparison to puppies not fed a prebiotic, higher levels of fecal

*Lactobacilli* and SCFAs were found in puppies who were fed a prebiotic, with reduced severity of clinical signs when infected with *Salmonella* [30]. Selective prebiotic supplementations are available in some therapeutic gastrointestinal diets that are formulated for growth.[1]

### 3.4.3 Non-maternal Colostrum

The addition of non-canine/feline mammalian colostrum in the diets of dogs and cats has been shown to stimulate the immune system in pets post-weaning. One study of 16-week-old kittens found the antibody response to a rabies vaccine to be quicker and stronger, with increased fecal IgA expression in those supplemented with bovine colostrum versus the control group [31]. Another demonstrated improvements in fecal quality in recently weaned puppies supplemented with bovine colostrum [32]. Potentially, supplementation of bovine colostrum could benefit weanlings during this stressful period and could be continued to be supplemented through the period when repeated vaccination boosters are occurring to help support the immune system (see Figure 3.4).

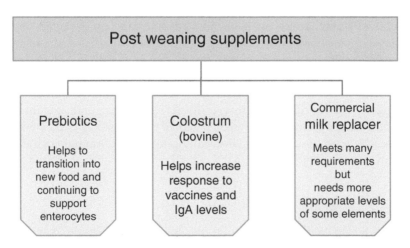

**Figure 3.4** Postweaning considerations for using different supplements.

---

1 e.g.: Hill's Healthy Advantage Kitten/Puppy Food, Rayne Clinical Nutrition Growth/Sensitive-GI, Royal Canin – Veterinary Exclusive Development Kitten/Puppy, Purina Pro Plan Veterinary Diets Gastrointestinal Health EN.

### 3.4.4 Commercial Milk Replacer

Milk replacers for companion animals are typically produced from the milk of other species and formulated to meet energy, essential protein, fatty acid, vitamin, and mineral requirements. Yet, one study that compared 15 commercial canine milk replacers with 5 canine maternal milk samples identified that all the milk replacers had numerous essential nutrients outside of the range of the dog milk samples, with most products needing more appropriate calcium, amino acids, and essential fatty acid concentrations along with the provision of more descriptive feeding directions [33]. Clearly, provision of canine or feline maternal milk is preferable to milk replacers produced from the milk of other mammals.

## 3.5 Chapter Summary

- Research has utilized the study of xenobiosis – creating a "germ-free state" – to evaluate the effects of the microbiome on developing animals
- Neonatal exposure to microbes may differ depending on presentation at birth, type of diet, method of feeding, age of the host, and health status
- In humans, disease states have been associated with early dysbiosis during development
- Age plays a role in the establishment of microbiomes, with early colonization in the GI tract being crucial in establishing resistance to invading pathogens
- Components of maternal milk shape the development of the neonatal microbiomes through a variety of nutrients and microbes that may not be provided through milk from other species or commercial formulations

## References

1 Tal, S., Tikhonov, E., Aroch, I. et al. (2021). Developmental intestinal microbiome alterations in canine fading puppy syndrome: a prospective observational study. *NPJ Biofilms and Microbiomes* 7 (1): https://doi.org/10.1038/s41522-021-00222-7.

**2** Blaser, M., Devkota, S., McCoy, K. et al. (2021). Lessons learned from the prenatal microbiome controversy. *Microbiome* 9 (8).

**3** Lyman, C., Holyoak, G., Meinkoth, K. et al. (2019). Canine endometrial and vaginal microbiomes reveal distinct and complex ecosystems. *PLoS One* 14 (1): e0210157.

**4** Pipan, M., Kajdic, L., Kalin, A. et al. (2020). Do newborn puppies have their own microbiota at birth? Influence of type of birth on newborn puppy microbiota. *Theriogenology* 152: 18–28.

**5** Fontaine, C., Skorupski, A., Vowles, C. et al. (2015). How free of germs is germ-free? Detection of bacterial contamination in a germ free mouse unit. *Gut Microbes* 6 (4): 225–233.

**6** Qv, L., Yang, Z., Yao, M. et al. (2020). Methods for establishment and maintenance of germ-free rat models. *Frontiers in Microbiology* 11.

**7** Wostmann, B. (1981). The germfree animal in nutritional studies. *Annual Review of Nutrition* 1: 257–279.

**8** Dubey, J., Buxton, D., and Wouda, W. (2006). Pathogenesis of bovine neosporosis. *Journal of Comparative Pathology* 134: 267–289.

**9** Guard, B., Mila, H., Steiner, J. et al. (2017). Characterization of the fecal microbiome during neonatal and early pediatric development in puppies. *PLoS One* 12 (4): e0175718.

**10** Spears, J., Vester Boler, B., Gardner, C., and Li, Q. (2017). Development of the oral microbiome in kittens. In: *Companion Animal Nutrition (CAN) Summit: The Nexus of Pet and Human Nutrition: Focus on Cognition and the Microbiome*, 4–7. Helsinki.

**11** Kačírová, J., Hornákocá, L., Madari, A. et al. (2021). Cultivable oral microbiota in puppies. *Folia Veterinaria* 65 (3): 69–74.

**12** Del Carro, A., Corrò, M., Bertero, A. et al. (2022). The evolution of dam-litter microbial flora from birth to 60 days of age. *BMC Veterinary Research* 18 (95): 1.

**13** Kelly, J., Nolan, L., and Good, M. (2021). Vaginal seeding after cesarean birth: can we build a better infant microbiome? *Med* 8: 889–891.

**14** Da Silva, S., Apparicio, M., Cardozo, M. et al. (2022). Colonization of canine intestinal microbiota and the effects of route of delivery and vaginal seeding: preliminary results. *Reproduction in Domestic Animals* 57: 50–50.

**15** Chong, C., Bloomfield, F., and O'Sullivan, J. (2018). Factors affecting gastrointestinal microbiome development in neonates. *Nutrients* 10: 274.

**16** Li, Y., Guo, Y., and Wen, Z. (2018). Weaning stress perturbs gut microbiome and its metabolic profile in piglets. *Nature* 8: 1–2.

**17** Stavroulaki, E., Suchodolski, J., Pilla, R. et al. (2022). The serum and fecal metabolomic profiles of growing kittens treated with amoxicillin/clavulanic acid or doxycycline. *Animals* 12: 330.

**18** Burton, E., O'Connor E, Ericsson A, Franklin C, Evaluation of fecal microbiota transfer as treatment for postweaning diarrhea in research-colony puppies. *Journal of the American Association for Laboratory Animal Science*, 2016. 55(5): p. 582–587.

**19** Deusch, O., O'Flynn C, Colyer A et al., Deep illumina-based shotgun sequencing reveals dietary effects on the structure and function of the fecal microbiome of growing kittens. *PLoS One*, 2014. 9(7) e101021.

**20** Hill, D. and Artis, D. (2010). Intestinal bacteria and the regulation of immune cell homeostasis. *Annual Review of Immunology* 28: 623–667.

**21** Gill, N. and Finlay, B. (2011). The gut microbiota: challenging immunology. *Nature Reviews Immunology* 11: 636–637.

**22** Vangoitsenhoven, R. and Cresci, G. (2020). Role of microbiome and antibiotics in autoimmune diseases. *Nutrition in Clinical Practice* 35 (3): 406–416.

**23** Hoffmann, A., Proctor, L., Surette, M., and Suchodolski, J. (2016). The microbiome: the trillions of microorganisms that maintain health and cause disease in humans and companion animals. *Veterinary Pathology* 53 (1): 10–21.

**24** Candon, S., Perez-Arroyo, A., Marquet, C. et al. (2015). Antibiotics in early life alter the gut microbiome and increase disease incidence in a spontaneous mouse model of autoimmune insulin-dependent diabetes. *PLoS One* 10 (5): e0125448.

**25** Uzan-Yulzari, A., Turta, O., Belogolovski, A. et al. (2021). Neonatal antibiotic exposure impairs child growth during the first six years of life by perturbing intestinal microbial colonization. *Nature Communications* 12: 1–2.

**26** Chastant-Maillard, S., Maillard, S., Aggouni, C. et al. (2017). Canine and feline colostrum. *Reproduction in Domestic Animals* 52 (Suppl. 2): 148–152.

**27** Rostami, S., Bénet, T., Spears, J. et al. (2014). Milk oligosaccharides over time of lactation from different dog breeds. *PLoS One* 9 (6): e99824.

**28** Milani, C., Mangifesta, M., Mancabelli, L. et al. (2017). Unveiling bifidobacterial biogeography across the mammalian branch of the tree of life. *The ISME Journal* 11: 2834–2847.

**29** Ge, Y., Zhu, W., Chen, L. et al. (2021). The maternal milk microbiome in mammals of different types and its potential role in the neonatal gut microbiota composition. *Animals* 11: 3349.

**30** Czarnecki-Maulden, G. (2008). Effect of dietary modulation of intestinal microbiota on reproduction and early growth. *Theriogenology* 70: 286–290.

**31** Gore, A., Satyaraj, E., Labuda, J. et al. (2021). Supplementation of diets with bovine colostrum influences immune and gut function in kittens. *Frontiers in Veterinary Science* 8: 675712.

**32** Giffard, C., Seino, M., Markwell, P., and Bektash, R. (2004). Benefits of bovine colostrum on fecal quality in recently weaned puppies. *Journal of Nutrition* 134: 2126S–2127S.

**33** Heinze, C., Freeman, L., Martin, C. et al. (2014). Comparison of the nutrient composition of commercial dog milk replacers with that of dog milk. *Journal of the American Veterinary Medical Association* 244 (12): 1413–1422.

# 4

# Factors Affecting the Diversity and Density of the Microbiomes

The composition of microbiomes are constantly shifting and adapting according to the changes within the host and their environment (Figure 4.1). Diversity and density are two ecologic properties used to describe communities in terms of the variety of organisms present and the quantity of each organism and the sum total of organisms [1]. Often, a simplistic view of "more is better" has been applied to both diversity and density;

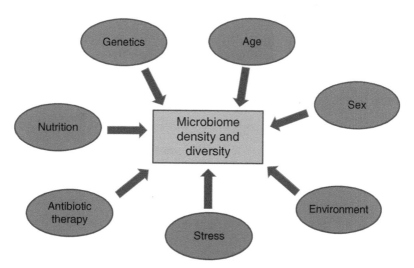

**Figure 4.1** The seven factors affecting the diversity and density of the microbiomes.

*Small Animal Microbiomes and Nutrition*, First Edition. Robin Saar and Sarah Dodd.
© 2024 John Wiley & Sons, Inc. Published 2024 by John Wiley & Sons, Inc.
Companion website: www.wiley.com/go/saar/1e

however, our limited understanding does not allow for definitive evaluation of the health of the community based exclusively on diversity and density, as these must be applied within context of the individual host animal. Diversity can be measured with different applications to describe the number of species present, their relative abundances, and relation to each other (see Chapter 6).

## 4.1 Physiological Factors

### 4.1.1 Genetics

While it is not always well understood how, it is recognized that the genetics of resident microbiota affect the host, and it would appear that host genetics also influence the composition of their microbiomes [2]. One study has demonstrated more similarity in the fecal microbiomes of genetically related dogs compared to unrelated dogs [3], and human studies have reported similar findings, with specific host gene elements associated with gastrointestinal microbiome heritability [4, 5]. For example, in humans, a significant association was detected between the presence of the LCT gene (providing instruction for making the enzyme lactase) and the richness of *Bifidobacterium* [6]. However, epigenetics play a role as well, as while this genetic component exists, it can be mediated by dietary influence – specifically lactose consumption. Further influence of host genetics is demonstrated in the heritability of GI microbiota, as demonstrated in humans [7] (Figure 4.2).

### 4.1.2 Age

Age is a factor in microbial composition, as changes in the microbiome are associated with different life stages – particularly during the growth and senior or geriatric years. The first stage of life includes the colonization of the host by microbiota and establishment of microbiomes (Chapter 3). This crucial time frame involves the development and maturation of the immune system as pioneer microbiota colonize and begin to influence some metabolic and immune functions [8–12]. Microbial populations are also influenced by changes in diet that occur during the growth phase as the neonate transitions from a maternal source of

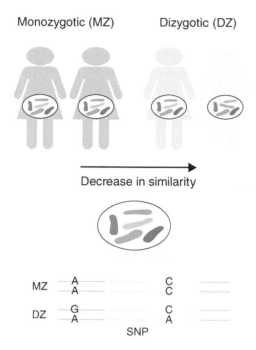

Monozygotic (MZ)    Dizygotic (DZ)

Decrease in similarity

MZ  A A    C C
DZ  G A    C A
         SNP

**Figure 4.2** Monozygotic twins show more microbial similarity, compared to dizygotic twins who show more diversity. *Source:* Hand et al. [3]. Creative Commons License: https://creativecommons.org/licenses/by/4.0.

**Table 4.1** Age difference on the stability and changes in the microbiome.

| Neonate | Adult | Senior |
|---------|-------|--------|
| Developing microbiota highly susceptible to changes | Relatively stable unless disrupted by influencing factors | Aging can affect absorption of nutrients and alter the microbiome. |

nutrition to solid foods [13]. The GI microbiome appears to stabilize and be similar to the composition of the dam as the dog or cat reaches approximately 5 months of age [10, 12].

Under normal circumstances, the GI microbiome is well established and stable during the adult life stage (Table 4.1) [14–16]. However, alterations or dysbiosis can occur secondary to environmental influences such as sudden dietary changes or pharmaceutical therapies [17]. As pets reach their senior life stage, there are age-related factors that may precede a change in the richness and function of the microbiomes. Changes in the ability to digest nutrients may influence the volume and type of nutrients provided to the microbial communities [18, 19]. One study has shown reduced density of beneficial *Bifidobacteria* and *Lactobacilli* with a corresponding increase in *Clostridium perfringens* in the feces of elderly dogs as compared to younger dogs of the same breed, fed the same diet [20]. In turn, changes in the microbiome may influence inflammation and immunity in aging dogs [21]. It is thus possible that support to enhance the microbiome and GI function may aid in prolonged optimal health and longevity, though further studies are required to determine precisely how to do so.

### 4.1.3 Sex

The GI microbiome can play a role in sex hormone homeostasis [22], and in some species, sex appears to impact by the microbiome [23]. Female mice have demonstrated similar microbiome composition pre- and post-puberty, while that of male mice differed, indicating that male sex hormones may influence the GI microbiota [23]. Furthermore, castrated male mice were found to have GI microbiota more similar to female mice than intact male mice in pre- or postpuberty states. When providing these castrated mice with testosterone, the microbiome composition more closely resembled that of postpuberty male mice. It has also been reported that transplanting fecal microbiota from a female donor mouse to male mice did not seem to have impact hormone status, whereas transferring microbiota from a postpuberty intact male donor to immature female mice resulted in higher testosterone levels in the females [24]. In cats, dogs, and horses, however, sex does not appear to impact microbiota of the gut or epithelium [16, 25].

### 4.1.4 Nutrition

Given that nutrients from the diet nourish the host animal and their microbiota, it is not surprising that the nutrient composition and digestibility of foods ingested by the host animal have a strong influence on the composition of the gut microbiome.

The macronutrient composition – protein, fat, carbohydrates – influences the type and metabolism of resident gut microbes [18, 26]. The metagenome, the combined genetic expression of the microbiota, can shift in response to alterations in diet in order to best utilize available substrate [27]. Additionally, the microbial populations themselves may change in favor of species more adapted at utilizing the available substrates [28–31]. As such, the microbial communities in animals with more omnivorous or varied dietary habits are often more diverse than those of animals with stricter and more homogenous dietary intake [1, 32]. Diets rich in animal tissues, including raw meat-based diets, tend to provide high proportions of protein and fat, resulting in increasing relative abundances of microbes associated with metabolism of protein and fat such as *Fusobacterium* and *Clostridium* spp., with a loss of microbes associated with carbohydrate fermentation [26, 33, 34]. In comparison, dogs fed diets with high plant-based fiber content demonstrated reductions in *Bacteroides, Clostridium,* and *Fusobacterium* relative abundances with increased *Bifidobacterium, Blautia, Lactobacillus, Helicobacter,* and *Megamonas* [31].

Not only is the nutritional composition a factor that drives the gut microbiome, but the digestibility of the ingested nutrients also plays a role. Digestible and absorbable nutrients may be taken up and utilized by the host in the more oral sections of the gut, while absorption of nutrients is reduced in the aboral gut, leaving less digestible nutrients to be fermented by resident microbes. These host indigestible, microbially fermentable compounds are utilized by the microbiota in the large intestine as a source of energy. This can encourage the growth of specific taxa and increased metabolite production. Depending on the taxa growth and metabolite(s) produced, these undigestible compounds may provide a benefit or be detrimental to the health of the host [32, 35, 36]. The quality of the nutrients may alter the quantity of host indigestible compounds that are unable to be absorbed in the small intestine. This has led to experimentation to manipulate the gut microbiome and its metabolite production via provision of indigestible ingredients, typically fiber, within their diet [37, 38].

Further discussion on the types and digestibility of nutrients can be found in Chapter 5.

### 4.1.5 Environment

The term "environment" is rather all-encompassing and includes all nonhost factors, such as dietary intake, as previously discussed, as well as physical contact and interactions with components in the host's surroundings: animals, soil, air, pollens, housing, living conditions, along with interactions with pathogens and parasites.

The environment likely has the most direct and rapid influence on the microbiome during the early colonization period of the neonate – discussed in Chapter 3. As newborn puppies and kittens are fairly immobile, most of their microbial exposure comes from maternal interaction [10, 12]. Once they reach the adult stage, the composition of the gut microbiome appears to be relatively stable and capable of withstanding most external environmental influences [14, 16]. Similarly, thanks to the dense coat that covers most of a dog or cat's external surface, healthy skin maintains a consistent microenvironment and microbiome [39]. Environmental variables such as presence or absence of fleas and time spent indoors vs. outdoors does not appear to have much impact on the skin microbiota of healthy dogs [40] (Box 4.1).

---

**Box 4.1   Antimicrobial Resistance**

The phenomenon of antimicrobial resistance allows for evolution of microbes to adapt to antimicrobial mechanisms of action and survive in the face of antimicrobial therapy that would inhibit or kill other microbes of the same species.

The World Health Organization has estimated the number of antimicrobial resistance-related deaths in humans could reach 10 million by 2050 [52]. A primary driver of this has been attributed to the inappropriate use of antimicrobials, both within humans and in nonhuman animals.

In 2015, the American College of Veterinary Internal Medicine (ACVIM) published a Consensus statement regarding therapeutic use of antimicrobials in animals, with respect to antimicrobial resistance [53]. In this document, actions to reduce the risk and occurrence of antimicrobial resistance are suggested, including preventing disease occurrence, reducing overall antimicrobial drug use, and improved antimicrobial drug use.

---

## 4.2  Pathophysiological Factors

### 4.2.1  Stress

Stress can be identified in many forms and for the context of this discussion; "stress" refers to a situation in which corresponding metabolic or hormonal reactions occur in response to a given "stressor." Stress can be physical arising from interaction with challenging activity or environmental conditions [41], or it can be psychological, such as a new environment, loud noises, and separation from family [42]. In dogs, anxiety and stress may precipitate gastrointestinal disorders, disrupt the gut barrier, induce inflammation and alteration in the gut microbiome [43, 44]. Manipulation of the microbiome through nutritional supplementation has been demonstrated to improve the abundance of fecal *Firmicutes* and *Lactobacillus* in puppies during periods of stress, resulting in higher fecal short-chain fatty acids and reduced incidence of diarrhea [43, 44]. Maternal stress may even impact the microbiome of neonates. In humans, infants of high-stress mothers had a higher abundance of *Proteobacteria* and lower abundances of *Lactobacillus* and *Bifidobacteria*, with these individuals experiencing potentially associated pathological conditions such as gut inflammation and the development of allergies [45].

Not only may the microbiome be affected by stress, but it would appear that the microbiome may itself contribute to psychological stress responses. Studies in "germ-free" mice have shown that the fecal microbiota transplant of colonic microbiota from anxious mice, or mice exposed to chronic unpredictable mild stress, into "germ-free" recipient mice resulted in higher levels of anxiety- and depression-like behaviors in the recipient mice [46]. Further discussion of this gut–brain axis can be found in Chapter 16.

### 4.2.2  Pharmaceutical Therapy

#### 4.2.2.1  Antimicrobials

Antimicrobials are commonly administered to companion animals for a variety of situations, ranging from prophylactic peri-operative antibiosis to acute treatment of infections and chronic management of antibiotic-responsive conditions such as antibiotic-responsive enteropathy (see Chapter 15). Regardless of administration, whether enteral

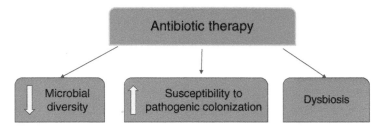

**Figure 4.3** Effects of antibiotic therapy on the microbiota.

or parenteral, systemic antimicrobial therapy can impact the GI microbiome. Antimicrobials do not exterminate all the microbiota within the GI tract, but selectively eliminate those susceptible to the mode of action of the particular agent used. This can lead to shifts in the growth of some species resulting in metabolic alterations and potentially increased susceptibility to pathogenic colonization [17] (Figure 4.3).

Even after therapy is discontinued, the alterations caused by antimicrobial agents may or may not readily return to the pre-treatment state, with long periods of dysbiosis possible, and the affected microbiome may not return to the exact state of colonization before treatment [47]. The ensuing dysbiosis may have negative impacts on the host's gut health, such as reduced microbial bile acid metabolism.

### Antimicrobial Use in Chronic Enteropathies

Metronidazole is an antibiotic and antiprotozoal medication commonly administered to pets with acute or chronic diarrhea [17, 48]. While therapy can result in acute resolution of symptoms, there are concerns associated with the overuse and misuse of this antibiotic. A study in dogs found a 14-day treatment plan with metronidazole caused significant alterations to the microbiome composition including the loss of key bacteria that are high producers of SCFA (*Firmicutes*) [47]. In treated dogs, the fecal dysbiosis index was significantly increased, and the dysbiotic state was still apparent 4 weeks after the antibiotic therapy was discontinued. Alterations in fecal metabolites were also apparent, with an increase in fecal total lactate and a decrease in secondary bile acids deoxycholic acid and lithocholic acid.

Tylosin is a bacteriostatic antibiotic that is also commonly used in dogs with acute or chronic diarrhea. As with metronidazole, clinical resolution of diarrhea is common with tylosin, though often signs will recur upon discontinuation, and long or repeat courses of treatment are often required [49]. Administration of tylosin has been demonstrated to impact the microbiome with dysbiosis and fecal metabolic alterations, characterized predominantly by losses of *Fusobateriacea* and *Veillonellaceae*, increases in *Enterococcus*-like organisms, *Pasteurella* spp., *Dietzia* spp., and *Escherichia coli*-like organisms, and reduced microbial bile acid metabolism, detectable for up to or more than 8 weeks after discontinuation [50, 51].

#### 4.2.2.2 Other Pharmaceuticals

Non-antimicrobial therapeutic agents may also have effects on microbiomes. Proton pump inhibitors, a class of gastroprotectants with a mechanism of action reducing hydrochloric acid secretion, alter the pH of gastric acid and can allow for increased survival of ingested bacteria and potential colonization and dysbiosis [54]. Furthermore, this disruption to the normal microbiome may increase the risk of enterocyte injury caused by non-steroidal anti-inflammatories. In cats, specific effects of omeprazole, a proton pump inhibitor, on the microbiome have been suggested [55].

## 4.3 Chapter Summary

- Host genes may exert some influence over the composition of the GI microbiome
- Changes in the microbiome are associated with different life stages, particularly during early growth and development
- Microbiomes within individuals of the same species may differ according to sex and reproductive status
- Host nutrition can directly impact the gut microbiome
- Stress may induce dysbiosis, even maternal stress may influence composition of a neonate's microbiome
- Systemic antimicrobial administration is associated with reduced GI microbiota diversity, even when used to treat GI disease
- Antimicrobials do not remove all the microbiota in the GI tract but selectively eliminate those susceptible to the antimicrobial's mechanism of action
- Microbes are able to evolve rapidly and have developed ways to elude the effects of antimicrobials

## References

**1** Reese, A. and Dunn, R. (2018). Drivers of microbiome biodiversity: a review of general rules, feces, and ignorance. *MBio* 9: e01294–e01218.

**2** Barko, P., McMichael, M., Swanson, K., and Williams, D. (2018). The gastrointestinal microbiome: a review. *Journal of Veterinary Internal Medicine* 32: 9–25.

**3** Hand, D., Wallis, C., Colyer, A., and Penn, C. (2013). Pyrosequencing the canine faecal microbiota: breadth and depth of biodiversity. *PLoS One* 8 (1): e53115.

**4** Khachatryan, Z., Ktsoyan, Z., Manukyan, G. et al. (2008). Predominant role of host genetics in controlling the composition of gut microbiota. *PLoS One* 3 (8): e3064.

**5** Goodrich, J., Davenport, E., Beaumont, M. et al. (2016). Genetic determinants of the gut microbiome in UK twins. *Cell Host & Microbe* 19: 731–743.

**6** Cahana, I. and Iraqi, F. (2020). Impact of host genetics on gut microbiome: take-home lessons from human and mouse studies. *Animal Models and Experimental Medicine* 3: 229–236.

**7** Kurilshikov, A., Wijmenga, C., Fu, J., and Zhernakova, A. (2017). Host genetics and gut microbiome: challenges and perspectives. *Trends in Immunology* 38 (9): 633–647.

**8** Tal, S., Tikhonov, E., Aroch, I. et al. (2021). Developmental intestinal microbiome alterations in canine fading puppy syndrome: a prospective observational study. *NPJ Biofilms and Microbiomes* 7 (1): 52.

**9** Pipan, M., Kajdic, L., Kalin, A. et al. (2020). Do newborn puppies have their own microbiota at birth? Influence of type of birth on newborn puppy microbiota. *Theriogenology* 152: 18–28.

**10** Guard, B., Mila, H., Steiner, J. et al. (2017). Characterization of the fecal microbiome during neonatal and early pediatric development in puppies. *PLoS One* 12 (4): e0175718.

**11** Spears, J.K., Vester Boler, B., Gardner, C., and Li, Q. (2017). Development of the oral microbiome in kittens. In: *Companion Animal Nutrition (CAN) Summit: The Nexus of Pet and Human Nutrition: Focus on Cognition and the Microbiome*, 4–7. Helsinki.

**12** Del Carro, A., Corrò, M., Bertero, A. et al. (2022). The evolution of dam-litter microbial flora from birth to 60 days of age. *BMC Veterinary Research* 18: 95.

**13** Deusch, O., O'Flynn, C., Colyer, A. et al. (2014). Deep illumina-based shotgun sequencing reveals dietary effects on the structure and function of the fecal microbiome of growing kittens. *PLoS One* 9 (7): e101021.

**14** Allaway, D., Haydock, R., Lonsdale, Z. et al. (2020). Rapid reconstitution of the fecal microbiome after extended diet-induced changes indicates a stable gut microbiome in healthy adult dogs. *Applied and Environmental Microbiology* 86 (13): e00562–e00520.

**15** Tizard, I. and Jones, S. (2018). The microbiota regulates immunity and immunologic diseases in dogs and cats. *Veterinary Clinics of North America: Small Animal Practice* 48: 307–322.

**16** Deusch, O., O'Flynn, C., Colyer, A. et al. (2015). A longitudinal study of the feline faecal microbiome identifies changes into early adulthood irrespective of sexual development. *PLoS One* 10 (12): e0144881.

**17** Suchodolski, J. (2016). Diagnosis and interpretation of intestinal dysbiosis in dogs and cats. *The Veterinary Journal* 215: 30–37.

**18** Bermingham, E., Young, W., Butowski, C. et al. (2018). The fecal microbiota in the domestic cat (felis catus) is influenced by interactions between age and diet; a five year longitudinal study. *Frontiers in Microbiology* 9: 1231.

**19** Jia, J., Frantz, N., Khoo, C. et al. (2011). Investigation of the faecal microbiota of geriatric cat. *Letters in Applied Microbiology* 53: 288–293.

**20** Simpson, J., Martineau, B., Jones, W. et al. (2002). Characterization of fecal bacterial populations in canines: effects of age, breed and dietary fiber. *Microbial Ecology* 44: 186–197.

**21** Gomes, M.D.O., Beraldo, M., Putarov, T. et al. (2011). Old beagle dogs have lower faecal concentrations of some fermentation products and lower peripheral lymphocyte counts than young adult beagles. *British Journal of Nutrition* 106: S187–S190.

**22** Koyasu, H., Takahashi, H., Yoneda, M. et al. (2022). Correlations between behavior and hormone concentrations or gut microbiome imply that domestic cats (felis silvestris catus) living in a group are not like 'groupmates'. *PLoS One* 17 (7): e0269589.

**23** Org, E., Mehrabian, M., Parks, B. et al. (2016). Sex differences and hormonal effects on gut microbiota composition in mice. *Gut Microbes* 7 (4): 313–322.

**24** Markle, J., Frank, D., Mortin-Toth, S. et al. (2013). Sex differences in the gut microbiome drive hormone-dependent regulation of autoimmunity. *Science* 339 (6123): 1084–1088.

**25** Ross, A., Müller, K., Weese, S., and Neufeld, J. (2018). Comprehensive skin microbiome analysis reveals the uniqueness of human skin and evidence for phylosymbiosis within the class mammalia. *Proceedings of the National Academy of Sciences of the United States of America* 115 (25): ES786–ES795.

**26** Butowski, C., Moon, C., Thomas, D. et al. (2022). The effects of raw-meat diets on the gastrointestinal microbiota of the cat and dog: a review. *New Zealand Veterinary Journal* 70 (1): 1–9.

**27** Young, W., Moon, C., Thomas, D. et al. (2016). Pre- and post-weaning diet alters the faecal metagenome in the cat with differences in vitamin and carbohydrate metabolism gene abundances. *Scientific Reports* 6: 1–6.

**28** Coelho, L., Kultima, J., Costea, P. et al. (2018). Similarity of the dog and human gut microbiomes in gene content and response to diet. *Microbiome* 6 (72): 1.

**29** Wakshlag, J., Simpson, K., Struble, A., and Dowd, S. (2011). Negative fecal characteristics are associated with pH and fecal flora alterations during dietary change in dogs. *International Journal of Applied Research in Veterinary Medicine* 9 (3): 278–283.

**30** Hang, I., Rinttila, T., Zentek, J. et al. (2012). Effect of high contents of dietary animal-derived protein or carbohydrates on canine faecal microbiota. *BMC Veterinary Research* 8: 90.

**31** Lin, C.-Y., Jha, A., Oba, P. et al. (2022). Longitudinal fecal microbiome and metabolite data demonstrate rapid shifts and subsequent stabilization after an abrupt dietary change in healthy adult dogs. *Animal Microbiome* 4: 46.

**32** Wernimont, S., Radosevich, J., Jackson, M. et al. (2020). The effects of nutrition on the gastrointestinal microbiome of cats and dogs: impact on health and disease. *Frontiers in Microbiology* 11: 1266.

**33** Schmidt, M., Unterer, S., Suchodolski, J. et al. (2018). The fecal microbiome and metabolome differs between dogs fed bones and raw food (barf) diets and dogs fed commercial diets. *PLoS One* 13 (8): e0201279.

**34** Kerr, K., Vester Boler, B., Morris, C. et al. (2012). Apparent total tract energy and macronutrient digestibility and fecal fermentative end-product concentrations of domestic cats fed extruded, raw beef-based, and cooked beef-based diets. *Journal of Animal Science* 90 (2): 515–522.

**35** Barry, K., Middelbos, I., Vester Boler, B. et al. (2012). Effects of dietary fiber on the feline gastrointestinal metagenome. *Journal of Proteome Research* 11: 5924–5933.

**36** Pilla, R. and Suchodolski, J. (2021). The gut microbiome of dogs and cats, and the influence of diet. *Veterinary Clinics of North America: Small Animal Practice* 51: 605–621.

**37** Fritsch, D., Wernimont, S., Jackson, M., and Gross, K. (2019). Select dietary fiber sources improve stool parameters, decrease fecal putrefactive metabolites, and deliver antioxidant and anti-inflammatory plant polyphenols to the lower gastrointestinal tract of adult dogs. *The FASEB Journal* 33 (S1): 587–581.

**38** Panasevich, M., Kerr, K., Dilger, R. et al. (2015). Modulation of the faecal microbiome of healthy adult dogs by inclusion of potato fibre in the diet. *British Journal of Nutrition* 113: 125–133.

**39** Cuscó, A., Belanger, J., Gershony, L. et al. (2017). Individual signatures and environmental factors shape skin microbiota in healthy dogs. *Microbiome* 5: 139.

**40** Hoffmann, A., Patterson, A., Diesel, A. et al. (2014). The skin microbiome in healthy and allergic dogs. *PLoS One* 9 (1): e83197.

**41** Bradley, D., Swaim, S., Vaughn, D. et al. (1996). Biochemical and histopathological evaluation of changes in sled dog paw skin associated with physical stress and cold temperatures. *Veterinary Dermatology* 7: 203–208.

**42** Part, C., Kiddie, J., Hayes, W. et al. (2013). Physiological, physical and behavioural changes in dogs (canis familiaris) when kennelled: testing the validity of stress parameters. *Physiology & Behavior* 133: 260–271.

**43** Cannas, S., Tonini, B., Belà, B. et al. (2021). Effect of a novel nutraceutical supplement (relaxigen pet dog) on the fecal microbiome and stress-related behaviors in dogs: a pilot study. *Journal of Veterinary Behavior* 42: 37–47.

**44** Yang, K., Deng, X., Jian, S. et al. (2022). Gallic acid alleviates gut dysfunction and boosts immune and antioxidant activities in puppies under environmental stress based on microbiome–metabolomics analysis. *Frontiers in Immunology* 12: 813890.

**45** Zijlmans, M., Korpela, K., Riksen-Walraven, J. et al. (2015). Maternal prenatal stress is associated with the infant intestinal microbiota. *Psychoneuroendocrinology* 53: 233–245.

**46** Li, N., Wang, Q., Wang, Y. et al. (2019). Fecal microbiota transplantation from chronic unpredictable mild stress mice donors affects anxiety-like and depression-like behavior in recipient mice via the gut microbiotainflammation-brain axis. *Stress* 22 (5): 592–602.

**47** Pilla, R., Gaschen, F., Barr, J. et al. (2020). Effects of metronidazole on the fecal microbiome and metabolome in healthy dogs. *Journal of Veterinary Internal Medicine* 34: 1853–1866.

**48** Hall, E. (2011). Antibiotic-responsive diarrhea in small animals. *Veterinary Clinics of North America: Small Animal Practice* 41 (2): 273–286.

**49** Westermarck, E., Skrzypczak, T., Harmoinen, J. et al. (2005). Tylosin-responsive chronic diarrhea in dogs. *Journal of Veterinary Internal Medicine* 19: 177–186.

**50** Suchodolski, J., Dowd, S., Westermarck, E. et al. (2009). The effect of the macrolide antibiotic tylosin on microbial diversity in the canine small intestine as demonstrated by massive parallel 16s rrna gene sequencing. *BMC Microbiology* 9: 210.

**51** Manchester, A., Webb, C., Blake, A. et al. (2019). Long-term impact of tylosin on fecal microbiota and fecal bile acids of healthy dogs. *Journal of Veterinary Internal Medicine* 33: 2605–1617.

**52** Bozkir, V. (2021). *High-Level Interactive Dialogue on Antimicrobial Resistance*. New York: United Nations.

**53** Weese, J., Giguère, S., Guardabassi, L. et al. (2015). Acvim consensus statement on therapeutic antimicrobial use inanimals and antimicrobial resistance. *Journal of Veterinary Internal Medicine* 29: 487–498.

**54** Marks, S., Kook, P., Papich, M. et al. (2018). Acvim consensus statement: support for rational administration of gastrointestinal protectants to dogs and cats. *Journal of Veterinary Internal Medicine* 32: 1823–1840.

**55** Schmid, S., Suchodolski, J., Price, J., and Tolbert, M. (2018). Omeprazole minimally alters the fecal microbial community in six cats: a pilot study. *Frontiers in Veterinary Science* 5: 79.

# 5

# Essential Nutrients and the Microbiota

The gastrointestinal (GI) tract, including the resident microbiota, interacts with and responds to nutrient provision. The composition of nutrients ingested can influence the microbiota diversity and density, along with the bacterial-derived metabolites, microbiota function, gene content, and influence of genes, along with host physiology and metabolism [1, 2]. Differences in canine and feline microbiome profiles can be seen between diet composition as well as the food form [3–12].

Changes to composition of the microbiome have been shown to respond rapidly to dietary intervention, particularly when there are changes in macronutrients, though changes may only be temporary if the diet change is not continued [1, 2]. For example, in a study in which healthy dogs were fed only purified amino acids and easily digestible starch for 32 weeks before returning to their control diet, the dogs' microbial taxa, and their genetic potential adapted rapidly to the purified diet, then returned again to their baseline state when the control diet was reinstated [13].

When considering nutrition to alter health status, a core concept to consider is that each nutrient can meet requirements or even provide benefits only when provided in the right volume and/or proportion for that individual's requirements; a greater volume does not always provide greater benefit and may even induce negative impacts on host health through the excessive production of nutrient-specific microbial metabolites.

## 5.1 Protein

While total protein is considered an essential nutrient in i's own right, in reality protein is provided in diets as a way to meet the amino acid requirements for the pet. Most foods for dogs and cats use animal protein sources as they contain a more complete amino acid profile, are in alignment with the physiology of carnivorous dogs and cats, and are a preferred ingredient of pet parents [14]. While protein sources may be evolving over the next few years, at present the majority of diets utilize animal protein predominantly, plant sources are often complementary, though there are a few completely plant-based diets, and there are some diets that include insect protein sources.

GI microbes are involved in digestion, absorption, and metabolism of dietary protein. Amino acids are absorbed in the small intestine by dogs and cats; undigested and/or unabsorbed proteins and amino acids reaching the hind gut are fermented by the resident microbiota [15].

Three main factors play a role in protein's influence on the GI microbiome: quantity (the total amount of protein ingested), quotient (the ratio of protein to other energy-containing ingredients like carbohydrates), and quality (the digestibility and amino acid composition) [2]. Finding a balance with these factors will result in the ideal provision of protein to ensure energy needs are adequately met by the host and the GI microbiota (Figure 5.1).

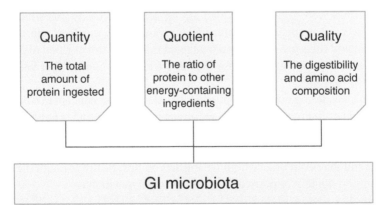

**Figure 5.1** Factors affecting the GI microbiota. Finding a balance with these factors will result in the ideal provision of protein to ensure energy needs are adequately met by the host and the GI microbiota.

### 5.1.1 Quantity

Though minimum protein requirements of dogs and have been determined [16], their "optimal" protein intake is as of yet unknown and likely varies between individuals based on a number of host-specific and environmental factors. At present, pet parents appear to have a preference for high-protein diets [17]. High-protein diets have been associated with higher abundance of *Proteobacteria* in canine and feline feces [18]. Depending on the specific microbial composition, this may be associated with dysbiosis with elevated counts of GI pathogens such as *Escherichia coli, Campylobacter jejuni, Klebsiella pneumoniae, Salmonella typhimurium,* and/or *Yersinia enterocolitica* – all species of the *Proteobacteria* phylum. Furthermore, elevated *Proteobacteria* abundance has been associated with GI inflammation in dogs and cats [19, 20]. High protein consumption, in one study determined as 45.77% on a dry matter basis, has been associated with increased microbial proteolytic activity and circulating levels of uremic toxins and inflammatory markers in otherwise healthy dogs [8]. Specifically, microbial fermentation of tryptophan and tyrosine results in the production of indole sulfates and *p*-cresol, respectively. It is possible that consumption of excess protein, or less digestible protein, or both, may contribute to chronic inflammation and specifically be detrimental to the animals' kidneys. However, just how much protein is too much is yet to be determined.

### 5.1.2 Quotient

The proportion of protein to nonprotein energy sources is another factor in creating a balance in the provision of protein. In particular, there is evidence that the protein to carbohydrate ratio can influence GI microbiome composition [4, 21]. Fecal microbial composition, blood metabolites, and blood hormones differed between kittens weaned onto a moderate-protein moderate-carbohydrate or high-protein low-carbohydrate diet [21]. Similar findings have been reported in dogs, with differential microbial composition and genetic potential between dogs fed a high-protein low-carbohydrate or moderate-protein high-carbohydrate diet [4]. Interestingly, effects were stronger in obese rather than lean dogs, suggesting potential for manipulation of the gut microbiome via dietary macronutrient composition to improve weight loss or weight maintenance. Ideally, finding a suitable ratio for the pet is preferred over the provision of protein in excess of the animal's needs, though as of yet, the ideal ratio of dietary protein to nonprotein energy sources is unknown.

### 5.1.3 Quality

Ingested protein must undergo proteolysis (hydrolysis) by gastric acid and proteolytic enzymes to digest it into peptides (amino acid chains), from which free amino acids, dipeptides (two amino acids bound together), or oligopeptides (short sequences of amino acids bound together) may be absorbed by the pet. Normally, this occurs as part of host digestion, though there are some therapeutic diets on the market that provide hydrolyzed protein compounds in smaller molecular weights.[1]

The goal of this process is to provide a protein source that can evade recognition by the intestinal immune system, aid in easier digestion, improve absorption, and support pets that experience an adverse response to intact proteins [22]. While hydrolyzed protein sources are more digestible, they do not appear to overly impact the GI microbiome [23].

The overall digestibility of the protein source and the amino acids contained within it may influence the composition of the GI microbiome. Moderate amounts of highly digestible, high-quality (meaning balanced amino acid composition, in relation to canine/feline requirements) protein can meet the needs of a pet with little undigested protein reaching the hind gut, while large amounts of poorly digestible protein (or highly digestible protein in a gut with poor absorptive capacity) become available for metabolism by microbiota in the lower GI tract. The process of microbial decomposition of amino acids is termed putrefaction, with a variety of potential metabolites produced, depending on the microbial taxa, their genetic capacity, and the specific amino acids present [11]. As discussed, some protein fermentation products may have detrimental effects to the host, so minimization of undigested protein reaching the hind gut is important to maintain animal health and well-being.

---

1 For example: Hill's Prescription Diet z/d, Purina Pro Plan Veterinary Diets Hydrolyzed HA, Royal Canin – Veterinary Exclusive Anallergenic, Royal Canin – Veterinary Exclusive Hypoallergenic Hydrolyzed Protein.

## 5.2 Carbohydrates

Carbohydrates, particularly indigestible carbohydrates (fiber), are a large focus of manipulation of the GI microbiome and host health, due to the positive effects of metabolites that are produced by some carbohydrate-fermenting microbes, including the short-chain fatty acids (SCFAs) butyrate, acetate, and propionate. Though not recognized as an essential nutrient for dogs or cats [16], the main function of digestible carbohydrates is to provide an energy source for cells. Carbohydrates consist of simple and complex forms, which can be further divided into four main categories based on molecular composition: monosaccharides, disaccharides, oligosaccharides, and polysaccharides. See Figure 5.2. Upon digestion, carbohydrates are reduced to simple sugars which may be oxidized or fermented to provide electrons and generate the energy-storing molecule adenosine triphosphate [24]. The term carbohydrate covers a broad spectrum of nutrients that provide energy to the host including host digestible sources (starches, sugars), sources that are indigestible by host enzymes but metabolizable by GI microbes (fermentable fiber) and those that are indigestible to both the host and microbes (non-fermentable fiber).

### 5.2.1 Simple Carbohydrates

Simple carbohydrates consist of monosaccharides and disaccharides – commonly known as sugars. Monosaccharides (e.g. glucose, galactose,

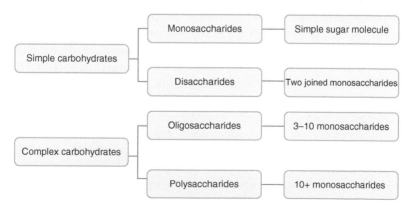

**Figure 5.2** Carbohydrate categories and molecular composition.

fructose) are the simplest carbohydrate molecule. They are readily absorbed in the small intestine via various transporters and directed to the liver via portal circulation [24]. Disaccharides (e.g. sucrose, lactose, maltose) are two joined monosaccharides that required hydrolysis by amylase, a pancreatic enzyme, to be broken down into monosaccharides and absorbed by the host. While the majority of simple carbohydrates may be absorbed by the host, unabsorbed sugars that reach the hind gut may be able to alter the composition of the GI microbiome. In rats, early life exposure to glucose and fructose altered the microbial composition, reducing *Prevotella* and *Lachnospiraceae* while increasing *Bacteroides*, *Alistipes*, *Lactobacillus*, *Clostridium* sensu stricto, *Bifidobacteriaceae*, and *Parasutterella* [25].

### 5.2.2 Complex Carbohydrates

Complex carbohydrates consist of oligosaccharides (3–9 sugar units) and polysaccharides (10 and greater sugar units) and are more resistant to rapid digestion by the host [24]. Complex carbohydrates include starch, glycogen, and non-starch polysaccharides, also known as fiber. While most conventional fiber sources come from plant materials, such as cellulose, peanut hulls, and beet pulp, there is growing interest into yeast cell wall components and "animal fibers," such as the chitinous exoskeleton of insects or hair and feathers, and their impact on the microbiome [26–28]. Starches may be digested by the host into their constituent sugars, though resistant starch may reach the hindgut undigested. Fiber is nearly completely indigestible to the host and most ingested fiber reaches the hindgut relatively unchanged. Fiber types are categorized based on their ability to be dissolved in water: insoluble fibers are unable to dissolve in water and soluble are; as well as the level of fermentability by GI microbes: fermentable or non-fermentable. These varying types of fibers interact with the GI microbes in different capacities. Often, commercial pet food products do not disclose the quantity of different types of dietary fibers added, with crude protein being the only requirement on pet food labels in North America [29]. Finding the right combination of fibers in the correct volume for each pet can be a challenge, particularly when fiber is being sought for therapeutic effects.

### 5.2.2.1 Solubility

Solubility is the capacity of the fiber to dissolve in water and has a profound effect on fiber functionality. Soluble fiber draws fluid into the GI tract and creates a gummy, viscous-like substance. The level of viscosity is directly proportional to the molecular weight or chain length of the fiber [10]. As a general rule, soluble fibers tend to be more fermentable [9]. Excess volumes of soluble fibers can create secretory (watery) diarrhea.

Insoluble fibers have strong cellular structures that resist enzymatic digestion. Examples of insoluble fibers are cellulose, lignin, and hemicellulose [10]. These fibers act as natural exfoliators, scraping along the GI tract [9]. This action increases mucus production and can enhance the GI barrier function [11] (Figure 5.3).

### 5.2.2.2 Fermentability

Fiber sources can also have varying levels of fermentability or metabolism by GI microbiota. Fermentability can occur rapidly or slowly. For example, oligosaccharides are highly fermentable by some GI microbes

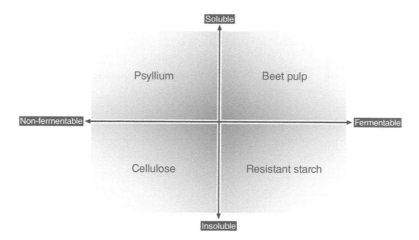

**Figure 5.3** Fermentability and solubility range of fiber and complex carbohydrate sources commonly found in the pet food industry. The left quadrants are less fermentable, right are more fermentable. Similarly, the upper quadrants are more soluble, and lower are less soluble. *Source:* Panasevich et al. [3]. Creative commons license: https://creativecommons.org/licenses/by/4.0/.

and rapidly produce SCFAs. The benefits of fiber metabolism by the GI microbes have been examined in numerous studies as the metabolites and metabolome from these interactions can provide beneficial health effects for the host.

1) Provide an energy source to microbes allowing for the growth of microbiota in the microbiomes.
2) Decrease in colon pH – this is a preferred environment for microbes that complete important processes like 7-α dehydroxylation, which is completed by specific bacteria in the conversion of primary to secondary bile acids.
3) Improve GI tract health by providing epithelial cells with energy sources.
4) Alter metabolic and neurological functions with some of these metabolites able to cross the blood–brain barrier.
5) Production of health beneficial metabolites by anaerobic microbes such as SCFAs. SCFAs have been shown to have numerous beneficial effects on the host including the inhibition of histone deacetylases, which regulate gene expression, and the activation of G-protein-coupled receptors that are receptors for SCFAs. These receptors aid in the regulation of metabolism and inflammation. SCFAs can alter chemotaxis and phagocytosis, induce reactive oxygen species, change cell proliferation and cell function, along with altering GI integrity. Additionally, SCFAs have anti-inflammatory, antitumorigenic, and antimicrobial effects on the host. *Firmicutes* are producers of SCFAs. Different types of SCFAs have different functions:
   1) Butyric acid (butyrate) is a primary source of energy for colonocytes and has potent anticancer activity. Additionally, there is evidence that butyrate can activate intestinal gluconeogenesis helping to regulate glucose and energy homeostasis. Predominant producers of butyrate are *Firmicutes* including some *Lachnospiraceae* and *Faecalibacterium prausnitzii* [7].
   2) Propionic acid (propionate) is an additional energy source for epithelial cells. Once converted to glucose in the intestine, it is transferred to the liver where it reduces hepatic glucose production. Propionate is produced by *Bacteroides species*, *Negativicutes*, and some *Clostridium species* [7].
   3) Acetic acid (acetate) is the most abundant SCFA and is used as energy for peripheral tissues, aids in the metabolism of cholesterol

and lipogenesis, and in mice has been shown to aid in appetite regulation [7, 12]. It is a co-factor and metabolite for other bacteria, where it is required for the growth of a bacteria species. For example, *F. prausnitzii* will not grow in a culture media unless acetate is present. Acetate is produced by many bacteria, whereas the former mentioned are produced by very specific bacteria in the intestinal tract [7].

Dietary fiber has many potential health-improving functions:

1) Inclusion of fermentable fiber in the diet of dogs with chronic enteritis may improve dysbiosis and influence the microbiome to appear more similar to that of dogs without GI disease [30, 31]
2) Fermentation of dietary fiber may reduce putrefactive branched SCFA (isobutyric, 2-methylbutyric, and isovaleric acids) and increase acetic acid and favor production of beneficial straight-chain SCFA (acetic, propionic, and butyric acids) [3, 30, 32, 33]
3) Addition of fiber to protein-rich diets may reduce putrefactive sulfides and indole, as well as ammonia [33]
4) Fermentation of fibers rich in polyphenols may yield anti-inflammatory postbiotics [30, 32]
5) Insoluble fiber can increase fecal output, moisture content, and frequency of defecation [34]
6) Mixtures of soluble and insoluble fibers can bind water and dilute calories in the diet, increase meal volume and potentially increase satiety and meal satisfaction – all of which may be beneficial for weight management and weight loss [35]
7) Dietary fiber may improve glycemic control, particularly in animals with impaired glucose regulation, potentially via altered carbohydrate absorption and/or augmentation of insulin sensitivity [36]
8) Some fiber types may affect gastric emptying and intestinal motility, decreasing the clinical signs of hairballs in cats [37]

Fiber also has negative health implications:

1) Excessive fermentation can lead to production of gas leading to marked borborygmus, flatulence, and abdominal discomfort
2) Soluble fiber in excess of an animal's tolerance may lead to increased soft, watery stool [38]

3) Excess of soluble and/or insoluble fiber can reduce macronutrient digestibility [39]

Non-absorbable synthetic disaccharides (lactulose and lactol) are commonly used to manage clinical signs of both constipation and hepatic encephalopathy [40]. The laxative effect of synthetic disaccharides may ameliorate constipation, while administration of synthetic disaccharides also results in a reduction in ammonia production, attributed to a prebiotic effect regulating GI microbiota.

## 5.3 Fat

The effects of dietary fat on the microbiome of dogs and cats has been understudied. In humans and mice, it would appear that a high-fat (45–60% of daily caloric intake) diet may have a negative impact on the GI microbiome, resulting in reduced diversity [2]. This has led to postulation that the pro-inflammatory nature of high levels of dietary fat may negatively impact the microbiome through host-microbiome immune-mediated mechanisms. This has yet to be demonstrated in dogs or cats.

Aside from total fat, individual fatty acids and their impact on GI bear consideration. At least some fatty acids may be considered prebiotics in a way as they have the potential to positively influence the health of the host through interactions with the GI microbiota. For example, one study in mice demonstrated production of a microbial metabolite of linoleic acid that benefitted epithelial barrier function and mitigated damage due to periodontopathic bacteria [41].

## 5.4 Vitamins and Minerals

Like macronutrients (proteins, fats, and carbohydrates), micronutrients (vitamins and minerals) may influence host microbiota. Though micronutrients may be recognized to play a role in host metabolism and normal tissue function in other species, little research has been performed specifically in dogs or cats.

### 5.4.1 Vitamins

Although GI microbes are well known for their production of vitamins, the interaction of injested vitamins and the microbiome are worth consideration as well. There are multiple ways in which ingested vitamins may impact the gut microbiome, including [42]:

1) Direct antimicrobial actions
2) Modulation of bacterial energy metabolism
3) Modification of host immune response

Furthermore, as producers of vitamins themselves, the microbiota themselves can contribute to their own vitamin requirements and thus modulate the composition of the microbiome to a degree.

#### 5.4.1.1 Fat-Soluble Vitamins

**Vitamin A:** Vitamin A has very high absorption efficiency, up to 90% in humans [42]. Provitamin A carotenoids such as beta-carotene may be less absorbed and thus more available to the GI microbiome. Evidence for direct effect of vitamin A or carotenoids on the microbiome is lacking; it is likely that compositional changes in the microbiome associated with vitamin A intake may be attributable to the impact of vitamin A on the host intestinal mucosal barrier [42]. Nevertheless, it is apparent that there is a requirement of vitamin A in order for individuals to maintain healthy gut microbial composition.

**Vitamin D:** Similar to vitamin A, vitamin D is efficiently absorbed in the small intestine and also plays a critical role in gut health. Though the main recognized function of vitamin D is related to calcium homeostasis and bone metabolism, vitamin D receptors are present in many nonbone tissues, including the intestine in the dog [43]. Indeed, it is through activation of intestinal vitamin D receptors that effects of ingested vitamin D are thought to influence the microbiome in humans [42]. In one study in which vitamin $D_3$ was compounded into a colonic-delivery capsule and dosed to humans, changes in the fecal microbiome were detected [44]. In another human study in which vitamin $D_3$ was dosed in a conventional format, not enterically coated or protected to prevent absorption in the small intestine, alterations to the microbiome of the upper GI tract but not the lower were reported [45]. This suggests that while changes to the microbiome may be due to absorption of vitamin D and activation of host vitamin D receptors, the vitamin may also directly impact the microbiota themselves.

One consideration to be born in mind is that dietary vitamin D may be provided as either vitamin $D_2$, ergocalciferol, derived from yeasts and fungi, or vitamin $D_3$, cholecalciferol, derived primarily from animal tissues or secretions, though also present in some algae and lichens [46, 47]. In one study in weanling piglets, dietary supplementation with vitamin $D_2$ resulted in decreased abundance of *Prevotella* and increased acetate, butyrate, and propionate [48], while another study in weanling piglets demonstrated decreased *Streptococcaceae* and increased *Lachnospiraceae* when diet was supplemented with 25-hydroxyvitamin $D_3$ [49]. It is thus possible that the impact of vitamin D on the gut microbiome may be dependent on the form ingested.

**Vitamin E:** Unlike vitamins A and D, vitamin E has a lower and more variable absorption in humans, potentially resulting in more luminal vitamin E for microbes to interact with [42]. Despite this, there is little conclusive evidence demonstrating an effect of vitamin E on the microbiome even in humans, further research in this area is required.

**Vitamin K:** Similar in a way to vitamin D, vitamin K can also be found in different forms – dietary vitamin K is predominantly in the form of phylloquinone from plant-based ingredients though menaquinone from microbial synthesis may also be found in fermented foods [42]. Menaquinones are also synthesized by gut microbiota, indeed, genes involved in the biosynthesis of vitamin K predominate in the canine gut metagenome [50]. Though production of vitamin K is a key role of gut microbes, the impact of vitamin K on the microbes themselves has received little attention. Within the human microbiome, quinones have been identified as co-factors supporting growth of specific microbial species, suggesting that ingested and endogenously synthesized vitamin K may influence microbial composition by selectively promoting growth of particular microbes [51].

### 5.4.1.2 Water-Soluble Vitamins

B-vitamin absorption at low concentrations is facilitated by active transport, while passive diffusion allows further absorption at high concentrations, primarily in the small intestine [52]. B-vitamins may be acquired through diet, though many are also synthesized by the gut microbiomes, primarily in the large intestine. Microbial B-vitamin synthesis is dependent on a number of factors, foremost being diet, with complex carbohydrate-rich diets resulting in greatest B-vitamin synthesis in human gut microbiomes [53]. Microbial synthesis can contribute greatly to the quantity of B-vitamins detected in feces, with fecal vitamin content even exceeding ingested vitamin quantity in some cases. It is not always well known what proportion of microbially synthesized B-vitamins are absorbed by the host, or what proportion of host requirements are met by these endogenously synthesized vitamins [42].

**Thiamine (B1):** Thiamine is produced by microbes in the gut, and although human colonocytes bear high-affinity thiamine transporters, microbially synthesized thiamine contributes little to their daily requirements [53, 54]. Deficiency reportedly occurs rapidly when mice are fed a thiamine-deficient diet, supporting the notion that microbial synthesis is inadequate for host requirements [55]. However, thiamine appears critical for growth of specific gut bacteria, suggesting a role in modulation of the composition of the gut microbiome [54].

**Riboflavin (B2):** Genetic capacity for riboflavin synthesis has been detected in over half of human gut microbes evaluated, and both mice and humans have functional riboflavin transporters in their large intestine [53, 54, 56]. It is suspected that microbial riboflavin synthesis may contribute meaningfully to host requirements, as well as regulating microbiota composition through selective growth and inhibition of various microbes [54].

**Niacin (B3):** Many mammalian species, including dogs, are capable of endogenous synthesis of niacin from tryptophan; notably, cats lack this capacity [16]. Gastrointestinal microbiota are also capable of conversion of tryptophan to niacin, and human colonocytes bear transporters capable of absorbing niacin [53]. Host intestinal barrier function is dependent on niacin, thus the vitamin exerts an effect upon the microbiota in this manner, and also directly via antioxidant, anti-inflammatory, and antiendotoxin activities [42]. Furthermore, microbe species lacking enzymes required for niacin synthesis rely on luminal niacin for growth, giving niacin a compositional-modifying effect on the microbiome.

**Pantothenic acid (B5) and Biotin (B7):** Mammalian colonocytes have a transporter capable of allowing absorption of both pantothenic acid and biotin (B7), with colonic uptake appearing to contribute significantly to host requirements [53, 57]. Pantothenic acid synthesis appears to be limited among a number of predominant phyla and individual species in the human GI microbiome, with these microbes appearing to rely heavily on synthesis from pantothenic-acid product in microbes [42]. In comparison, biotin appears to be widely synthesized by nearly 40% of human gut microbes evaluated [56]. However, biotin-dependent microbes were also present, suggesting a modulating effect of biotin on the gut microbiome as well.

**Pyridoxine (B6):** Pyridoxine is also synthesized in large quantities by the human gut microbiota, likely contributing markedly toward host requirements [56]. This vitamin appears to have a modulatory effect on intestinal inflammation and is a critical co-factor for riboflavin and niacin metabolism [42].

**Folate (B9):** Similar to pyridoxine, around 40% of human gut microbes evaluated maintain genes coding for folate synthesis, with folate transporters present in the colon of multiple mammalian species and microbial synthesis considered likely to contribute greatly to host requirements [42, 56]. In dogs and cats, however, it has been considered that folate absorption occurs primarily in the proximal small intestine, so much so that increased folate absorption, evidenced by high serum folate levels, are suggested to indicate pathogenic accumulation of folate-producing microbes in the small intestine [58]. Among the microbiota, folate appears to act on microbe function independent of host folate status [42].

**Cobalamin (B12):** In dogs and cats, cobalamin is exclusively absorbed via a complex, receptor-mediated mechanism located in the ileum [59]. Thus, microbial synthesis of cobalamin distal to the ileum is unavailable to the host in these species. In human GI microbes, approximately 40% of genomes included coding for the biosynthetic pathway for cobalamin, yet over 80% encode cobalamin-dependent enzymes [56, 60]. Cobalamin may have the ability to alter the density and diversity of the GI microbiome as bacteria compete to take up and metabolize the vitamin [61] (Table 5.1).

### 5.4.2 Minerals

Minerals, sometimes also referred to as electrolytes, particularly in solution, may also interact with gut microbes. For example, zinc oxide has long been used to reduce stress-associated diarrhea in weanling piglets. Zinc oxide has direct toxicity to bacteria while being relatively harmless

**Table 5.1** Functions of vitamins on the GI microbiota.

| Vitamin | Role |
| --- | --- |
| A, D, E, B2, and beta-carotene | Increase commensal abundance |
| A, B2, B3, C, and K | Increase or maintain microbial diversity |
| D | Alter diversity of microbiome |
| C | Increases production of SCFAs |
| B2 and E | Increase the species that produces SCFAs |

to mammalian cells [62], so addition of the mineral compound to diets for weanling piglets can reduce dysbiosis and proliferation of pathogenic bacteria during this challenging time, with both transient and long-lasting effects on the microbiome reported [48, 63, 64]. Zinc has also been shown to modulate microbiomes regulate gut epithelial barriers both in humans and other animals [65]. In another case, iron status has been demonstrated to affect the microbiome in mice. *Lactobacillus* species may be able to sense iron levels within the intestinal milieu communicate to the host to attenuate host iron absorption [66].

## 5.5 Processing and Digestibility of Nutrients

Digestibility is a key factor in the provision nutrients for the health of both the host animal and the microbiota. Highly digestible ingredients are more easily broken down and absorbed by the host, leaving little within the lumen to interact with the gut microbes, especially in more aboral sections of the gut. In comparison, indigestible portions of the diet will continue to the large colon where they may provide a source of energy and nutrients for the GI microbiota [1, 3, 7, 67]. As a result, diet digestibility plays a role in the density and diversity of the gut microbiome.

The digestibility of a diet is determined by the types of ingredients, ingredient and diet processing, and interactions between the two. Fiber, as previously discussed, provides indigestible carbohydrates that may be fermented by colonic microbes. Starches, typically digestible, may become more digestible through gelatinization with moisture and heat but may also be rendered indigestible, known as resistant starch, through processing such as high-temperature and high-pressure extrusion or retorting [24]. Less-intensive processing methods, such as "human-grade" cooking, may result in a different balance of digestibility, nutrient availability, denaturation of anti-nutritional factors, and safety through sterilization of potentially pathogenic microbes [10].

Though processing is typically employed to improve digestibility, nutrient availability and safety of pet foods, there may also be drawbacks. The term advanced glycation end products (AGEs) refers to compounds resulting from binding of reducing sugars to amino groups in proteins, nucleic acids, or lipids [68]. Some AGEs, such as Maillard complexes (from protein amino acids, commonly lysine), may be absorbed (but not utilized) by the host while excess may escape absorption and be degraded by colonic microbes [69]. In rats, AGEs have been shown to reduce the diversity and richness of the gut microbiome, particularly for some species of SCFA-producing carbohydrate-metabolizing species, while concurrently increasing the abundance of potentially pathogenic species and metabolites, including *Desulfovibrio* and *Bacteroides*, ammonia, and branched-chain fatty acids [68]. Cumulatively, these alterations to the microbiome and metabolome may impair colonic mucosal integrity and have been postulated to have associations with chronic inflammation [68–70]. Research is required to determine the possible implications to pet health from dietary AGEs and possible solutions to reduce AGEs in canine and feline food products.

## 5.6 Chapter Summary

- Differences in microbiome profiles can be seen between diets of different compositions and processing types
- Changes to the microbiome taxa have been shown to respond quickly to dietary intervention
- Gastrointestinal microbes are involved in protein digestion including absorption and metabolism of dietary protein. Undigested amino acids can be metabolized into numerous microbial-derived metabolites
- Indigestible fiber may be fermented by colonic microbes, resulting in the production of beneficial short-chain fatty acids
- A diet with a high inclusion (45–60% of daily caloric intake) of fat may have negative impacts on the gut microbiome

- Like macronutrients, micronutrients (vitamins and minerals) are associated with alterations in the microbiota
- Indigestible portions of the diet may be fermented by the gut microbes, thus potentially effecting the microbial density and diversity

## References

1  Pilla, R. and Suchodolski, J. (2021). The gut microbiome of dogs and cats, and the influence of diet. *Veterinary Clinics of North America: Small Animal Practice* 51: 605–621.
2  Wernimont, S., Radosevich, J., Jackson, M. et al. (2020). The effects of nutrition on the gastrointestinal microbiome of cats and dogs: impact on health and disease. *Frontiers in Microbiology* 11: 1266.
3  Panasevich, M., Kerr, K., Dilger, R. et al. (2015). Modulation of the faecal microbiome of healthy adult dogs by inclusion of potato fibre in the diet. *British Journal of Nutrition* 113: 125–133.
4  Li, Q., Lauber, C., Czarnecki-Maulden, G. et al. (2016). Effects of the dietary protein and carbohydrate ratio on gut microbiomes in dogs of different body conditions. *MBio* 8: e01703–e01716.
5  Sandri, M., Monego, S.D., Conte, G. et al. (2017). Raw meat based diet influences faecal microbiome and end products of fermentation in healthy dogs. *BMC Veterinary Research* 13: 65.
6  Schmidt, M., Unterer, S., Suchodolski, J. et al. (2018). The fecal microbiome and metabolome differs between dogs fed bones and raw food (barf) diets and dogs fed commercial diets. *PLoS one* 13 (8): e0201279.
7  Coelho, L., Kultima, J., Costea, P. et al. (2018). Similarity of the dog and human gut microbiomes in gene content and response to diet. *Microbiome* 6: 72.
8  Ephraim, E., Cochrane, C.-Y., and Jewell, D. (2020). Varying protein levels influence metabolomics and the gut microbiome in healthy adult dogs. *Toxins* 12: 517.
9  Ephraim, E. and Jewell, D. (2020). Effect of added dietary betaine and soluble fiber on metabolites and fecal microbiome in dogs with early renal disease. *Metabolites* 10: 370.
10  Do, S., Phungviwatnikul, T., de Godoy, M., and Swanson, K. (2021). Nutrient digestibility and fecal characteristics, microbiota, and

metabolites in dogs fed human-grade foods. *Journal of Animal Science* 99 (2): skab028.

11 Bermingham, E., Maclean, P., Thomas, D. et al. (2017). Key bacterial families (clostridiaceae, erysipelotrichaceae and bacteroidaceae) are related to the digestion of protein and energy in dogs. *PeerJ* 5: e3019.

12 Bermingham, E., Young, W., Butowski, C. et al. (2018). The fecal microbiota in the domestic cat (*felis catus*) is influenced by interactions between age and diet; a five year longitudinal study. *Frontiers in Microbiology* 9: 1231.

13 Allaway, D., Haydock, R., Lonsdale, Z. et al. (2020). Rapid reconstitution of the fecal microbiome after extended diet-induced changes indicates a stable gut microbiome in healthy adult dogs. *Applied and Environmental Microbiology* 86 (13): e00562–e00520.

14 Dodd, S., Cave, N., Abood, S. et al. (2020). An observational study of pet feeding practices and how these have changed between 2008 and 2018. *Veterinary Record* 186: 643.

15 Hendriks, W. and Sritharan, K. (2002). Apparent ileal and fecal digestibility of dietary protein is different in dogs. *Journal of Nutrition* 132: 1692S–1694S.

16 National Research Council (2006). *NRC, Nutrient Requirements of Dogs and Cats*. Washington, DC: National Research Council.

17 Okin, G. (2017). Environmental impacts of food consumption by dogs and cats. *PLoS One* 12 (8): e0181301.

18 Moon, C., Young, W., Maclean, P. et al. (2018). Metagenomic insights into the roles of proteobacteria in the gastrointestinal microbiomes of healthy dogs and cats. *Microbiology Open* 7: e00677.

19 Vázquez-Baeza, Y., Hyde, E., Suchodolski, J., and Knight, R. (2016). Dog and human inflammatory bowel disease rely on overlapping yet distinct dysbiosis networks. *Nature Microbiology* 1: 1–5.

20 Suchodolski, J., Markel, M., Garcia-Mazcorro, J. et al. (2012). The fecal microbiome in dogs with acute diarrhea and idiopathic inflammatory bowel disease. *PLoS One* 7 (12): e51907.

21 Hooda, S., Boler, B.V., Kerr, K. et al. (2013). The gut microbiome of kittens is affected by dietary protein:carbohydrate ratio and associated with blood metabolite and hormone concentrations. *British Journal of Nutrition* 109: 1637–1646.

22 Cave, N. (2006). Hydrolyzed protein diets for dogs and cats. *Veterinary Clinics of North America: Small Animal Practice* 36: 1251–1268.

**23** Pilla, R., Guard, B., Steiner, J. et al. (2019). Administration of a synbiotic containing enterococcus faecium does not significantly alter fecal microbiota richness or diversity in dogs with and without food-responsive chronic enteropathy. *Frontiers in Veterinary Science* 6: 277.

**24** Rankovic, A., Adolphe, J., and Verbrugghe, A. (2019). The role of carbohydrates in the health of dogs. *Journal of the American Veterinary Medical Association* 255 (5): 546–554.

**25** Noble, E., Hsu, T., Jones, R. et al. (2017). Early-life sugar consumption affects the rat microbiome independently of obesity. *Journal of Nutrition* 147: 20–28.

**26** Jarett, J., Carlson, A., Serao, M. et al. (2019). Diets with and without edible cricket support a similar level of diversity in the gut microbiome of dogs. *PeerJ* 7: e7661.

**27** de Oliveira Matheus, L., Risolia, L., Ernandes, M. et al. (2021). Effects of saccharomyces cerevisiae cell wall addition on feed digestibility, fecal fermentation and microbiota and immunological parameters in adult cats. *BMC Veterinary Research* 17: 351.

**28** Depauw, S., Hesta, M., Whitehouse-Tedd, K. et al. (2013). Animal fibre: the forgotten nutrient in strict carnivores? First insights in the cheetah. *Journal of Animal Physiology and Animal Nutrition* 97: 146–154.

**29** AAFCO, Official Publication (2020). *Champaign.* Illinois: Association of American Feed Control Officials.

**30** Jackson, M. and Jewell, D. (2019). Balance of saccharolysis and proteolysis underpins improvements in stool quality induced by adding a fiber bundle containing bound polyphenols to either hydrolyzed meat or grain-rich foods. *Gut Microbes* 10 (3): 298–320.

**31** Rossi, G., Cerquetella, M., Gavazza, A. et al. (2020). Rapid resolution of large bowel diarrhea after the administration of a combination of a high-fiber diet and a probiotic mixture in 30 dogs. *Veterinary Sciences* 7: 21.

**32** Fritsch, D., Wernimont, S., Jackson, M., and Gross, K. (2019). Select dietary fiber sources improve stool parameters, decrease fecal putrefactive metabolites, and deliver antioxidant and anti-inflammatory plant polyphenols to the lower gastrointestinal tract of adult dogs. *The FASEB Journal* 33 (S1): 587.

**33** Simpson, J., Martineau, B., Jones, W. et al. (2002). Characterization of fecal bacterial populations in canines: effects of age, breed and dietary fiber. *Microbial Ecology* 44: 186–197.

**34** Loureiro, B., Sakomura, N., Vaconcellos, R. et al. (2016). Insoluble fibres, satiety and food intake in cats fed kibble diets. *Journal of Animal Physiology and Animal Nutrition* 101: 824–834.

**35** Weber, M., Bissot, T., Servet, E. et al. (2007). A high-protein, high-fiber diet designed for weight loss improves satiety in dogs. *Journal of Veterinary Internal Medicine* 21: 1203–1208.

**36** Nelson, R., Scott-Moncrieff, J., Feldman, E. et al. (2002). Effect of dietary insoluble fiber on control of glycemia in cats with naturally acquired diabetes mellitus. *Journal of the American Veterinary Medical Association* 216: 1082–1088.

**37** Dann, J., Adler, M., Duffy, K., and Giffard, C. (2004). A potential nutritional prophylactic for the reduction of feline hairball symptoms. *Journal of Nutrition* 134: 2024S–2125S.

**38** Sunvold, G., Fahey, G., and Reinhart, G. (1995). Dietary fiber for cats: in vitro fermentation of selected fiber sources by cat fecal inoculum and in vivo utilization of diets containing selected fiber sources and their blends. *Journal of Animal Science* 73 (8): 2329–2339.

**39** Kienzle, E., Meyer, H., and Schneider, R. (1991). Investigations on palatability, digestibility and tolerance of low digestible food components in cats. *Journal of Nutrition* 121 (11): S56–S57.

**40** Ding, J.-H., Jin, Z., Yang, X.-X. et al. (2020). Role of gut microbiota via the gut-liver-brain axis in digestive diseases. *World Journal of Gastroenterology* 26 (40): 6141–6142.

**41** Yamada, M., Takahashi, N., Matsuda, Y. et al. (2018). A bacterial metabolite ameliorates periodontal pathogen-induced gingival epithelial barrier disruption via gpr40 signaling. *Scientific Reports* 8: 1–2.

**42** Pham, V., Dold, S., Rehman, A. et al. (2021). Vitamins, the gut microbiome and gastrointestinal health in humans. *Nutrition Research* 95: 35–53.

**43** Cartwright, J., Gow, A., Milne, E. et al. (2018). Vitamin d receptor expression in dogs. *Journal of Veterinary Internal Medicine* 32: 764–774.

**44** Pham, V., Fehlbaum, S., Seifert, N. et al. (2021). Effects of colon-targeted vitamins on the composition and metabolic activity of the human gut microbiome – a pilot study. *Gut Microbes* 13 (1): 1875774.

**45** Bashir, M., Prietl, B., Tauschmann, M. et al. (2016). Effects of high doses of vitamin d3 on mucosa-associated gut microbiome vary between regions of the human gastrointestinal tract. *European Journal of Nutrition* 55: 1479–1489.

**46** Ljubic, A., Thulesen, E., Jacobsen, C., and Jakobsen, J. (2021). Uvb exposure stimulates production of vitamin d3 in selected microalgae. *Algal Research* 59: 102472.

**47** Wang, T., Bengtsson, G., Kärnefelt, I., and Björn, L. (2001). Provitamins and vitamins d2 and d3 in cladinia spp. Over a latitudinal gradiet: possible correlation with uv levels. *Journal of Photochemistry and Photobiology B: Biology* 62: 118–122.

**48** Dowley, A., Sweeney, T., Conway, E. et al. (2021). Effects of dietary supplementation with mushroom or vitamin d2-enriched mushroom powders on gastrointestinal health parameters in the weaned pig. *Animals* 11: 3603.

**49** Zhang, L., Yang, M., and Piao, X. (2021). Effects of 25-hydroxyvitamin d3 on growth performance, serum parameters, fecal microbiota, and metabolites in weaned piglets fed diets with low calcium and phosphorus. *Journal of the Science of Food and Agriculture* 102 (2): 597–606.

**50** Swanson, K., Dowd, S., Suchodolski, J. et al. (2011). Phylogenetic and gene-centric metagenomics of canine intestinal microbiome reveals similarities with humans and mice. *The ISME Journal* 5: 639–649.

**51** Fenn, K., Strandwitz, P., Stewart, E. et al. (2017). Quinones are growth factors for the human gut microbiota. *Microbiome* 5: 1.

**52** Zeisel, S. (1998). *Dietary Reference Intakes for Thiamin, Riboflavin, Niacin, Vitamin b6, Folate, Vitamin b12, Pantothenic Acid, Biotin, and Choline*. Washington, DC: Food and Nutrition Board, Institute of Medicine.

**53** Said, H. (2013). Recent advances in transport of water-soluble vitamins in organs of the digestive system: a focus on the colon and the pancreas. *American Journal of Physiology Gastrointestinal and Liver Physiology* 305 (9): G601–G610.

**54** Uebanso, T., Shimohata, T., Mawatari, K., and Takahashi, A. (2020). Functional roles of b-vitamins in the gut and gut microbiome. *Molecular Nutrition & Food Research* 64: 2000426.

**55** Kunisawa, J., Sugiura, Y., Wake, T. et al. (2015). Mode of bioenergetic metabolism during b cell differentiation in the intestine determines the distinct requirement for vitamin b1. *Cell Reports* 13: 122–131.

**56** Magnúsdóttir, S., Ravcheev, D., de Crécy-Lagard, V., and Thiele, I. (2015). Systematic genome assessment of b-vitamin biosynthesis suggests co-operation among gut microbes. *Frontiers in Genetics* 6: 148.

**57** Ghosal, A., Lambrecht, N., Subramanya, S. et al. (2012). Conditional knockout of the slc5a6 gene in mouse intestine impairs biotin absorption. *American Journal of Physiology Gastrointestinal and Liver Physiology* 304 (1): G64–G71.

**58** Suchodolski, J. (2016). Diagnosis and interpretation of intestinal dysbiosis in dogs and cats. *The Veterinary Journal* 215: 30–37.

**59** Ruaux, C., Steiner, J., and Williams, D. (2005). Early biochemical and clinical responses to cobalamin supplementation in cats with signs of gastrointestinal disease and severe hypocobalaminemia. *Journal of Veterinary Internal Medicine* 19: 155–160.

**60** Degnan, P., Barry, N., Mok, K. et al. (2014). Human gut microbes use multiple transporters to distinguish vitamin b12 analogs and compete in the gut. *Cell Host & Microbe* 15 (1): 47–57.

**61** Xu, Y., Xiang, S., Ye, K. et al. (2018). Cobalamin (vitamin b12) induced a shift in microbial composition and metabolic activity in an in vitro colon simulation. *Frontiers in Microbiology* 9: 2780.

**62** Xie, Y., He, Y., Irwin, P. et al. (2011). Antibacterial activity and mechanism of action of zinc oxide nanoparticles against *campylobacter jejuni*. *Applied and Environmental Microbiology* 77 (7): 2325–2331.

**63** Li, Y., Guo, Y., Wen, Z. et al. (2018). Weaning stress perturbs gut microbiome and its metabolic profle in piglets. *Nature* 8: 1–2.

**64** Starke, I., Pieper, R., Neumann, K. et al. (2013). The impact of high dietary zinc oxide on the development of the intestinal microbiota in weaned piglets. *FEMS Microbiology Ecology* 87: 416–427.

**65** Usama, U., Khan, M., and Fatima, S. (2018). Role of zinc in shaping the gut microbiome; proposed mechanisms and evidence from the literature. *Journal of Gastrointestinal & Digestive System* 8 (1): 548.

**66** Das, N., Schwartz, A., Barthel, G. et al. (2020). Microbial metabolite signaling is required for systemic iron homeostasis. *Cell Metabolism* 31: 115–130.

**67** Middelbos, I., Boler, B., Qu, A. et al. (2010). Phylogenetic characterization of fecal microbial communities of dogs fed diets with or without supplemental dietary fiber using 454 pyrosequencing. *PLoS one* 5 (3): e9768.

**68** Qu, W., Yuan, X., Zhao, J. et al. (2017). Dietary advanced glycation end products modify gut microbial composition and partially increase colon permeability in rats. *Molecular Nutrition & Food Research* 61 (10): 1700118.

**69** van Rooijen, C., Bosch, G., Poel, A.v. et al. (2013). The maillard reaction and pet food processing: effects on nutritive value and pet health. *Nutrition Research Reviews* 26: 130–148.

**70** Teodorowicz, M., Hendriks, W., Wichers, H. et al. (2018). Immuno-modulation by processed animal feed: the role of maillard reaction products and advanced glycation end-products (ages). *Fronteirs in Immunology* 9: 2088.

# 6

# Current Methods for Microbiome Analysis

## 6.1 Introduction

In this chapter, some of the current methods used to characterize the microbiome in companion animals will be reviewed. Methods matter in the study of the microbiome and using different methods allows different questions to be answered.

Methodological innovations help drive scientific advances and this is exemplified in the field of microbiology. When the father of microbiology Antonie van Leeuwenhoek made the very first observations of "wee animalcules" (bacteria and other microbes) in 1676, he introduced us to the microscopic world. Cultivation methods followed in the nineteenth century, allowing microbiologists to isolate and describe bacteria, fungi, protozoa, and viruses that were host-associated, ultimately advancing medicine through the diagnosis and treatment of infectious disease. These cultivation-based approaches allowed many pathogens to be identified based on phenotypic measures, including responses to stains, culture requirements, and phenotypic growth characteristics. Indeed, cultivation-based approaches are still used today as a mainstay for first-line diagnosis of many infectious conditions in veterinary patients.

A revolution in microbiology began in the mid-1970s when Carl Woese and George Fox proposed using ribosomal RNA as genetic markers to characterize microbial life. By sequencing 16S ribosomal RNA, they [1] built the first phylogenetic trees to describe evolutionary relationships

*Small Animal Microbiomes and Nutrition*, First Edition. Robin Saar and Sarah Dodd.
© 2024 John Wiley & Sons, Inc. Published 2024 by John Wiley & Sons, Inc.
Companion website: www.wiley.com/go/saar/1e

and distinguish convergent similarities from homologous ones. Combined with the invention of automated sequencing technology [2], this approach revolutionized the study and classification of microbes. Culture-independent sequencing methods began to be used to describe environmental and host-associated microbial communities that could not be cultivated, starting with a relatively simple microbial community found in the Octopus hot spring in Yellowstone National Park [3]. The invention of the polymerase chain reaction (PCR) by Kary Mullis in 1983, along with other advances in molecular techniques and sequencing technologies further advanced our ability to characterize the hidden world of microorganisms that had resisted cultivation.

Marker genes such as the 16S ribosomal RNA (or 16S rRNA) gene are useful markers because they contain regions of DNA with slow rates of evolution that are adjacent to regions with high rates of evolution. Other commonly used marker genes are 18S ribosomal RNA (rRNA) gene for eukarya (eukaryotes) and the nuclear ribosomal internal transcribed spacer (ITS) gene for fungi. The proximity between these conserved and highly variable regions allows PCR primers to be designed for the conserved regions that can be used to amplify and sequence neighboring variable regions in order to detect a signal of the evolutionary history of the organism (Figure 6.1).

By sequencing marker genes such as the 16S rRNA gene locus and comparing it to a reference database, bacteria can be phylogenetically typed (or identified) and the number of copies of sequencing reads matching that identification can be counted, all based on nucleotide sequences. Thus, DNA sequencing can be used to catalog and describe different kinds of microbes, almost like a field guide for microbial life [4]. Phylogenetic methods built upon this foundational research are used today to characterize highly diverse microbial communities, including the gut microbiome.

Though the best way to understand the biology of a microbe may be to isolate it, it is now widely recognized that classical microbiological methods are not the best ways to determine the taxonomic or phylogenetic identity of a microbe. This is particularly true for those organisms that are not well characterized, phenotypically variable, or difficult to cultivate. By surmounting the need for isolation, DNA sequencing allows these problems to be overcome and it facilitates the discovery of new microbes based on their genetic material. It has been estimated that for

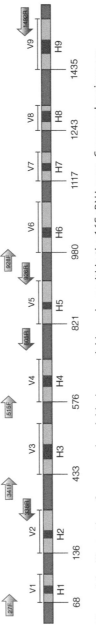

**Figure 6.1** Illustration of conserved, variable, hypervariable regions within the 16S rRNA gene. Conserved regions are indicated in blue, the nine variable regions (V1–V9) in gray, and hypervariable regions in red (H1–H9). Commonly used forward and reverse primers are presented in arrows.

each bacterial species that has been cultivated in a laboratory, there are at least 100 more in the world that have not yet been isolated and that the isolates we recognize today are the tip of the microbial iceberg.

## 6.2    Why is it Important to Characterize the Microbiome?

Microbiome analysis assesses the breadth of microbes within a specific sample, such as feces, skin and oral scrapings or swabs, and blood. Characterization of the entirety of a microbiome using the phylogenetic methods mentioned above allows for the detection of specific pathogens and additionally provides information on commensal microbes that may be missing or in differential abundances compared with those found in healthy individuals. Today, we still face challenges in determining what a "healthy" population and abundance is for any particular individual as there as a great number of factors influencing the microbiome even within animals of the same species (see Chapter 4).

While microbiome analyses have been performed in academic research for decades, their application in veterinary medicine is relatively new. Studies in both human and veterinary medicine have noted patterns of alteration in microbial communities associated with a number of disease states, suggesting that microbiome testing is a promising diagnostic tool (e.g. [5]). In addition, the microbiome has the possibility to be manipulated and can be rapidly responsive to changes such as dietary intervention and fecal microbiota transplantation (FMT).

Microbial diversity, functional redundancy across different microbes and metabolic flexibility within the gut microbiome contribute to its resilience in response to disruptions such as antibiotic therapy [6]. However, microbial diversity and functional richness of the gut microbiome can be depleted by exposure to antibiotics [7] and other medications [8]. Non-targeted adverse effects on beneficial bacteria in the gut microbiome may arise from such necessary therapies, so identification of these effects may allow for restorative measures to be taken.

From a clinical perspective, prediction of how an individual might respond to a perturbation, such as a course of antibiotics, as well as how they may respond to restorative measures, such as the addition of prebiotic fibers to the diet, probiotics, or FMT, could be useful to specifically target individual therapies to maximize benefit and minimize harm. As individuals can vary greatly in their responses to such interventions, therapeutic approaches to microbiome restoration may benefit from personalized assessment, including evaluation of microbiome compositions.

## 6.3 Sample Collection and Preservation Methods

The National Institutes of Health (NIH) sponsored Human Microbiome Project helped reveal more details than had previously been known about how the human body has many different niches with each having a somewhat characteristic set and amount of microbes [9]. These different niches require different collection techniques. For example, dry swabs are common for sample collection from skin [10], otic [11], oral [12], ocular [13], and vaginal surfaces. Dental samples are typically collected using paper points. Dry swab samples of low biomass regions of the body and dental samples must be processed promptly or frozen [14]. When low amounts of bacterial DNA are expected, such as in blood [15], contamination arising from the collection site (needle penetration through the skin surface), as well as the hospital and lab environment must be selectively minimized. Blood samples can be stored either frozen or using blood tubes containing EDTA (ethylenediaminetetraacetic acid).

Fecal samples are often used as a noninvasive diagnostic specimen to assess the gut microbiome. Though some changes in microbial composition may be attributable to differences in storage conditions, storage duration, and sample preservation method used in humans [16], this may not be as relevant in veterinary species [17]. Nevertheless, the gold standard for capturing a snapshot of the gut microbiome is a fresh fecal sample that is processed immediately or within a ~4-hour window at room temperature and within 48 hours under refrigeration. Given that this is usually not practical, sample preservation methods are often employed, including drying the sample, using preservation buffers, and freezing.

Ethanol is an economical agent that provides stability and reproducibility for fecal samples. In a study comparing different preservation methods [18], it was found that fecal preservation using 70% ethanol with homogenization yielded DNA concentrations and bacterial composition closest to that of fresh samples, highlighting its potential utility in field, laboratory, and clinical settings without access to a laboratory freezer. This ethanol concentration (70%) was also reported to provide effective preservation for spider monkey feces [19], while 95% ethanol for dog feces was found to be preferable when used without homogenization by ([20]). Some fecal preservation buffers contain Tris-EDTA, which dissolves cellular membranes to solubilize the DNA and chelates the metal cations that catalyze DNase respectively. However, due to concerns about toxicity [21], EDTA is not ideal for in-home use by clients and its use in-clinic requires hazardous waste disposal.

## 6.4 Current Methods for Microbiome Analysis

Current methods for microbiome analysis range from microscopy, laboratory cultivation, PCR panels using quantitative PCR (qPCR), amplicon sequencing, metagenomic shotgun sequencing, RNA sequencing, and metabolomics (Table 6.1). The selection of the best method depends on the data intended to be collected. Bacteria are typically the focus of gut microbiome analysis partly because the gut microbiome is dominated by

**Table 6.1** Current methods used to characterize the microbiome

| Method | Description |
| --- | --- |
| Microscopy | Study of microbial phenotypes, which are not reliable for distinguishing between taxa. Molecular probes have been developed for fluorescent in situ hybridization (FISH). Limitations: Their use requires prior knowledge of targets of interest and works best for communities living on a flat surface, such as an oral biofilm |
| Cultivation | Liquid or solid growth media used to grow single cells of microbes in isolation. Essential for assessing the organism's biology and physiology. Continues to have relevance for pathogen and antimicrobial resistance screening. Limitations: Not necessarily representative of activity in vivo and not all microbes can be cultivated |
| qPCR | Some panels have been developed to target a small number of microbes in the microbiome, including the Dysbiosis Index (DI). Affordable and rapid (few hours), and analysis of results is straight-forward. Limitations: Like FISH, qPCR panels work best when the targets are well known and few in number. Typically the panels are optimized for a specific condition, such as chronic enteropathy in the case of the DI, and as such have a more narrow application than discovery-based methods like amplicon sequencing and metagenomics. Unlike digital PCR, quantification is not absolute and requires careful titration of standard curves |

*(Continued)*

Table 6.1    (Continued)

| Method | Description |
| --- | --- |
| Amplicon sequencing | PCR primers are designed for one or more of the hypervariable regions of the bacterial 16S ribosomal RNA (rRNA) gene (V1–V9) for bacteria and archaea), 18S rRNA gene (for eukaryotes), or nuclear ribosomal internal transcribed spacer (ITS, for fungi). PCR is used to make billions of copies (amplicons) of all the gene variants found in the sample. Sequencing followed by phylogenetic analysis allows the genes to be identified using reference databases. The numbers of each type found are estimated from the number of times each is found in the sequence data. Affordable and rapid (a few days). Limitations: Results limited to amplicon target (e.g. 16S rRNA gene for bacteria and archaea, ITS gene for fungi). PCR amplification introduces bias. Using short-read sequencing methods (Illumina), not all of the variable regions are sequenced, limiting interpretation to genus level. However, long-read sequencing (PacBio and Oxford Nanopore) allows the full gene to be sequenced for species-level identification. Assesses relative abundances rather than absolute abundances, which may be more relevant for pathogens. Copy number of 16S rRNA gene is variable among bacterial species |
| Metagenomics | Shotgun metagenomic sequencing yields sequence data for all genomic DNA in a sample, including DNA viruses, fungi, protists, bacteria, archaea, as well as host DNA. Samples can be prepared without amplification, reducing PCR bias. Useful for taxonomic profiling to the strain level and genetic capacity for metabolic functions and antimicrobial resistance. Limitations: Cost is much greater than amplicon sequencing and sample preparation is involved, with a much higher rate of samples failing due to high DNA input requirements and sensitivity to inhibitors in the sample. Samples with appreciable amounts of host DNA require deeper sequencing for microbiome analysis. May not yield reliable results for parasites, including *Giardia* and *Toxoplasma gondii* |
| Metabolomics | Analytical chemistry used to measure metabolites, such as short-chain fatty acids (SCFAs) and bile acids (primary and secondary) in the case of gut health. Methods include liquid chromatography-mass spectrometry (LCMS), gas chromatography-mass spectrometry (GCMS), and nuclear magnetic resonance spectroscopy (NMR). Limitations: Does not describe taxonomic composition but measures metabolic function. Samples require careful storage, typically at $-80\,°C$. Preservation methods associated with strong storage effects |

bacteria, and partly because, at present, bacteria have been better described and cataloged than fungi, protozoa, or viruses. However, there is growing support for the idea that key groups of fungi can play important roles in gastrointestinal disease, especially *Saccharomycetes* and *Candida* spp. in humans [22]. Analyses of gut fungi have been performed in dogs as well, with potentially congruent findings [23, 24].

### 6.4.1 Microscopy

Microscopy maintains relevance because PCR and sequencing do not provide information about morphology, spatial distribution, and the cellular environment of microbes. Spatial interactions between the microbiome and the host can be visualized using fluorescent in situ hybridization (FISH) [25], which combines the precision of molecular biology with the visual information provided by microscopy. Using fluorescently labeled probes designed for specific targets, such as the 16S rRNA genes for specific groups of bacteria found in vaginal biofilms [26], FISH allows microbial cells to be visualized, identified, and counted within a biofilm or tissue. This method involves fixing the specimen, sample preparation, hybridization with probes for detecting specific target sequences, followed by washing to remove unbound probes. Still it is relatively fast and affordable compared to sequencing. The biggest limitations with using FISH to characterize the microbiome are autofluorescence of nontarget microorganisms, and that the number of probes that can be used is limited. As with all of these methods, controls are essential. At this point, access to FISH technology remains limited in veterinary medicine and it is primarily used by specialists and academics as a research tool.

### 6.4.2 Cultivation

Microbial cultivation maintains relevance for testing for pathogens as well as screening for antimicrobial resistance (AMR) and a variety of other purposes including for use in experimental manipulations. It is also possible to assess the presence of AMR genes in metagenomes [27, 28]. However, because genomic sequencing requires disassembly and reassembly, it can be challenging to ascribe the presence of an AMR gene to a specific organism. To combat this, there are a few elaborate and expensive tagging techniques for metagenomic sample preparation to help identify which genomes belong together. The current gold standard for identifying the presence of AMR genes in a microbe is to first isolate it and then sequence its genome. Clinical microbiology laboratories may provide screening for pathogens and some AMR genes using cultivation methods as well as PCR panels. They do not typically assess microbiome composition of commensal bacteria, focusing on pathogenic species instead.

### 6.4.3 Molecular Methods

Molecular methods for microbiome characterization include quantitative PCR panels (qPCR), amplicon sequencing (sequencing of amplified targets), and metagenomic sequencing (Figure 6.2) [29]. PCR panels provide a relatively fast way to assess the presence and abundance of known targets, such as pathogens that are well characterized, and are less commonly used to characterize commensal bacteria. This is in part due to the tremendous diversity of commensals in the microbiome, high levels of variation in their representation (prevalence) across populations, as well as a lack of knowledge about their biology. Amplicon and metagenomic sequencing are discovery-based approaches to catalog all known microbes found in the sample using reference databases. In addition to these DNA-based methods, mRNA present in a sample can be characterized using sequencing to assess levels of gene expression (transcriptomics) and protein expression can be described using proteomics. However, such methods are primarily used as research tools in veterinary science for describing disease etiology [30] and biomarker discovery and will not be discussed further in this chapter.

#### 6.4.3.1 Quantitative PCR Panels

Designed to target, amplify, and quantify known microbial targets, qPCR panels include the more familiar panels offered by veterinary diagnostic laboratories, which traditionally have focused on screening for parasites (protozoa and helminths) and pathogens (bacteria, fungi, and viruses) [29]. Assessment of microbiome composition using PCR panels depends on the identification of a relatively small number of taxa associated with a specific type of imbalance or dysbiosis. For example, the Texas A&M Gut Dysbiosis Indices (DI) are panels of qPCR assays that report a single numerical value indicating normobiosis versus dysbiosis associated with chronic enteropathy in dogs and cats. The dog DI panel utilizes a universal bacterial primer and primers specific for *Blautia*, *Clostridium hiranonis*, *Escherichia coli*, *Faecalibacterium*, *Fusobacterium*, *Streptococcus*, and

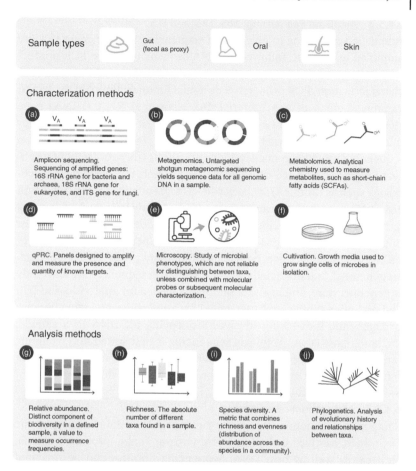

**Figure 6.2** Current techniques used to characterize and analyze microbial communities in host-associated microbiomes.

*Turicibacter* [31] with a 74% sensitivity and 95% specificity separating chronic enteropathy from healthy dogs. The cat DI panel likewise measures total bacteria and the seven bacterial taxa: *Bacteroides, Bifidobacterium, Clostridium hiranonis, Escherichia coli, Faecalibacterium, Streptococcus,* and *Turicibacter* [32] sensitivity and 96% specificity separating chronic enteropathy from healthy cats. These qPCR panels work best when the targets are relatively well known and few in number and are typically optimized for a specific condition, such as chronic enteropathy in the case of these Dysbiosis Indices.

### 6.4.3.2 Amplicon Sequencing: 16S, 18S, and ITS

Amplicon sequencing is a method of sequencing specific genes that are amplified using PCR, followed by DNA sequencing of the PCR product or amplicon [29]. When amplicon sequencing is used for microbial characterization, PCR primers are designed for one or more of the hyper-variable regions of the bacterial 16S ribosomal RNA (rRNA) gene (V1–V9 for bacteria and archaea), 18S rRNA gene (for eukaryotes), or nuclear ribosomal internal transcribed spacer (ITS, for fungi). Amplicon sequencing provides genus-level identifications (for sequences of a sub-set of regions of the 16S rRNA gene using a short-read sequencing technology such as Illumina) or species-level (for sequences of the full length 16S rRNA gene, which can be accomplished with long-read sequencing technologies such as Pacific Biosystems and Oxford Nanopore). The cost of amplicon sequencing is significantly less expensive than the cost of metagenomic sequencing, both computationally, given the smaller data-set generated, and financially because amplicon sequences are less costly to generate, store, and analyze. Samples collected for analysis of the skin and oral microbiome are better suited for amplicon sequencing because metagenomic sequencing involves sequencing all DNA in a sample, including host DNA. Amplicon sequencing is best suited for taxonomic profiling of microbiome samples (who is there) but does not provide information about metabolic function (what they are doing).

### 6.4.3.3 Metagenomic Sequencing

Shotgun metagenomic sequencing yields sequence data for all genomic DNA in a sample, including DNA viruses, fungi, protists, bacteria, archaea, as well as host DNA. Sequencing libraries can be prepared without amplification, eliminating PCR bias [29]. For samples with low biomass, PCR still needs to be performed (whole genome amplification) in order to yield results, generating amplification bias.

The numbers of each type of microbe found are estimated from the number of times each is found in the sequence data. Depending on sequencing depth and the reference database, metagenomic sequencing can identify taxa to species or strain-level taxonomic resolution. In addition to taxonomic profiling, metagenomic databases allow for the identification and annotation of genes associated with metabolic functions.

A major limitation from the perspective of diagnostic testing is that the cost of metagenomic sequencing is currently from 10 to 50× greater than amplicon sequencing, with a much higher rate of samples failing due to high DNA input requirements and sensitivity to inhibitors in the sample.

In addition to sequencing cost, metagenomic libraries take longer to sequence and are costly in terms of computational analysis and storage of large datasets. Shallow sequencing is not advised for clinical samples because it does not yield consistent results. Samples with appreciable amounts of host DNA, such as skin and oral samples, will lose a lot of sequencing reads to the host genome, requiring deeper sequencing.

In addition, this approach for identifying the presence of certain parasites, including *Giardia* and *Toxoplasma gondii,* does not yield reliable results because these organisms form cysts that are resistant to standard DNA extraction methods and require specific approaches to optimize yield. For these reasons, other approaches such as antigen testing and microscopy may be more reliable for detecting these parasites.

### 6.4.3.4 Metabolomics

After cataloging members of microbial communities, a potentially valuable next step is to characterize the metabolic functions of the community in order to help assess what the microbes are doing [33, 34]. Metabolomics uses analytical chemistry to describe and quantify metabolites found in a sample using targeted or untargeted (discovery-based) approaches. Although not yet widely available as a veterinary diagnostic tool, high-throughput, high-resolution, and wide metabolite coverage is available by liquid chromatography-mass spectrometry (LCMS) platforms with the advent of ultra-performance liquid chromatography (UPLC) and ionization switching systems. Using minimal sample preparation, detecting SCFAs by LCMS is often difficult because their masses are in the lower mass range, where peaks from solvents and additives interfere, their hydrophilicity results in poor chromatographic separation and insufficient ionization in electrospray ionization. These challenges can be overcome by introducing specific derivatization steps ([35]). Other common techniques to analyze SCFAs include gas chromatography-mass spectrometry (GCMS) and nuclear magnetic resonance spectroscopy (NMR).

Fecal SCFAs are often reduced in chronic enteropathy dogs [36]. This change has been attributed to decreased *Faecalibacterium* and *Bacteroides* species [37]. Untargeted fecal metabolomics performed on samples of dogs with chronic enteropathy revealed differences in the short- and medium-chain fatty acids, amino acids, and bile acid metabolism [38]. Similarly, untargeted fecal metabolomics comparing fecal samples from cats with chronic enteropathy versus those from healthy cats revealed differences in an inflammation-associated polyunsaturated fatty acid, amino acids, and vitamins [39].

## 6.5 Chapter Summary

- Microbiome analyses are used to assess the diversity and abundance of microbes within a sample
- Amplicon and metagenomic sequencing are the most commonly used methods and are untargeted, discovery-based methods that provide a snapshot of the whole community
- Amplicon sequencing is useful for profiling who is in the community, and metagenomics adds functional predictions
- Older methods including qPCR, cultivation, and microscopy continue to provide useful insights
- PCR-based diagnostic panels have been developed for chronic enteropathies

## References

1 Woese, C.R. and Fox, G.E. (1977). Phylogenetic structure of the prokaryotic domain: the primary kingdoms. *Proceedings of the National Academy of Sciences of the United States of America* 74 (11): 5088–5090.

2 Sanger, F., Nicklen, S., and Coulson, A.R. (1977). DNA sequencing with chain-terminating inhibitors. *Proceedings of the National Academy of Sciences* 74 (12): 5463–5467.

3 Stahl, D.A., Lane, D.J., Olsen, G.J., and Pace, N.R. (1985). Characterization of a yellowstone hot spring microbial community by 5S rRNA sequences. *Applied and Environmental Microbiology* 49 (6): 1379–1384.

4 Eisen, J.A. (2007). Environmental shotgun sequencing: its potential and challenges for studying the hidden world of microbes. *PLoS Biology* 5 (3): e82.

5 Pilla, R. and Suchodolski, J.S. (2019). The role of the canine gut microbiome and metabolome in health and gastrointestinal disease. *Frontiers in Veterinary Science* 6: 498.

6 Fassarella, M., Blaak, E.E., Penders, J. et al. (2021). Gut microbiome stability and resilience: elucidating the response to perturbations in order to modulate gut health. *Gut* 70 (3): 595–605.

7 Pilla, R., Gaschen, F.P., Barr, J.W. et al. (2020). Effects of metronidazole on the fecal microbiome and metabolome in healthy dogs. *Journal of Veterinary Internal Medicine/American College of Veterinary Internal Medicine* 34 (5): 1853–1866.

**8** Le Bastard, Q., Al-Ghalith, G.A., Grégoire, M. et al. (2018). Systematic review: human gut dysbiosis induced by non-antibiotic prescription medications. *Alimentary Pharmacology & Therapeutics* 47 (3): 332–345.

**9** Zhou, Y., Gao, H., Mihindukulasuriya, K.A. et al. (2013). Biogeography of the ecosystems of the healthy human body. *Genome Biology* 14 (1): R1.

**10** Bradley, C.W., Morris, D.O., Rankin, S.C. et al. (2016). Longitudinal evaluation of the skin microbiome and association with microenvironment and treatment in canine atopic dermatitis. *The Journal of Investigative Dermatology* 136 (6): 1182–1190.

**11** Tang, S., Prem, A., Tjokrosurjo, J. et al. (2020). The canine skin and ear microbiome: a comprehensive survey of pathogens implicated in canine skin and ear infections using a novel next-generation-sequencing-based assay. *Veterinary Microbiology* 247 (August): 108764.

**12** Oba, P.M., Carroll, M.Q., Alexander, C. et al. (2021). Microbiota populations in supragingival plaque, subgingival plaque, and saliva habitats of adult dogs. *Animal Microbiome* 3 (1): 38.

**13** Banks, K.C., Ericsson, A.C., Reinero, C.R., and Giuliano, E.A. (2019). Veterinary ocular microbiome: lessons learned beyond the culture. *Veterinary Ophthalmology* 22 (5): 716–725.

**14** Marotz, C., Cavagnero, K.J., Song, S.J. et al. (2021). Evaluation of the effect of storage methods on fecal, saliva, and skin microbiome composition. *mSystems* 6 (2): https://doi.org/10.1128/mSystems. 01329-20.

**15** Scarsella, E., Sandri, M., Dal Monego, S. et al. (2020). Blood microbiome: a new marker of gut microbial population in dogs? *Veterinary Science in China* 7 (4): https://doi.org/10.3390/vetsci7040198.

**16** Vogtmann, E., Chen, J., Amir, A. et al. (2017). Comparison of collection methods for fecal samples in microbiome studies. *American Journal of Epidemiology* 185 (2): 115–123.

**17** Tal, M., Verbrugghe, A., Gomez, D. et al. (2017). The effect of storage at ambient temperature on the feline fecal microbiota. *BMC Veterinary Research* 13 (256): 1–8.

**18** Horng, K.R., Ganz, H.H., Eisen, J.A., and Marks, S.L. (2018). Effects of preservation method on canine (Canis Lupus Familiaris) fecal microbiota. *PeerJ* 6 (May): e4827.

**19** Hale, V.L., Tan, C.L., Knight, R., and Amato, K.R. (2015). Effect of preservation method on spider monkey (Ateles Geoffroyi) fecal microbiota over 8 weeks. *Journal of Microbiological Methods* 113 (June): 16–26.

**20** Song, S.J., Amir, A., Metcalf, J.L. et al. (2016). Preservation methods differ in fecal microbiome stability, affecting suitability for field studies, mSystems. 1 (3): https://doi.org/10.1128/mSystems.00021-16.

**21** Lanigan, R.S. and Yamarik, T.A. (2002). Final report on the safety assessment of EDTA, calcium disodium EDTA, diammonium EDTA, dipotassium EDTA, disodium EDTA, TEA-EDTA, tetrasodium EDTA, tripotassium EDTA, trisodium EDTA, HEDTA, and trisodium HEDTA. *International Journal of Toxicology* 21 (Suppl 2): 95–142.

**22** Sciavilla, P., Strati, F., Di Paola, M. et al. (2021). Gut microbiota profiles and characterization of cultivable fungal isolates in IBS patients. *Applied Microbiology and Biotechnology* 105 (8): 3277–3288.

**23** Handl, S., Dowd, S., Garcia-Mazcorro, J. et al. (2011). Massive parallel16S rRNA gene pyrosequencing reveals highly diverse fecal bacterial and fungal communities in healthy dogs and cats. *FEMS Microbiology Ecology* 76: 301–310.

**24** Suchodolski, J., Morris, E., Allenspach, K. et al. (2008). Prevalence and identification of fungal DNA in the small intestine of healthy dogs and dogs with chronic enteropathies. *Veterinary Microbiology* 132: 379–388.

**25** Moter, A. and Göbel, U.B. (2000). Fluorescence in situ hybridization (FISH) for direct visualization of microorganisms. *Journal of Microbiological Methods* 41 (2): 85–112.

**26** Hardy, L., Jespers, V., Dahchour, N. et al. (2015). Unravelling the bacterial vaginosis-associated biofilm: a multiplex Gardnerella Vaginalis and Atopobium Vaginae fluorescence in situ hybridization assay using peptide nucleic acid probes. *PLoS One* 10 (8): e0136658.

**27** Chawnan, N., Lampang, K., Mektrirat, R. et al. (2021). Cultivation of bacterial pathogens and antimicrobial resistance in canine periapical tooth abscesses. *Veterinary Integrative Sciences* 19 (3): 513–525.

**28** Skarżyńska, M., Leekitcharoenphon, P., Hendriksen, R. et al. (2020). A metagenomic glimpse into the gut of wild and domestic animals: quantification of antimicrobial resistance and more. *PLoS One* 15 (12): e0242987.

**29** Suchodolski, J. (2021). Analysis of the gut microbiome in dogs and cats. *Veterinary Clinical Pathology* 50 (Suppl. 1): 6–17.

**30** Klopfleisch, R. and Gruber, A.D. (2012). Transcriptome and proteome research in veterinary science: what is possible and what questions can be asked? *The Scientific World Journal* 2012 (January): https://doi.org/10.1100/2012/254962.

**31** AlShawaqfeh, M.K., Wajid, B., Minamoto, Y. et al. (2017). A dysbiosis index to assess microbial changes in fecal samples of dogs with chronic inflammatory enteropathy. *FEMS Microbiology Ecology* 93 (11): https://doi.org/10.1093/femsec/fix136.

**32** Sung, C.-H., Marsilio, S., Chow, B. et al. (2022). Dysbiosis index to evaluate the fecal microbiota in healthy cats and cats with chronic enteropathies. *Journal of Feline Medicine and Surgery* 24 (6): e1–e12.

**33** Gika, H., Theodoridis, G., Plumb, R., and Wilson, I. (2014). Current practice of liquid chromatography–mass spectrometry in metabolomics and metabonomics. *Journal of Pharmaceutical and Biomedical Analysis* 87: 12–25.

**34** Moore, R., Anturaniemi, J., Velagapudi, V. et al. (2020). Targeted metabolomics with ultraperformance liquid chromatography-mass spectrometry (UPLC-MS) highlights metabolic differences in healthy and atopic staffordshire bull terriers fed two different diets, a pilot study. *Frontiers in Veterinary Science* 7: https://doi.org/10.3389/fvets.2020.554296.

**35** Song, H.E., Lee, H.Y., Kim, S.J. et al. (2019). A facile profiling method of short chain fatty acids using liquid chromatography-mass spectrometry. *Metabolites* 9 (9): https://doi.org/10.3390/metabo9090173.

**36** Minamoto, Y., Minamoto, T., Isaiah, A. et al. (2019). Fecal short-chain fatty acid concentrations and dysbiosis in dogs with chronic enteropathy. *Journal of Veterinary Internal Medicine/American College of Veterinary Internal Medicine* 33 (4): 1608–1618.

**37** Suchodolski, J.S., Markel, M.E., Garcia-Mazcorro, J.F. et al. (2012). The fecal microbiome in dogs with acute diarrhea and idiopathic inflammatory bowel disease. *PLoS One* 7 (12): e51907.

**38** Pilla, R., Guard, B.C., Blake, A.B. et al. (2021). Long-term recovery of the fecal microbiome and metabolome of dogs with steroid-responsive enteropathy. *Animals: An Open Access Journal from MDPI* 11 (9): https://doi.org/10.3390/ani11092498.

**39** Marsilio, S., Chow, B., Hill, S.L. et al. (2021). Untargeted metabolomic analysis in cats with naturally occurring inflammatory bowel disease and alimentary small cell lymphoma. *Scientific Reports* 11 (1): 9198.

# 7

# Microbiome-Centric Management of Dysbiosis

This chapter describes microbiome-focused methods to address dysbiosis or imbalances in the gastrointestinal (GI) microbiome. Research over the past decade has led to increasing recognition of the unintended consequences of modern medicine and diets on microbiome composition and function [1–3]. These findings are fueling a shift toward approaches that restore balance to better support diversity and function in the microbiome. Common microbiome problems include the presence or overgrowth of pathobionts, such as *Escherichia coli* or *Clostridioides difficile*, absence or low representation in the microbiome of key groups of beneficial bacteria, and imbalances in the community with a small number of taxa dominating [4–9]. In order to assess whether a microbiome is "dysbiotic" or considered unhealthy, the range of microbiomes in healthy populations must first be assessed, and then deviations from healthy can be defined.

Deviations in microbiome composition may be a consequence rather than cause of disease. By its nature, most microbiome research is observational, rather than experimentally inducing disease. Consequently, we often do not know if an altered microbiome is a sign or a cause of another condition. However, as discussed in Chapter 4, contributors to imbalances or dysbiosis in the microbiome include many commonly used antibiotics that can reduce beneficial gut bacteria, along with the pathogen of interest. Other approaches, such as dietary management, probiotics,

*Small Animal Microbiomes and Nutrition*, First Edition. Robin Saar and Sarah Dodd.
© 2024 John Wiley & Sons, Inc. Published 2024 by John Wiley & Sons, Inc.
Companion website: www.wiley.com/go/saar/1e

fecal microbial transplantation, or bacteriophage therapy, may be less harmful to native gut bacteria and warrant consideration for management of gut dysbiosis.

Regardless of whether dysbiosis is a sign of a condition or its cause, the GI microbiome is a promising target for interventions to restore function and alleviate signs associated with associated conditions. The gut microbiome can be rapidly responsive to diet and other interventions aimed at shifting microbial composition and function.

## 7.1 Key Nutritional Factors

Diet is been discussed in Chapter 4, yet is also mentioned here to reinforce its centrality in supporting not just host nutrition but also microbiome composition, gut barrier function, and overall host health. In the case of dysbiosis and gastrointestinal conditions, dietary interventions are an important approach, though their impact on intestinal microbiota can be variable [10–15]. In healthy individuals, the gut microbiome responds rapidly to changes in diet [16], putting a whole new spin on the aphorism that "we are what we eat." We are also what we provide to the multitudes of microorganisms that live inside of us and support our complex physiology, and this is also true for companion animals [17]. Feeding a diet that supports a diversity of microbes and a diversity of function in the gut appears to be essential for maintaining microbiome health. While there are nutritional standards governing production of commercial pet food in North America[1] and Europe,[2] there is a broad range of what constitutes a "complete and balanced" diet, and these standards were not developed with the microbiome in mind. Today, our understanding of how the microbiome responds to diet remains simplistic due to the complexities of the diversity of the microbiome community as well as the complexities of

---

1 Association of American Feed Control Officials AAFCO (2020). *Official Publication*. Champaign, Illinois: Association of American Feed Control Officials.
2 European Pet Food Industry Federation FEDIAF (2020). *Nutritional Guidelines for Complete and Complementary Pet Food for Cats and Dogs*. Bruxelles, Belgium: The European Pet Food Industry Federation.

chemistry affecting the composition and availability of nutrients in food that may be raw, fresh, cooked, extruded, freeze-dried, or fermented [18–20]. The three main macronutrients in food are carbohydrates, protein, and fat, and at the macronutrient level, we are finding strong effects on microbial diversity and composition [13, 21]. For example, after overweight cats previously fed a diet low in protein and high in carbohydrates were switched to a diet-rich in protein but low in carbohydrates, their fecal microbiomes showed an increase in protein-metabolizing bacteria in the genus *Fusobacterium*, reaching levels similar to that of lean cats [22]. In addition, numerous studies have also shown effects of fiber on the gut microbiome [23–26].

## 7.2 Probiotics

Probiotics are live microbes (typically bacteria and fungi) intended to provide health benefits [27]. In some cases, there is evidence for their use as an alternative to antibiotics for management of some conditions [28–33]. In veterinary medicine, probiotics are most frequently used in dogs with atopic dermatitis or gastrointestinal diseases. For example, supplementation with the yeast probiotic, *Saccharomyces boulardii,* significantly improved intestinal health (measured by a decrease in fecal calprotectin Immunoglobulin A) as well as stress (decrease in fecal cortisol) in healthy dogs [34]. In humans, probiotics have also been reported to also have benefits for oral health, colorectal cancer, controlling diabetes mellitus and glucose control, and to have immune-stimulating properties (reviewed by [35]. Probiotics may provide functional benefits that are missing in an impaired microbiome, such as reducing levels of pathobionts like *Clostridium perfringens* [36], and some probiotics contain bacterial groups such as *Lactobacillus* or *Bifidobacterium* that are more common in young animals. It should be noted that the vast majority of probiotics do not contain the gut-associated anaerobic bacteria that are reduced or eliminated by exposure to antibiotics.

Probiotics are commonly prescribed following antibiotic exposure. Following antibiotic treatment, the potential benefits of probiotics may be offset by compromising microbiome recolonization in hosts whose gastrointestinal tracts were perturbed by antibiotics.

## 7.3 Fecal Microbiota Transplantation

Fecal microbiota transplantation (FMT) is perhaps the most effective approach for microbiome manipulation and is currently being explored for use across a wide range of health conditions [37–39]. In companion animal medicine, FMT is an emerging treatment modality for acute and chronic gastrointestinal conditions [10]. FMT involves taking fecal material from a healthy donor and translocating it into an ailing recipient. FMT is most often delivered orally via capsule or rectally via enema (Figure 7.1). Fecal material used can be fresh, frozen, or lyophilized. FMT can also be delivered to different parts of the gastrointestinal tract, such as using a nasal-jejunal tube guided by an endoscope. Studies in dogs and cats are needed to analyze efficacy of the different administration routes, though the route of delivery does not appear to affect efficacy in people with *Clostrioides difficile* infections (e.g., [40]). While antibiotic therapies were previously used to treat patients with Crohn's disease, it is

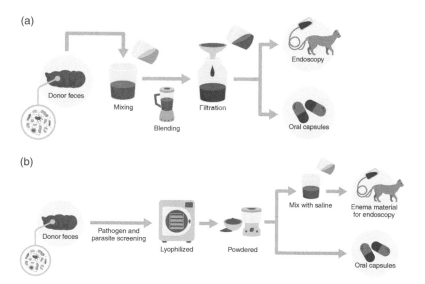

**Figure 7.1** Fecal microbiota transplantation can be performed with two different approaches: (a) Fresh or frozen material that is mixed with saline and delivered via enema (sometimes guided by endoscopy) or orally. (b) Lyophilized fecal powder can also be used and delivered in oral capsules or mixed with saline and delivered via enema.

now recognized that there is no clinical benefit. Instead, a growing number of clinical trials are now investigating the therapeutic effect of fecal microbiota transplantation (FMT) in human patients with IBD and related conditions [41].

FMTs are thought to restore fecal microbiome composition, diversity, and homeostasis by increasing microbiome diversity, enhancing the numbers of beneficial microbes, and outcompeting pathogens [37–39]. FMTs are sometimes used as an alternative to conventional treatment methods, or they can supplement these treatment methods for an enhanced resolution of clinical signs, as in the case of canine parvovirus [42–46]. Recent studies have found the use of FMT-accelerated recovery of microbiome composition after antibiotic administration, proving more useful than probiotics for this application [47, 48].

In veterinary medicine, FMT procedures have been used since at least the eighteenth century to successfully treat cattle, horses, sheep, and other animals suffering from rumination disorders, indigestion, inappetence, and colitis [49, 50]. A study in puppies that were administered maternal fecal inoculum during the weaning period exhibited decreased incidence of diarrhea [51]. These lines of evidence suggest that microbes can be introduced from a donor into the gut microbiome of a recipient, where they can be maintained for a period of time, potentially leading to improved health outcomes. Research also shows that complete microbiome engraftment is not necessary for resolution of disease, thus, even one or a few rounds of FMT treatment could be beneficial [52, 53].

In domestic dogs, FMTs are now being used to treat or as an adjuvant to treatment for acute diarrhea [42–46], relapsing chronic diarrhea [54], inflammatory bowel disease [42–46], atopic dermatitis [55], canine parvovirus [46] and diabetes mellitus [56]. Despite facing similar conditions, far fewer studies have been published so far on the application of FMT in domestic cats. FMT treatment led to long-term resolution of vomiting and diarrhea in a six year old cat [57], and successfully resolved chronic ulcerative colitis in an adult cat [58]. In a study on the application of oral delivery of FMT capsules containing lyophilized stool in 68 cats with diagnosed or suspected IBD, Rojas et al. [59] found that 77% of cats were reported to show improvement in their clinical signs and that microbiome responses were associated with the recipient's initial presenting clinical signs, prior IBD diagnoses, recent antibiotic use, and diet.

## 7.4 Bacteriophages

As discussed in Chapter 4, antimicrobials are pharmaceutical compounds used to treat infectious diseases, and they can also be used to modulate the gut microbiome – for better or for worse. While essential to the practice of medicine, their overuse has been linked to dysbiosis in gut microbiota, impairment in gut function, the spread of antimicrobial resistant strains, and may contribute to the development of chronic disease and some cancers [60]. Some antibiotics can stimulate the growth of beneficial bacteria but given all of the known deleterious effects, the range of applications for their use is becoming increasingly narrow. One application involves the treatment of uncomplicated urinary tract infections where nitrofurantoin administration was associated with increases in *Bifidobacterium* [61] and *Faecalibacterium* [62], which are both health associated. In a murine model for colitis-associated colorectal cancer, gut microbial manipulation using antibiotics affected tumorigenesis [63]. Antibiotics are also sometimes used to prepare a patient for a fecal transplant in human medicine, particularly for treatment of recurrent *Clostidioides difficile* infections. However, few studies have examined whether this improves patient outcomes. Using a mouse model, Freitag et al. [64] found that pre-treatment with broad-spectrum antibiotics did not improve the overall engraftment of donor microbiota but did improve the engraftment of a few specific taxa.

Bacteriophages offer another possible means to modulate gut microbiota. Bacteriophages are viruses that specialize in infecting bacteria and are named for their ability to lyse or consume bacteria [65]. They may also be used as an alternative to antibiotics. Compared to most antibiotics, bacteriophages are narrow spectrum and can target a single species or even strain of bacteria. The range of bacteria that a phage can lyse and kill is called the host range and varies from one bacteriophage to another. Growing concerns about antimicrobial resistance have sparked renewed efforts to discover and develop new bacteriophage cocktails in the United States. Initially these cocktails have targeted food safety organisms (*Salmonella enterica*, *Escherichia coli* (*E. coli*), and *Listeria monogenes*). The phage cocktail, PreForPro, targets *E. coli* and was clinically shown to reduce *E. coli* and *Clostridium perfringens* and to increase butyrate production [66] and to synergistically improve gut health responses to probiotics, specifically by reducing inflammatory markers and increasing short-chain fatty acid-producing bacteria [67] in people. More phage cocktails are in development and recent preclinical studies suggest that phage therapies have promise. Phages targeting adherent-invasive *E. coli* was found to be beneficial for colitis in people and another found that phages against cytolysin-positive *Enterococcus faecalis* reduced ethanol-induced liver disease [68].

At present, bacteriophages are not commonly used in clinical veterinary practice. Promising research regarding use of phages for treatment of infectious diseases in companion animals has been undertaken (review by [69]), yet there are many challenges to overcome before widespread veterinary application can be expected.

## 7.5 Chapter Summary

- The microbiome is a promising target for interventions to restore function and alleviate signs associated with dysbiosis.
- While critical for treating infections, antibiotics also harm host-associated commensal gut bacteria and can induce lasting dysbiosis.
- Probiotics may provide a less harmful alternative to antibiotics in certain circumstances
- A growing body of research is providing evidence to support the use of FMT in companion animal medicine to reduce dysbiosis and alleviate signs for a range of conditions.

## References

1 Manchester, A.C., Webb, C.B., Blake, A.B. et al. (2019). Long-term impact of tylosin on fecal microbiota and fecal bile acids of healthy dogs. *Journal of Veterinary Internal Medicine/American College of Veterinary Internal Medicine* 33 (6): 2605–2617.

2 Pilla, R., Gaschen, F.P., Barr, J.W. et al. (2020). Effects of metronidazole on the fecal microbiome and metabolome in healthy dogs. *Journal of Veterinary Internal Medicine/American College of Veterinary Internal Medicine* 34 (5): 1853–1866.

3 Suchodolski, J.S., Dowd, S.E., Westermarck, E. et al. (2009). The effect of the macrolide antibiotic tylosin on microbial diversity in the canine small

intestine as demonstrated by massive parallel 16S rRNA gene sequencing. *BMC Microbiology* 9 (October): 210.

**4** AlShawaqfeh, M.K., Wajid, B., Minamoto, Y. et al. (2017). A Dysbiosis index to assess microbial changes in fecal samples of dogs with chronic inflammatory enteropathy. *FEMS Microbiology Ecology* 93 (11): https://doi.org/10.1093/femsec/fix136.

**5** DeGruttola, A., Low, D., Mizoguchi, A., and Mizoguchi, E. (2016). Current understanding of dysbiosis in disease in human and animal models. *Inflammatory Bowel Diseases* 22 (5): 1137–1150.

**6** Minamoto, Y., Minamoto, T., Isaiah, A. et al. (2019). Fecal short-chain fatty acid concentrations and dysbiosis indogs with chronic enteropathy. *Journal of Veterinary Internal Medicine* 33: 1608–1618.

**7** Suchodolski, J. (2016). Diagnosis and interpretation of intestinal dysbiosis in dogs and cats. *The Veterinary Journal* 215: 30–37.

**8** Sung, C.-H., Marsilio, S., Chow, B. et al. (2022). Dysbiosis index to evaluate the fecal microbiota in healthy cats and cats with chronic enteropathies. *Journal of Feline Medicine and Surgery* 24 (6): e1–e2.

**9** Vázquez-Baeza, Y., Hyde, E., Suchodolski, J., and Knight, R. (2016). Dog and human inflammatory bowel disease rely on overlapping yet distinct dysbiosis networks. *Nature Microbiology* 1: 1–5.

**10** Schmitz, S.S. (2022). Modifying the gut microbiota – an update on the evidence for dietary interventions, probiotics, and fecal microbiota transplantation in chronic gastrointestinal diseases of dogs and cats. *Advances in Small Animal Care* 3 (1): 95–107.

**11** Allaway, D., Haydock, R., Lonsdale, Z. et al. (2020). Rapid reconstitution of the fecal microbiome after extended diet-induced changes indicates a stable gut microbiome in healthy adult dogs. *Applied and Environmental Microbiology* 86 (13): e00562–e00520.

**12** Coelho, L., Kultima, J., Costea, P. et al. (2018). Similarity of the dog and human gut microbiomes in gene content and response to diet. *Microbiome* 6: 72.

**13** Li, Q., Lauber, C., Czarnecki-Maulden, G. et al. (2016). Effects of the dietary protein and carbohydrate ratio on gut microbiomes in dogs of different body conditions. *MBio* 8: e01703–e01716.

**14** Lin, C.-Y., Jha, A., Oba, P. et al. (2022). Longitudinal fecal microbiome and metabolite data demonstrate rapid shifts and subsequent stabilization after an abrupt dietary change in healthy adult dogs. *Animal Microbiome* 4 (46): 1–21.

**15** Pilla, R. and Suchodolski, J. (2021). The gut microbiome of dogs and cats, and the influence of diet. *Veterinary Clinics of North America: Small Animal Practice* 51: 605–621.

**16** David, L.A., Maurice, C.F., Carmody, R.N. et al. (2014). Diet rapidly and reproducibly alters the human gut microbiome. *Nature* 505 (7484): 559–563.

**17** Wernimont, S.M., Radosevich, J., Jackson, M.I. et al. (2020). The effects of nutrition on the gastrointestinal microbiome of cats and dogs: impact on health and disease. *Frontiers in Microbiology* 11 (June): 1266.

**18** Sandri, M., Dal Monego, S., Conte, G. et al. (2017). Raw meat based diet influences faecal microbiome and end products of fermentation in healthy dogs. *BMC Veterinary Research* 13 (1): 65.

**19** Bermingham, E., Young, W., Butowski, C. et al. (2018). The fecal microbiota in the domestic cat (Felis catus) is influenced by interactions between age and diet; a five year longitudinal study. *Frontiers in Microbiology* 9: 1231.

**20** Do, S., Phungviwatnikul, T., de Godoy, M., and Swanson, K. (2021). Nutrient digestibility and fecal characteristics, microbiota, and metabolites in dogs fed human-grade foods. *Journal of Animal Science* 99 (2): https://doi.org/10.1093/jas/skab028.

**21** Hooda, S., Vester Boler, B., Kerr, K. et al. (2013). The gut microbiome of kittens is affected by dietary protein:carbohydrate ratio and associated with blood metabolite and hormone concentrations. *British Journal of Nutrition* 109: 1637–1646.

**22** Li, Q. and Pan, Y. (2020). Differential responses to dietary protein and carbohydrate ratio on gut microbiome in obese vs. lean cats. *Frontiers in Microbiology* 11 (October): 591462.

**23** Ephraim, E. and Jewell, D. (2020). Effect of added dietary betaine and soluble fiber on metabolites and fecal microbiome in dogs with early renal disease. *Metabolites* 10: 370.

**24** Hall, J., Jackson, M., Jewell, D., and Ephraim, E. (2020). Chronic kidney disease in cats alters response of the plasma metabolome and fecal microbiome to dietary fiber. *PLoS One* 15 (7): e0235480.

**25** Middelbos, I., Boler, B., Qu, A. et al. (2010). Phylogenetic characterization of fecal microbial communities of dogs fed diets with or without supplemental dietary fiber using 454 pyrosequencing. *PLoS One* 5 (3): e9768.

**26** Panasevich, M., Kerr, K., Dilger, R. et al. (2015). Modulation of the faecal microbiome of healthy adult dogs by inclusion of potato fibre in the diet. *British Journal of Nutrition* 113: 125–133.

**27** Pandey, K., Naik, S., and Vakil, B. (2015). Probiotics, prebiotics and synbiotics- a review. *Journal of Food Science and Technology* 52 (12): 7577–7587.

**28** Bybee, S., Scorza, A., and Lappin, M. (2011). Effect of the probiotic enterococcus faecium SF68 on presence of diarrhea in cats and dogs housed in an animal shelter. *Journal of Veterinary Internal Medicine* **25** (4): 856–860.

**29** Gómez-Gallego, C., Junnila, J., Männikkö, S. et al. (2016). A canine-specific probiotic product in treating acute or intermittent diarrhea in dogs: a double-blind placebo-controlled efficacy study. *Veterinary Microbiology* 197: 122–128.

**30** Kim, H., Rather, I., Kim, H. et al. (2015). A double-blind, placebo controlled-trial of a probiotic strain lactobacillus sakei probio-65 for the prevention of canine atopic dermatitis. *Journal of Microbiology and Biotechnology* 25 (11): 1966–1969.

**31** Rossi, G., Cerquetella, M., Gavazza, A. et al. (2020). Rapid resolution of large bowel diarrhea after the administration of a combination of a high-fiber diet and a probiotic mixture in 30 dogs. *Veterinary Sciences* 7: 21.

**32** Sauter, S., Benyacoub, J., Allenspach, K. et al. (2006). Effects of probiotic bacteria in dogs with food responsive diarrhoea treated with an elimination diet. *Journal of Animal Physiology and Animal Nutrition* 90: 269–277.

**33** Aktas, M., S., Borku, M.K., and Ozkanlar, Y. (2007). Efficacy of *Saccharomyces boulardii* as a probiotic in dogs. *Bulletin of the Veterinary Institute in Pulawy = Biuletyn Instytutu Weterynarii W Pulawach* 51: 365–369.

**34** Meineri, G., Martello, E., Atuahene, D. et al. (2022). Effects of *Saccharomyces boulardii* supplementation on nutritional status, fecal parameters, microbiota, and mycobiota in breeding adult dogs. *Veterinary Science in China* 9 (8): https://doi.org/10.3390/vetsci9080389.

**35** Sivamaruthi, B.S., Kesika, P., and Chaiyasut, C. (2021). Influence of probiotic supplementation on health status of the dogs: a review. *NATO Advanced Science Institutes Series E: Applied Sciences* 11 (23): 11384.

**36** Park, H.-E., Kim, Y.J., Do, K.-H. et al. (2018). Effects of queso blanco cheese containing *Bifidobacterium longum* KACC 91563 on the intestinal microbiota and short chain fatty acid in healthy companion dogs. *Korean Journal for Food Science of Animal Resources* 38 (6): 1261–1272.

**37** Niederwerder, M.C. (2018). Fecal microbiota transplantation as a tool to treat and reduce susceptibility to disease in animals. *Veterinary Immunology and Immunopathology* 206 (December): 65–72.

**38** Tuniyazi, M., Xiaoyu, H., Yunhe, F., and Zhang, N. (2022). Canine fecal microbiota transplantation: current application and possible mechanisms. *Veterinary Science in China* 9 (8): https://doi.org/10.3390/vetsci9080396.

**39** Zheng, L., Ji, Y.-Y., Wen, X.-L., and Duan, S.-L. (2022). Fecal microbiota transplantation in the metabolic diseases: current status and perspectives. *World Journal of Gastroenterology: WJG* 28 (23): 2546–2560.

**40** Jiang, Z.-D., Jenq, R.R., Ajami, N.J. et al. (2018). Safety and preliminary efficacy of orally administered lyophilized fecal microbiota product compared with frozen product given by enema for recurrent clostridium difficile infection: a randomized clinical trial. *PLoS One* 13 (11): e0205064.

**41** Gubatan, J., Boye, T.L., Temby, M. et al. (2022). Gut microbiome in inflammatory bowel disease: role in pathogenesis, dietary modulation, and colitis-associated colon cancer. *Microorganisms* 10 (7): https://doi.org/10.3390/microorganisms10071371.

**42** Chaitman, J., Ziese, A.-L., Pilla, R. et al. (2020). Fecal microbial and metabolic profiles in dogs with acute diarrhea receiving either fecal microbiota transplantation or oral metronidazole. *Frontiers in Veterinary Science* 7 (April): 192.

**43** Collier, A. (2022). Fecal microbiota alterations in illness and efficacy of fecal microbiota transplantation in treatment of inflammatory bowel disease in dogs. University of Guelph. https://atrium.lib.uoguelph.ca/xmlui/handle/10214/26622 (accessed 20 November 2022).

**44** Gal, A., Barko, P.C., Biggs, P.J. et al. (2021). One dog's waste is another dog's wealth: a pilot study of fecal microbiota transplantation in dogs with acute hemorrhagic diarrhea syndrome. *PLoS One* 16 (4): e0250344.

**45** Niina, A., Kibe, R., Suzuki, R. et al. (2021). Fecal microbiota transplantation as a new treatment for canine inflammatory bowel disease. *Bioscience of Microbiota, Food and Health* 40 (2): 98–104.

**46** Pereira, G.Q., Gomes, L.A., Santos, I.S. et al. (2018). Fecal microbiota transplantation in puppies with canine parvovirus infection. *Journal of Veterinary Internal Medicine/American College of Veterinary Internal Medicine* 32 (2): 707–711.

**47** Suez, J., Zmora, N., Zilberman-Schapira, G. et al. (2018). Post-antibiotic gut mucosal microbiome reconstitution is impaired by probiotics and improved by autologous FMT. *Cell* 174 (6): 1406–23.e16.

**48** Taur, Y., Coyte, K., Schluter, J. et al. (2018). Reconstitution of the gut microbiota of antibiotic-treated patients by autologous fecal microbiota transplant. *Science Translational Medicine* 10 (460): https://doi.org/10.1126/scitranslmed.aap9489.

**49** DePeters, E.J. and George, L.W. (2014). Rumen transfaunation. *Immunology Letters* 162 (2 Pt A): 69–76.

**50** Mandal, R.S., Joshi, V., and Balamurugan, B. (2017). Rumen transfaunation an effective method for treating simple indigestion in ruminants. *North East Veterinarian* 17: 31–33. https://www.cabdirect.org/cabdirect/abstract/20183074200.

**51** Burton, E.N., O'Connor, E., Ericsson, A.C., and Franklin, C.L. (2016). Evaluation of fecal microbiota transfer as treatment for postweaning diarrhea in research-colony puppies. *Journal of the American Association for Laboratory Animal Science: JAALAS* 55 (5): 582–587.

**52** Niederwerder, M.C., Constance, L.A., Rowland, R.R.R. et al. (2018). Fecal microbiota transplantation is associated with reduced morbidity and mortality in porcine circovirus associated disease. *Frontiers in Microbiology* 9 (July): 1631.

**53** Wang, J.-W., Kuo, C.-H., Kuo, F.-C. et al. (2019). Fecal microbiota transplantation: review and update. *Journal of the Formosan Medical Association = Taiwan Yi Zhi* 118 (Suppl 1): S23–S31.

**54** Cerquetella, M., Marchegiani, A., Rossi, G. et al. (2022). Case report: oral fecal microbiota transplantation in a dog suffering from relapsing chronic diarrhea-clinical outcome and follow-up. *Frontiers in Veterinary Science* 9 (July): 893342.

**55** Kerem, U. (2022). Fecal microbiota transplantation capsule therapy via oral route for combatting atopic dermatitis in dogs. *Ankara Üniversitesi Veteriner Fakültesi Dergisi* 69 (2): 211–219.

**56** Gal, A., Brown, R., Barko, P. et al. (2022). Abstract EN11: interim analysis of a prospective clinical trial of fecal microbial transplantation in diabetic dogs. 2022 ACVIM Hybrid Forum.

**57** Weese, J.S., Costa, M.C., and Webb, J.A. (n.d.). Preliminary clinical and microbiome assessment of stool transplantation in the dog and cat. *Journal of Atomic and Molecular Physics* 27: 705.

**58** Furmanski, S. and Mor, T. (n.d.). First case report of fecal microbiota transplantation in a cat in Israel. *Israel Journal of Veterinary Medicine* 12: 35–41. http://www.ijvm.org.il/sites/default/files/fecal_microbiota_transplantation.pdf.

**59** Rojas, C.A., Entrolezo, Z., Jarett, J.K. et al. (2022). Abstract G131: microbiome responses to fecal microbiota transplantation in cats. 2022 ACVIM Hybrid Forum.

**60** Sanyaolu, L.N., Oakley, N.J., Nurmatov, U. et al. (2020). Antibiotic exposure and the risk of colorectal adenoma and carcinoma: a systematic review and meta-analysis of observational studies. *Colorectal Disease: The Official Journal of the Association of Coloproctology of Great Britain and Ireland* 22 (8): 858–870.

**61** Vervoort, J., Xavier, B.B., Stewardson, A. et al. (2015). Metagenomic analysis of the impact of nitrofurantoin treatment on the human faecal microbiota. *The Journal of Antimicrobial Chemotherapy* 70 (7): 1989–1992.

**62** Stewardson, A.J., Gaïa, N., François, P. et al. (2015). Collateral damage from oral ciprofloxacin versus nitrofurantoin in outpatients with urinary tract infections: a culture-free analysis of gut microbiota. *Clinical Microbiology and Infection: The Official Publication of the European Society of Clinical Microbiology and Infectious Diseases* 21 (4): 344.e1–344.e11.

**63** Lee, J.G., Eun, C.S., Jo, S.V. et al. (2019). The impact of gut microbiota manipulation with antibiotics on colon tumorigenesis in a murine model. *PLoS One* 14 (12): e0226907.

**64** Freitag, T.L., Hartikainen, A., Jouhten, H. et al. (2019). Minor effect of antibiotic pre-treatment on the engraftment of donor microbiota in fecal transplantation in mice. *Frontiers in Microbiology* 10 (November): 2685.

**65** Sulakvelidze, A., Alavidze, Z., and Morris, J. Jr. (2001). Bacteriophage therapy. *Antimicrobial Agents and Chemotherapy* 45 (3): 649–659.

**66** Febvre, H.P., Rao, S., Gindin, M. et al. (2019). PHAGE study: effects of supplemental bacteriophage intake on inflammation and gut microbiota in healthy adults. *Nutrients* 11 (3): https://doi.org/10.3390/nu11030666.

**67** Grubb, D.S., Wrigley, S.D., Freedman, K.E. et al. (2020). PHAGE-2 study: supplemental bacteriophages extend *Bifidobacterium Animalis*

*Subsp. Lactis* BL04 benefits on gut health and microbiota in healthy adults. *Nutrients* 12 (8): 10.3390/nu12082474.

**68** Duan, Y., Young, R., and Schnabl, B. (2022). Bacteriophages and their potential for treatment of gastrointestinal diseases. *Nature Reviews. Gastroenterology & Hepatology* 19 (2): 135–144.

**69** Squires, R. (2018). Bacteriophage therapy for management of bacterial infections in veterinary practice: what was once old is new again. *New Zealand Veterinary Journal* 66 (5): 229–235.

# Section II

# The Microbiome's Involvement in Body Systems

# 8

# The Immune System

## 8.1 Innate and Adaptive Immunity

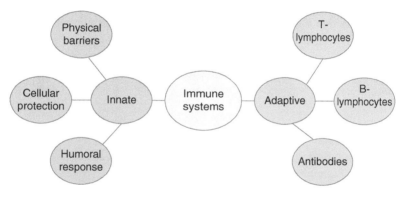

**Figure 8.1** Components of the innate and adaptive immune responses.

### 8.1.1 Innate Immune System

The innate immune system is the body's first line of defense against foreign substances (bacteria, viruses, and other infectious agents that are perceived to cause harm to the host) that enter the body. It responds to each detection quickly, using the same mode of action, and is limited in its capabilities to stop the spreading of infection. This system offers protection through the use of physical barriers, cellular (immune cells and proteins) protection, and humoral response [1].

*Small Animal Microbiomes and Nutrition*, First Edition. Robin Saar and Sarah Dodd.
© 2024 John Wiley & Sons, Inc. Published 2024 by John Wiley & Sons, Inc.
Companion website: www.wiley.com/go/saar/1e

### 8.1.1.1 Physical Barriers

Barrier protection, the closed surface of the skin, and mucous membranes offer a physical barrier against foreign substances. Additionally, the body has physical structures such as cilia in the bronchi, intestinal villa, intestinal contractions in the gastrointestinal tract, and the production of mucous, tears, sweat, and urine to help protect and remove unwanted substances from the body [2]. The mucosal barrier in the GI tract plays a vital role in preventing microbes from contacting epithelial cells and inducing an immune response. Lamina propria is a loose connective tissue located in mucosal barriers that consist of three layers (deep, intermediate, and superficial). In healthy animals, lamina propria contains immune cells and secrete cytokines. In this capacity, the role of the lamina propria is to secrete cytokines that are anti-inflammatory mediators such as transforming growth factor β [TGF-β] and interleukin (IL)-10, which downregulate immune responses. The lamina propria, along with macrophages completing phagocytosis, prevent excessive translocation of intestinal microbiota and defend against pathogens [3, 4]. This relationship results in a homeostatic balance maintained between regulatory T (Treg) cells and effector T helper cells (Th1, Th2, and Th17) [3].

### 8.1.1.2 Cellular Protection

Cellular protection is activated through special immune system cells and proteins if foreign substances get past physical barriers. These cells travel to the area of invasion (infection) and release substances into the immediate area which dilates blood vessels causing inflammation in the area. Different types of immune cells will act in different ways. Leukocytes, phagocytes (commonly known as scavenger cells), engulf the foreign substance, digesting them, with any remains of the foreign substance moving to the surface of the phagocyte, which may stimulate the adaptive immune system [2]. Other types of immune system cells release substances that kill bacteria. Nine protein enzymes work in conjunction with each other to increase the level of the immune response. The enzymes specifically identify the foreign substances for phagocytes, attract immune cells from the bloodstream, and kill bacteria and viruses by weakening cell wall structure. Some cells specialize in identifying changes to the cell surface's structure and destroy these abnormal cells using toxins [2].

### 8.1.1.3 Humoral Immune Response

The presence of antigens along with helper T cells activates B cells that can proliferate and evolve into plasma cells that can secrete antibodies. These antibodies will break down the extracellular area of microorganisms to help prevent the spread of intracellular infections [5]. Antibodies protect the host by (i) Neutralization – inhibiting the toxic effect or bind to pathogens, (ii) Opsonization – coating pathogens, ingesting, and killing the pathogen, or (iii) Compliment proteins – enhance opsonization and can directly kill some bacteria cells [5]. The humoral response has components in both the innate and adaptive immune systems.

## 8.1.2 Adaptive Immune System

The adaptive immune system initiates if the innate immune response cannot remove the foreign substance, specifically targeting the organism causing the infection. This system is slower though more accurate and creates memory to respond to recurrent infections more rapidly. The adaptive system is made up of T lymphocytes, B lymphocytes, and antibodies [2].

### 8.1.2.1 Lymphocytes

T lymphocytes (T cells – T = *thymus*) are produced in the bone marrow and then stored in the thymus to mature. Different types of T cells work to initiate and support the adaptive immune response. T helper cells utilize chemical messengers (small proteins produced in the body known as cytokines) to activate the adaptive immune responses such as stimulating B cells. Cytotoxic T cells detect and kill cells infected by viruses or tumors. Memory T cells develop from T cells that have killed foreign substances (antigens). T cells can produce specific cells to match the antigen much like a lock and key. Once a substance locks to the surface of a T cell, the T cell can multiply, creating an immune response to that specific antigen [2].

B lymphocytes (B cells – B = *bone marrow*) are produced and stored in the bone marrow. When activated by T helper cells, matching B cells rapidly multiply and transform into plasma cells, which can produce large amounts of specific antibodies that are released into the blood. Some B cells become memory cells [2].

### 8.1.2.2 Antibodies

Antibodies are produced by plasma cells and attach to specific antigens. Antibodies support both the innate and the adaptive immune response. The main functions of antibodies are to neutralize antigens by attaching to the cell surface or surface of antigen toxin preventing the antigen from attaching to other cells in the body. They activate proteins and attach to other immune cells such as phagocytes, enabling them to better fight antigens [2].

### 8.1.3 Immune System Maturation

Commensal GI microbiota have a fundamental role in the induction, education, and function of the host's immune system, which allows for an evolved symbiotic relationship. The original colonizing microbiota plays a role in intestinal epithelial cell maturation, angiogenesis (maturation of new blood vessels), and tolerance of antigens produced by pioneer colonizing microbiota to become part of regulatory pathways while teaching the immune system to recognize and develop protective actions against the colonization of future pathogens [6]. Both the innate and adaptive immune systems are needed to initiate an appropriate response to pathogens through conserved microbial-associated molecular patterns (MAMPs) that are present in bacterial antigens, such as lipopolysaccharides (LPS), peptidoglycans, flagella, or unmethylated bacterial DNA CpG motifs [3]. Neonates' cells express Toll-like receptors ligands, and their response to microbial ligands is distinct compared to adult cells. This early response to microbial ligands conditions the epithelial cells that line the GI tract to decrease their response to subsequent exposure to those specific pioneer colonizers [6]. Additionally, neonatal cells do not have the same ability to produce inflammatory mediators such as oxygen radicals though their production of some regulatory cytokines is increased [6].

## 8.2 The Microbiome's Involvement in Immunity

The GI microbiota and the host's immune system are closely intertwined with the same mechanisms utilized to maintain a commensal relationship between the GI microbiota and the host, and to also manage the risk of potential pathogens. The ability of the microbiota to initiate disease depends on the host's genetic predisposition, how prepared the system is to react, and the localization of particular microbes [6].

### 8.2.1 Germ-Free Animals

"Germ-free" animals have helped to understand the role of the microbiota in the GI microbiome, including the necessity of their presence in the GI tract for the normal maturation of the immune system. "Germ-free" mice have reduced development of gut-associated lymphoid tissue (GALT), decreased numbers of T cells, B cells, and antimicrobial peptides, along with thinner mucous layer, and fewer Peyer's patches resulting in less immunotolerance [7]. Additionally, "germ-free" mice have an abnormally developed spleen and lymph nodes with decreased numbers of both T and B cells in the germinal centers (a specialized microstructure that forms in secondary lymphoid tissues, producing long-lived antibody-secreting plasma cells and memory B cells) [7, 8].

### 8.2.2 Intestinal Permeability's Association with the Immune System

There is an association with an increase in intestinal permeability preceding most autoimmune diseases [7]. In a healthy host, contact between the microbiota and GI epithelial cell surface is minimized through the actions of mucus, IgA, immune cells, antimicrobial peptides, and epithelial cells in the GI tract. On the skin, microbes are regulated by keratinocytes that secrete antibacterial peptides. These "protective firewalls" limited contact and prevent tissue inflammation and microbial translocation [6]. GI dysbiosis and secondary intestinal inflammation are several factors that contribute to increased bacterial exposure, which start with the breakdown of the "protective firewall" (see Figure 8.2). This includes disruptions to the mucous layer and dysregulation of the epithelial tight junctions resulting in increased intestinal permeability and bacterial adherence to the epithelial cells [3]. The exposure of bacteria to the epithelial cells is recognized by the microbial-associated molecular patterns, which stimulates Toll-like receptors resulting in pro-inflammatory stimulation. The response of the innate immune system (secretion of cytokines, chemokines, dendritic cells) starts when

## Healthy microbiome

High biodiversity of microorganisms provide
nutrient competition and production of valuable
metabolites to benefit the microbiome and host

## Afflicted host

Low biodiversity (i.e. dysbiosis) hinders the
production of beneficial metabolites, increasing
stress to GI epithelial cells and helpful microfauna

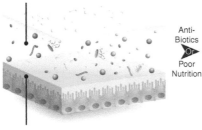
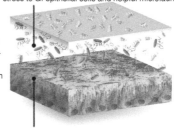

Anti-
Biotics

Or

Poor
Nutrition

"Protective Firewall" of mucus, IgA, immune cells.
Antimicrobial peptides limit contact, preventing
tisssue inflammation and microbial translocation.

Breakdown of the "protective firewall." Increased
bacterial exposure from dysbiosis to the GI epithelial
cells results in secondary intestinal inflammation

**Figure 8.2** Intestinal permeability in a healthy host and an afflicted host. The
"protective firewall" acts as a barrier between the microbiota and GI epithelial
cells to help reduce the impact of the bacteria on the cells. In an afflicted host
this barrier breaks down causing inflammation in the epithelial cells. *Source:*
George Andrew Abernathy, https://orcid.org/0000-0002-1336-3631, last
accessed 8 December 2022 / Licensed under CC0 license.

Toll-like receptors and MAMPs contact. Dendritic cells travel to
mesenteric lymph nodes, exposing T cells to an antigen resulting in the
development of Treg and Th17 cells. Treg cells produce immunosuppressive cytokines and stimulate epithelial cells to secrete antimicrobial
proteins. Additionally, they attract neutrophils from the circulatory system to the intestine [3]. The adaptive immune response consists of tumor
necrosis factor α, IL-1β, IL-6, IL-12, IL-23, and chemokines, which may
be stimulated if the innate response is ineffective. An early study found
that alteration in the GI microbiota in both mothers and/or neonates
may predispose the neonate to diseases such as asthma, which are associated with a dysfunctional barrier [6].

### 8.2.3 Cancer's Association with the Immune System and GI Microbiome

Cancer is a complex disease, and it is estimated that 15–20% of cancers
involve microorganisms, with dysbiosis in the microbiomes being associated with gastric, esophageal, hepatobiliary, pancreatic, lung, colorectal,
and lymphoma in dogs [3]. Microorganisms are found inside the tumor

and in adjacent healthy tissue. The development, progression, and interactions between the tumor and these or other microorganisms can influence the development of neoplasia [3]. There are four main mechanisms by which microorganisms can contribute to carcinogenesis at the molecular level:

1) Genomic integration – integration of a virus into the host genome [3].
2) Genotoxicity – alteration of phenotypes [3].
3) Metabolic programming – alteration of circulating metabolites [3].
    a) Tumor-suppressive metabolites – Short-chain fatty acids (SCFAs) and phytochemicals
    b) Harmful metabolites – Bile acids where secondary bile acids (deoxycholic acid and lithocholic acid) that have pro and anticancer activity [3].
4) Promotion of immunological modification – the use of proinflammatory and immunosuppressive pathways to disrupt the host cancer immunosurveillance. A loss of homeostasis can result in chronic inflammation, a by-pass of an immune response, or immune suppression, which may create a pro-neoplastic inflammatory environment [3].

The role of the immune system is to prevent or slow cancer growth. Cancer cells can be genetically altered to be less visible to the immune system, attach to proteins that disable the immune cells, and they can alter normal cells around the tumor to interfere with how the immune system responds to the neoplastic cells [9].

### 8.2.3.1 Immunotherapy

Immunotherapy helps the immune system to better respond to immune-mediated disease [9]. Several types of immunotherapies are used to treat cancer including:

1) Immune checkpoint inhibitors – drugs that block immune checkpoints and allow immune cells to respond more strongly [9]. There is evidence that the GI microbiota are effective immune checkpoint inhibitors [3].
2) T-cell transfer therapy (adoptive cell therapy, immunotherapy, or immune cell therapy) – dendric cells are used to enhance the response of T cells to act against cancer cells [9].

3) Monoclonal antibodies (therapeutic antibodies) – mark cancer cells so they are more easily identified by the immune system [9].
4) Treatment vaccines – improve the immune system's response to cancer cells. [3, 9].
5) Immune system modulators – specifically or generally enhance the body's immune response [9].

## 8.3 Supportive Nutrients

### 8.3.1 Prebiotics

Prebiotics are food for beneficial GI microbiota that will allow for these bacteria to flourish and produce healthy beneficial metabolites. These metabolites have multiple functions including strengthening enterocytes through the provision of SCFAs, which will help strengthen the GI mucosal barrier. For example, phytochemicals (polyphenols) have biological effects associated with reduced risk of disease, including cancer where they can also have an antioxidant effect by modulating xenobiotic detoxification pathways, cell proliferation, apoptosis (program cell death), and inflammation [3] (Figure 8.3).

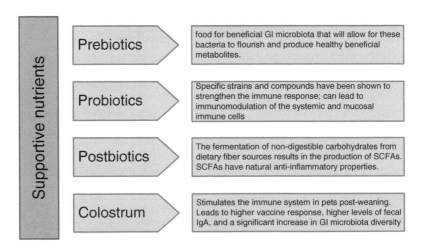

**Figure 8.3** Supportive nutrients for the microbiota and their effect on the immune system.

## 8.3.2 Probiotics

Specific strains and compounds derived from probiotics have been shown to strengthen the immune response [10, 11]. The two major mechanisms of probiotic action are the regulation of gene expression and signaling pathways in the host cells. These mechanisms can lead to immunomodulation of the systemic and mucosal immune cells along with the intestinal epithelial cells [11]. Probiotic bacteria interact with intestinal epithelial cells, or dendritic cells and follicle-associated epithelial cells. These communicate with macrophages, and T and B lymphocytes to initiate an immune response [11].

There are a few studies in animals looking at the effects of probiotics on the immune system, which have revealed increased immune defenses (lymphocytes) and lessened morbidity compared to non-treated animals [12, 13].

## 8.3.3 Postbiotics

### 8.3.3.1 Short Chain Fatty Acids

The fermentation of non-digestible carbohydrates from dietary fiber sources results in the production of SCFAs including acetate, butyrate, formate, lactate, and propionate. SCFAs are becoming well known for being influential in the immune system by having natural anti-inflammatory properties, playing a role in epithelial integrity, and having antiproliferative tumor-suppressive effects [3]. In particular, butyrate is rapidly absorbed from the gut lumen and is the preferred energy source of colonocytes. Additionally, this metabolite can alter cytokine production and influence Treg cells that play a role in intestinal inflammation [3]. Butyrate production is associated with Firmicutes, *Eubacterium rectale, Roseburia* spp., *Eubacterium hallii, Coprococcus catus, and Faecalibacterium prausnitzii* [3].

### 8.3.3.2 Colostrum (Bovine)

The addition of mammalian colostrum in the diets of dogs and cats has been shown to stimulate the immune system in pets post-weaning. One study in adult dogs (Satyaraj et al. [14]) found a significantly higher vaccine response, higher levels of fecal IgA, and a significant increase in GI microbiota diversity in dogs supplemented with bovine colostrum compared to the control group [14]. Similarly, a study in 16-week-old kittens (Gore et al. [15]) found the antibody response to a rabies vaccine to be quicker and stronger, increased fecal IgA expression, with a 91% stabilization of the fecal microbiota in those supplemented with bovine colostrum versus the control group that had some microbiota stabilization (65%) [15]. The supplementation of bovine colostrum could benefit weanlings during this stressful period.

## 8.4 Chapter Summary

- The immune system consists of innate and adaptive immune systems.
- The innate immune system is the body's first line of defense against foreign substances (bacteria, viruses, and other infectious agents that are perceived to cause harm to the host) that enter the body.
- Barrier protection, the closed surface of the skin and mucous membranes, offers a physical barrier against foreign substances.
- Cellular protection is activated through special immune system cells and proteins if foreign substances get past physical barriers.
- The development of antibodies will break down the extracellular area of microorganisms to help prevent the spread of intracellular infections.
- The adaptive immune system initiates if the innate immune response cannot remove the foreign substance, specifically targeting the organism causing the infection.
- Commensal GI microbiota have a fundamental role in the induction, education, and function of the host's immune system, which allows for an evolved symbiotic relationship.
- "Germ-free" mice have reduced development of gut-associated lymphoid tissue (GALT), decreased numbers of T cells, B cells, antimicrobial peptides, along with thinner mucous layer, and fewer Peyer's patches resulting in less immunotolerance.
- There is an association with an increase in intestinal permeability preceding most autoimmune diseases.
- Cancer is a complex disease, and it is estimated that 15–20% of cancers involve microorganisms, with dysbiosis in the microbiomes being

associated with gastric, esophageal, hepatobiliary, pancreatic, lung, colorectal, and lymphoma in dogs.

- Supportive nutrients such as prebiotics, probiotics, and postbiotics, along with colostrum have shown to be beneficial in enhancing immune function.

## References

1 Smith, N.C., Rise, M.L., and Christian, S.L. (2019). A comparison of the innate and adaptive immune systems on cartilaginous fish, ra-finned fish, and lobe-finned fish. *Frontiers in Immunology* 10: 2292. https://doi.org/10.3389/fimmu.2019.02292.

2 InformedHealth.org [Internet] (2006). Cologne, Germany: Institute for Quality and Efficiency in Health Care (IQWiG). The Innate and Adaptive Immune Systems (accessed 20 July 20 2022).

3 Epiphanio, T.M.F. and Santos, A. (2021). Small animals gut microbiome and its relationship with cancer. In: *Canine Genetics, Health and Medicine* (ed. C. Rutland). IntechOpen https://doi.org/10.5772/intechopen.95780.

4 Santaolalla, R., Fukata, M., and Abreu, M.T. (2011). Innate immunity in the small intestine. *Current Opinion in Gastroenterology* 27 (2): 125–131. https://doi.org/10.1097/MOG.0b013e3283438dea.

5 Janeway, C.A. Jr., Travers, P., Walport, M., *et al.* (2001)The Humoral Immune Response. In Immunobiology: The Immune System in Health and Disease. 5. New York: Garland Science. https://www.ncbi.nlm.nih.gov/books/NBK10752 (accessed 20 July 2022)

6 Belkaid, Y. and Hand, T.W. (2014). Role of the microbiota in immunity and inflammation. *Cell* 157 (1): 121–141. https://doi.org/10.1016/j.cell.2014.03.011.

7 Vangoitsenhoven, R. and Cresci, G.A. (2020). Role of microbiome and antibiotics in autoimmune diseases. *Nutrition in Clinical Practice* 35 (7): https://doi.org/10.1002/ncp.10489.

8 Stebegg, M., Kumar, S.D., Silva-Cayetano, A. et al. (2018). Regulation of the germinal center response. *Frontiers in Immunology* 9: 2469. https://doi.org/10.3389/fimmu.2018.02469.

9 Gonzalez, H., Hagerling, C., and Werb, Z. (2018). Roles of the immune system in cancer: from tumor initiation to metastatic progression. *Genes & Development* 32 (19–20): 1267–1284. https://doi.org/10.1101/gad.314617.118.

**10** Hardy, H., Harris, J., Lyon, E. et al. (2013). Probiotics, prebiotics and immunomodulation of gut mucosal defences: homeostasis and immunopathology. *Nutrients* 5 (6): 1869–1912. https://doi.org/10.3390/nu5061869.

**11** Yan, F. and Polk, D.B. (2011). Probiotics and immune health. *Current Opinion in Gastroenterology* 27 (6): 496–501. https://doi.org/10.1097/MOG.0b013e32834baa4d.

**12** Lappin, M.R., Veir, J.K., Satyaraj, E. et al. (2009). Pilot study to evaluate the effect of oral supplementation of *Enterococcus faecium* SF68 on cats with latent feline herpesvirus 1. *Journal of Feline Medicine and Surgery* 11 (8): 650–654. https://doi.org/10.1016/j.jfms.2008.12.006.

**13** Veir, J.K., Knorr, R., Cavadini, C. et al. (2007). Effect of supplementation with *Enterococcus faecium* (SF68) on immune functions in cats. *Veterinary Therapeutics* 8 (4): 229–238.

**14** Satyaraj, E., Reynolds, A., Pelker, R. et al. (2013). Supplementation of diets with bovine colostrum influences immune function in dogs. *British Journal of Nutrition* 110 (12): 2216–2221. https://doi.org/10.1017/S000711451300175X.

**15** Gore, A.M., Satyaraj, E., Labuda, J. et al. (2021). Supplementation of diets with bovine colostrum influences immune and gut function in kittens. *Frontiers in Veterinary Science* 8: 675712. https://doi.org/10.3389/fvets.2021.675712.

# 9

# The Endocannabinoid System

## 9.1 Endocannabinoid System

The endocannabinoid system is a regulatory system located in many parts of the body [1]. It is composed of several bioactive lipids (*N*-acylethanolamines and 2-acylglycerols) and works on a chemical-receptor function [1, 2]. The chemicals work on both cannabinoid CB1 and CB2 receptors. When they bond there is a response. They are designed to respond to the body and initiate changes [1]. They increase when there is exercise, stress, pain, at certain times of day, and is involved with appetite, coping, stress, and anxiety [1]. Ross [3] compared this function to cortisol in a Ted talk "Demystifying the endocannabinoid system". She described that unlike cortisol levels that decrease in response to repetitive high stress situations, the endocannabinoid system will continually increase (see Figure 9.1). Normally, this intrinsic system works in the right place at the right time; it is precise, responsive, and highly controlled [1]. Endocannabinoid tone describes the overall functioning of the endocannabinoid system including the function or density of cannabinoid receptors, levels of endocannabinoids, and their metabolic enzymes [4].

The endocannabinoid system is involved in energy regulation through CB1 receptors [5]. CB1 receptors are located in many regions of the body including the hypothalamus, limbic system, gastrointestinal tract, adipose tissue, pancreas, and in the liver [5]. These receptors are also involved in the control of body weight [5]. CB2 receptors are mainly

*Small Animal Microbiomes and Nutrition*, First Edition. Robin Saar and Sarah Dodd.
© 2024 John Wiley & Sons, Inc. Published 2024 by John Wiley & Sons, Inc.
Companion website: www.wiley.com/go/saar/1e

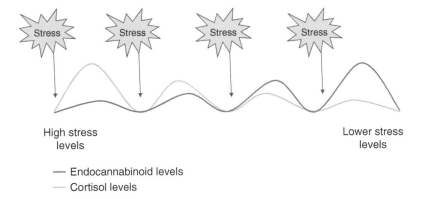

High stress
levels

Lower stress
levels

— Endocannabinoid levels
— Cortisol levels

**Figure 9.1** Change in endocannabinoid and cortisol levels in response to stress.

found in immune tissues and have an influence over inflammation and inflammatory disease [6]. Further investigation is still needed to fully understand the role and influence CB2 receptors have on brain functions, immune cells, and inflammation [6]. In dogs, cannabinoid receptors have been identified in the skin, the gastrointestinal tract, central and peripheral nervous system, joints, and embryo, while in cats cannabinoid receptors are located in the brain, skin, ovary, and oviduct 7. The endocannabinoid system is involved in multiple functions including memory, learning, and coordination of motor functions [7]. It can manipulate appetite and the regulation of sleep, as well as perform pain-relieving, anti-inflammatory, antioxidant, immunosuppressive, hypotensive, and antiemetic activity, and play a role in reproductive functions [7].

## 9.2 The Endocannabinoidome Axis

The complex signaling system with more than 100 lipid mediators and 50 protein metabolites of the endocannabinoid system is referred to as the endocannabinoidome [8]. When perturbations occur in one system, it can cause alterations in the other physiological systems leading to health consequences in organs including the brain [8]. For example, dysbiosis in the GI microbiome is accompanied by alterations in the endocannabinoid and endocannabinoidome signaling in the gut. These signals participate in mediating the negative effects of GI dysbiosis [8]. The same effect can be observed with the administration of prebiotics or probiotics where the restoration of "normal" in the GI microbiome results in a return to normal endocannabinoidome signaling [8]. GI microbiota are able to modulate the endocannabinoidome, pharmacological or genetic manipulation of endocannabinoidome signaling can modify the composition of gut microbiota and change its molecular signaling structure [8]. This axis can be used in part to prevent negative metabolic effects, including systemic inflammation induced by dysbiosis [8] (see Figure 9.2).

It has also been proposed that GI microbiota may respond to endocannabinoidome mediators and/or metabolize them [8]. There is evidence that commensal bacteria may influence the endocannabinoidome in its function also by producing endocannabinoid-like molecules that are capable of binding the same receptors as their host counterparts [8]. A recent study in germ-free mice showed alterations of endocannabinoidome signaling in the small intestine post a fecal microbiota transplant. Changes in the mRNA expression of some endocannabinoidome receptors including CB1 were increased, while two G-protein-coupled receptors were decreased [8].

Another function of the GI microbiome-endocannabinoid axis involves a change in GI microbial diversity that can contribute to anhedonia (the ability to feel pleasure), and amotivation (the lack of motivation) behaviors, via the endocannabinoid system [9, 10]. These conditions are associated with multiple mental health issues in humans,

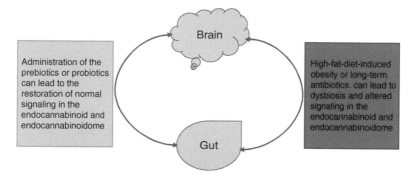

**Figure 9.2** The state of the endocannabinoidome is closely associated with the gut microbiome and has a bidirectional effect on the brain in response to changes.

including chronic fatigue and depression. An alteration, usually a decrease, in microbial diversity has been associated with a variety of mood disorders. A study in mice using unpredictable chronic mild stress showed phenotypic alteration, which successfully transferred via fecal microbiota transplantation to naive recipient mice [11]. Cellular and behavioral changes were observed in the recipient mice along with a decrease in endocannabinoid signaling. These changes were then reversed or and the behaviors were alleviated by selectively enhancing the central endocannabinoid or through the addition of a strain of the *Lactobacilli* genus [11]. This study represented a scenario for how chronic stress, diet, and GI microbiota generate a pathological feed-forward loop that contributes to depressive type behaviors via the central endocannabinoid system [11] (Figure 9.3).

Obesity has also been correlated with an altered GI microbiota, chronic low-grade inflammation, and endocannabinoid system tone (Figure 9.4) [12]. While further research is needed, one study revealed the ability to control gut permeability and adipogenesis through plasma lipopolysaccharide levels by interfering with the endocannabinoid system using CB1 agonist and antagonist in lean and obese mice. Through lipopolysaccharide-endocannabinoid system regulatory loops, the GI microbiota were able to determine adipose tissue physiology [12]. Alterations in microbiota via prebiotic treatment, and antibiotics reversed obesity-induced changes in endocannabinoid tone in adipose tissue [5]. Novel mechanisms such as the impacts of glucagon-like peptide-2 and specific probiotic bacteria

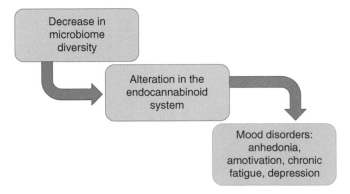

**Figure 9.3** Effect of the GI-microbiome – endocannabinoid axis on behavioral disorders.

(e.g. Bifidobacterium spp.) have been investigated to be involved in the control of the gut barrier in mice and humans [13].

Several recent studies support the concept that the GI microbiome and endocannabinoidome signaling manipulate lipid and glucose metabolism under both physiological and dysmetabolic conditions in gastrointestinal tissues, along with adipose tissue and in the brain [8]. Several microbiota metabolites typically such as SCFA and indole derivatives profoundly affect the host metabolism, with these molecules possibly indirectly affecting endocannabinoidome signaling [8]. The molecular mechanisms and functional importance of such communication require further studies [8].

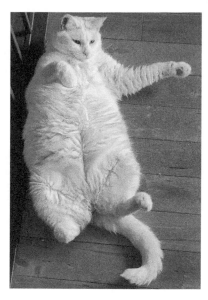

**Figure 9.4** Example of an obese cat.

## 9.3 Chapter Summary

- The endocannabinoid system is a regulatory system located in many parts of the body.
- The chemicals work on both cannabinoid CB1 and CB2 receptors.
- When a stressful situation is repeated, cortisol levels will decrease over time, while in an endocannabinoid system, it continually increases in response to the situation.
- The complex signaling system with more than 100 lipid mediators and 50 protein metabolites of the endocannabinoid system is referred to as the endocannabinoidome.
- Another function of the GI-microbiome – endocannabinoid axis involves a change in GI microbial diversity that can contribute to anhedonia (the ability to feel pleasure), and amotivation (the lack of motivation) behaviors, via the endocannabinoid system.

- Several recent studies support the concept that the GI microbiome and endocannabinoidome signaling manipulate lipid and glucose metabolism under both physiological and dysmetabolic conditions in gastrointestinal tissues, along with adipose tissue and in the brain.

## References

1 Silver, R.J. (2019). The endocannabinoid system of animals. *Animals* 9 (9): 686. https://doi.org/10.3390/ani9090686.

2 Rastelli, M., Cani, P.D., and Knauf, C. (2019). The gut microbiome influences host endocrine functions. *Endocrine Reviews* 40 (5): 1271–1284. https://doi.org/10.1210/er.2018-00280.

3 Ross, R. (2019). Demystifying the endocannabinoid system. *Ted Talks Mississauga*. TedTalks.com. https://www.ted.com/talks/ruth_ross_demystifying_the_endocannabinoid_system.

4 Russo, E.B. (2016). Clinical endocannabinoid deficiency reconsidered: current research supports the theory in migraine, fibromyalgia, irritable bowel, and other treatment-resistant syndromes. *Cannabis and Cannabinoid Research* 1 (1): 154–165. https://doi.org/10.1089/can.2016.0009.

5 Cluny, N.L., Keenan, C.M., Reimer, R.A. et al. (2015). Prevention of diet-induced obesity effects on body weight and gut microbiota in mice treated chronically with Δ9-Tetrahydrocannabinol. *PLoS One* 10 (12): e0144270. https://doi.org/10.1371/journal.pone.0144270.

6 Turcotte, C., Blanchet, M.R., Laviolette, M. et al. (2016). The CB2 receptor and its role as a regulator of inflammation. *Cellular and Molecular Life Sciences* 73 (23): 4449–4470. https://doi.org/10.1007/s00018-016-2300-4.

7 Della, R.G. and Di Salvo, A. (2020). Hemp in veterinary medicine: from feed to drug. *Frontiers in Veterinary Science* 7: 387. https://doi.org/10.3389/fvets.2020.00387.

8 Iannotti, F.A. and Di Marzo, V. (2021). The gut microbiome, endocannabinoids and metabolic disorders. *The Journal of Endocrinology* 248 (2): R83–R97. https://doi.org/10.1530/JOE-20-0444.

9 Minichino, A., Jackson, M.A., Francesconi, M. et al. (2021). Endocannabinoid system mediates the association between gut-microbial diversity and anhedonia/amotivation in a general population cohort. *Molecular Psychiatry* 26: 6269–6276. https://doi.org/10.1038/s41380-021-01147-5.

**10** Lee, J.S., Jung, S., Park, I.H. et al. (2015). Neural basis of anhedonia and amotivation in patients with schizophrenia: the role of reward system. *Current Neuropharmacology* 13 (6): 750–759. https://doi.org/10.2174/1570159x13666150612230333.

**11** Chevalier, G., Siopi, E., Guenin-Macé, L. et al. (2020). Effect of gut microbiota on depressive-like behaviors in mice is mediated by the endocannabinoid system. *Nature Communications* 11: 1–15. 10.1038/s41467-020-19931-2.

**12** Muccioli, G.G., Naslain, D., Bäckhed, F. et al. (2010). The endocannabinoid system links gut microbiota to adipogenesis. *Molecular Systems Biology* 6: 392. https://doi.org/10.1038/msb.2010.46.

**13** Cani, P.D. and Delzenne, N.M. (2011). The gut microbiome as therapeutic target. *Pharmacology & Therapeutics* 130 (2): 202–212. https://doi.org/10.1016/j.pharmthera.2011.01.012.

# 10

# Respiratory System Microbiome

## 10.1 The Respiratory System Microbiome

The main functions of the upper respiratory system are to act as a filter and provide heat and humidity to the air before it reaches the lungs [1]. Historically, the lungs were considered sterile and any microbial colonization was synonymous with pathology, though new capabilities in microbial identification has challenged the long-held belief [2]. The upper respiratory system includes the nostrils, rhino-pharynx, oropharynx, larynx, and the middle cavity of the ear through the Eustachian tube [1, 3]. The mucous surfaces of the respiratory system are colonized by a wide range of bacteria belonging to the genera *Firmicutes, Actinobacteria, Bacteroidetes, Proteobacteria,* and *Fusobacteria* in humans [1]. Each area in this system have their own features such as humidity, temperature, relative oxygen concentration, and specific type of epithelial cells, along with individualized diversity of microbiota colonizing each area [2]. As the initial site for the introduction of microbes through respiration and ingestion, the commensal bacteria in these areas are the first responders against pathogens [3]. For example, in humans during normal respiration, the lower airways are exposed to 105 microbiota per day [3].

Resident microbiota of the upper airway includes many pathogenic bacteria. These bacteria may colonize asymptomatically in the upper respiratory tract though these same organisms can be aspirated into the lower respiratory tract resulting in infection. Examples of potentially pathogenic bacteria are *Streptococcus pneumoniae, Staphylococcus*

*Small Animal Microbiomes and Nutrition*, First Edition. Robin Saar and Sarah Dodd.
© 2024 John Wiley & Sons, Inc. Published 2024 by John Wiley & Sons, Inc.
Companion website: www.wiley.com/go/saar/1e

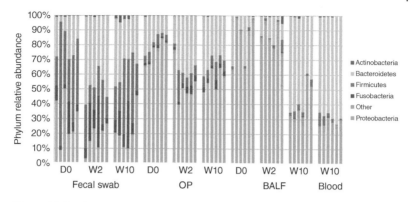

**Figure 10.1** Bacterial diversity in the oropharyngeal (OP) and bronchoalveolar systems (BAL) in cats. Relative abundance of bacteria at the phylum level taken at day 0, week 2, and week 10 of the study. Samples were collected from feces, oropharyngeal, bronchoalveolar lavage fluid, and blood. *Source:* Vientós-Plotts et al. [2] / PLOS / Public Domain CC BY 4.0.

*aureus, Moraxella catarrhalis, and Haemophilus influenzae,* along with antibiotic-resistant microbiota and virulence genes (genes that have an ability to infect the host and cause disease) [3].

Microbial identification through metagenomics has identified rich and diverse communities of microbiota in the lungs of healthy humans, mice, dogs, sheep, and pigs. In dogs, four major phyla are commonly identified, including *Proteobacteria, Actinobacteria, Firmicutes,* and *Bacteroidetes* [4]. Cats have fewer studies, with one study identifying *Proteobacteria* as the most abundant phylum in the upper and lower airways, and *Proteobacteria, Bacteroidetes, and Firmicutes* as the most commonly identified phylum (see Figure 10.1) [2, 5]. Studies on healthy dogs reveal microbiota of the lower airway being distinct from other sites including the upper respiratory tract and the GI tract [2]. One challenge in identifying microbiota in the lower airway is the risk or possible risk of contamination of the sample during bronchoscopy, which could lead to questioning samples' accuracy [3].

## 10.2 Factors Affecting Diversity and Density

As discussed in Chapter 3, colonization of the respiratory tract beings at birth with the mode of delivery (vaginal or caesarian), environmental influences (habitat, diet), and antibiotic treatments as the three main modalities that are associated with the development of the original microbiome and the causation of alterations to the original microbiome [1]. During the establishment of both the GI and lung microbiomes, their encoded signals affect the maturity of both the epithelium of airways and the immune system [1]. Thus, there is an importance in ensuring the integrity of the composition and proper maturation of the microbiomes early in life. Studies have shown how this influences the prevention of certain lung diseases [1]. Dynamic changes in the commensal flora occur during the first year and final stages of life. These changes combined with an immature or weakened immune system can lead to a higher susceptibility to infection or disease [3, 5].

The external environment can affect the diversity and density of respiratory microbiomes. A study in horses found changes in the lower (lung) and upper (oral and nasal) communities based on environmental changes and exposures [6]. Mice can have very predictable microbes associated with lower respiratory (lung) microbial communities. These "normal" communities are highly variable depending on the mice origin (breeder/vendor), mode of shipment, and habitat [7]. A 2017 study (Dorn et al. [5]) on cats, looked at how both age and environment influence the respiratory microbiome state in both healthy and disease-affected cats [5]. Interestingly, they found a higher number of species in indoor cats compared to outdoor cats with *Proteobacteria* sp. being the predominant bacterial phylum in both healthy and diseased cats [5]. There were distinct differences in the nasal microbial composition in the healthy cats depending on their age. This may be identified as a barrier in studies, as growth is a period of change and development in respiratory microbiomes and can create inappropriate data if comparing data from subjects in varying life stages. Another interesting common finding was the identification of the *Moraxellaceae* family in both healthy cats and cats with feline upper respiratory tract disease. *Moraxella* spp. has a history of being associated with respiratory diseases. In humans, presence of this species is linked as a risk factor for childhood asthma, bronchitis, pneumonia, and acute infections in the first year of life. In cats, *Moraxella* spp. has been identified as a core species of the oral and nasal microbiomes [5]. The results in this study indicated that the bacterial communities in the respiratory tract are influenced by both age and different environment factors (see Figure 10.2) [5].

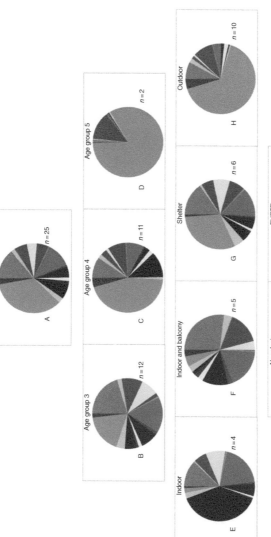

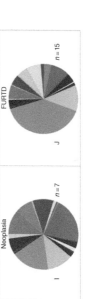

**Figure 10.2** Nasal samples from cats in different ages, environments, and health status. The most prevalent bacterial phyla and families found in healthy cats (charts A–H) and cats with feline upper respiratory tract disease and nasal neoplasia. *Source:* Dorn et al. [5] / PLOS / Public Domain CC BY 4.0.

In dogs, one study found that the breed was another influencer on respiratory microbial communities [4]. There were distinct microbial differences in West Highland terriers compared to other healthy domestic dogs, regardless of the West Highland terrier being healthy or experiencing canine idiopathic pulmonary fibrosis [4].

## 10.3 Diseases Associated with Dysbiosis

As commonly found with other disease states, a loss of beneficial microbiota, a decrease in diversity, and/or an increase in potentially pathogenic bacteria are the characteristics associated with dysbiosis in the respiratory tract. In humans, asthma, chronic obstructive pulmonary disease (COPD), and cystic fibrosis are the commonly associated dysbiotic-induced disease states [2]. Dogs may be used as comparable models for humans as they have similar anatomy, physiology, and immune system functions. Dogs are also commonly exposed to similar environmental stimuli and have similar respiratory diseases as the humans they live with [8] (Figure 10.3).

In the above-mentioned study on horses, while the external environment has strong influence on the density and diversity, true dysbiosis was observed in the lower (lung) respiratory tract in asthmatic horses when compared to healthy horses and was thought to be the result of inflammation associated with the disease [6]. Additionally, inflammation involving IL-1α and IL-4 (inflammatory cytokines) are correlated with altered diversity of lower respiratory microbial communities of mice [7]. Similarly, antibiotic administration will alter the community in a microbially predictable manner. Dogs under

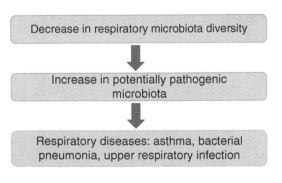

**Figure 10.3** Changes in the respiratory tract microbiota can lead to common diseases.

antimicrobial treatment have a relative increase in *Pseudomonas* genera that are also involved in chronic infections, particularly in humans on ventilators and those affected with chronic lung diseases. Conversely, the high ability for *Pseudomonas* to grow aids in the prevention of other potentially pathogen bacteria to flourish. In addition, *Pseudomonas* spp. can benefit the host as they have the capacity to produce and degrade multiple compounds including materials that may be toxic to the host [4].

### 10.3.1 Asthma

Pathologically, asthma is the result of an inflammatory response to a particular stimulus including allergic and nonallergic sources. This is a chronic condition that causes inflammation of the bronchial, tightening of the chest muscles, and increasing mucous production [9]. Dogs are not known to develop asthma but may develop an eosinophilic airway inflammatory syndrome, Canine Eosinophilic Bronchopneumopathy [10]. Eosinophilic inflammation is also associated with bronchitis (asthma) in cats where an allergic component is similar to models in human allergic asthma [2, 9].

### 10.3.2 Bacterial Pneumonia

In dogs, bacterial pneumonia is one of the most common diagnosis when a dog is in acute or chronic respiratory distress [11]. This disorder can occur as either a primary or be a secondary disease from aspiration, viral infections, a result of an immune dysfunction, foreign body, or a nosocomial event [11, 12]. Community-acquired pneumonia is usually observed acutely post an exposure to a contagious pathogen such as *Bordetella bronchiseptica, Yersinia pestis, Mycoplasma* spp., *Streptococcus cania,* and *Streptococcus equi* subspecies *zooepidemicus* [12, 13]. Secondary bacterial pneumonia in dogs occurs secondary to a predisposed condition being either an anatomic or physiological condition. For example, dysfunction of the upper respiratory or GI tract may result in bacterial translocation or aspiration of microbes or foreign matter into the lower respiratory tract. Conditions associated with secondary bacterial pneumonia in dogs are megaesophagus, laryngeal paralysis, ciliary dyskinesia, and neoplasias [12, 13]. Dysbiosis in the lower respiratory track has been identified as a relative increase of a specific taxa, along with a

**Table 10.1** Sources and common microbes found in primary and secondary bacterial pneumonia in dogs and cats.

| Bacterial pneumonia | |
| --- | --- |
| Primary | • Acquired through exposure to a contagious pathogen in the community<br>• *Bordetella bronchiseptica, Yersinia pestis, Mycoplasma* spp., *Streptococcus cania, Streptococcus equi* subspecies *zooepidemicus* |
| Secondary | • Acquired secondary to a predisposed condition such as megaesophagus or laryngeal paralysis.<br>• *E. coli, Pasturella* spp., *Streptococcus* spp., *B. bronchiseptica, Enterococcus* spp., *Mycoplasma* spp., *S. pseudintermedius.* |

decrease in the normal taxa found in healthy dogs [12]. Common microbes identified in dogs and cats with secondary associated lower respiratory disease are *E. coli, Pasteurella* spp., *Streptococcus* spp., *B. bronchiseptica, Enterococcus* spp., *Mycoplasma* spp., *Staphylococcus pseudintermedius* and other coagulase-positive *Staphylococcus* spp., and *Pseudomonas* spp. [13] (Table 10.1).

### 10.3.3 Upper Respiratory Infection

Feline upper respiratory tract disease is a syndrome consisting of clinical signs that can include both ocular and nasal discharges, epistaxis, sneezing, and conjunctivitis and are directly associated with one or more of the known pathogenic viral (feline herpesvirus 1, or calicivirus), bacterial (*Staphylococcus* spp., *Streptococcus* spp., *Pasteurella multocida, E. coli, Chlamydia felis, B. bronchiseptica, S. canis, S. equi sub* spp. *zooepidemicus, and Mycoplasma* spp., and anaerobes), or fungal organisms [13].

In cats with upper respiratory tract disease, viable bacterial cultures can be difficult to obtain, as bacteria that may be cultured from the nasal cavity of healthy animals, can include multi-drug-resistant bacteria that is part of the "normal" community and is not causing illness. While treatment in these cats may provide some relief from severe clinical signs, these cats are predisposed to opportunist infections from antimicrobial-resistant bacteria [13]. The use of antimicrobials in cats with upper respiratory tract disease should be reserved for severe clinical cases [13].

## 10.4 Key Nutritional Factors

### 10.4.1 Probiotics

Probiotics have been shown to influence the immune system and provide benefit to a compromised respiratory system. The common mucosal immune system enables cross talk between the GI and respiratory tracts. In a study in humans, the immune response in the lungs was modulated by the administration of oral probiotics. This response promoted a more tolerant response to allergic triggers [14].

A 2009 study by Lappin et al. look at using the probiotic *Enterococcus faecium* strain SF68 to enhance the immune response in cats with feline herpesvirus 1 [15]. Cats who received the probiotic had fecal microbial diversity maintained throughout the study, while cats fed a placebo saw a decrease in diversity. There was an overall lessened morbidity associated with chronic feline herpesvirus-1 in cats that were administered the probiotic [16].

Other suggest that there is a systemic effect on the host's cytokine concentrations with the use of oral probiotics, thus indicating a positive effect on immune function [14].

### 10.4.2 Minerals, Vitamins, and Antioxidants

Some minerals, vitamins, and nutrients that are considered to have antioxidant properties have shown to positively influence the immune system that may benefit a patient experiencing respiratory microbial dysbiosis. Antioxidants have the potential to assist the immune system where there is a deficiency and the potential to boost the immune system with supplementation [16]. Studies in humans identify the benefit of utilizing antioxidants with respiratory diseases including the use of vitamins C, D, E, and β-carotene [17]. Additionally, selenium is a notable antioxidant as it is a component of glutathione peroxidase and has been shown to enhance immune function in animal studies, along with minerals zinc and copper that are additionally known to influence immune function [18]. Polyphenols have the potential to act not only as an antioxidant, anti-inflammatory agents, and possibly increase the efficacy of glucocorticoids in some respiratory diseases [17].

### 10.4.3 Omega 3 Fatty Acids

While there are few to no studies on the effects of omega 3 fatty acids on animals with respiratory diseases, omega 3 fatty acids are well known to decrease overall body inflammation. A study in cats did see some improvement in asthmatic cats that were supplemented with both omega 3 fatty acids and luteolin, a polyphenolic flavone found in many herbs, fruits, and vegetables that is traditionally used in Chinese medicine and is known to have anti-inflammatory properties. In this study, there was a decrease in the airway hyper-responsiveness with no significant decrease in inflammation [19].

## 10.5 Chapter Summary

- The main functions of the upper respiratory system are to act as a filter and provide heat and humidity to the air before it reaches the lungs.
- Being the initial site for the introduction of microbes through respiration and ingestion, the commensal bacteria in these areas are the first responders against pathogens.
- Resident microbiota of the upper airway includes many pathogenic bacteria.
- Colonization of the respiratory tract beings at birth with the mode of delivery (vaginal or caesarian), environmental influences (habitat, diet), and antibiotic treatments as the three main modalities that are associated with the development of the original microbiome and the causation of alterations to the original microbiome.
- As commonly found with other disease states, a loss of beneficial microbiota and a decrease in diversity including an increase in potentially pathogenic bacteria are the characteristics associated with dysbiosis in the respiratory tract.
- Pathologically, asthma is the result of an inflammatory response to a particular stimulus including allergic and nonallergic sources.
- Probiotics have shown to positively influence the influence the immune system that may benefit pets suffering with respiratory conditions.

# References

1 Santacroce, L., Charitos, I.A., Ballini, A. et al. (2020). The human respiratory system and its microbiome at a glimpse. *Biology (Basel)* 9 (10): 318. https://doi.org/10.3390/biology9100318.

2 Vientós-Plotts, A.I., Ericsson, A.C., Rindt, H. et al. (2017). Dynamic changes of the respiratory microbiota and its relationship to fecal and blood microbiota in healthy young cats. *PLoS One* 12 (3): e0173818. https://doi.org/10.1371/journal.pone.0173818.

3 Hoffman, A.R., Proctor, L.M., Surette, M.G. et al. (2015). The microbiome: the trillions of microorganisms that maintain health and cause disease in humans and companion animals. *Veterinary Pathology* 53 (1): 10–21. https://doi.org/10.1177/0300985815595517.

4 Fastrès, A., Roels, E., Vangrinsven, E. et al. (2020). Assessment of the lung microbiota in dogs: influence of the type of breed, living conditions and canine idiopathic pulmonary fibrosis. *BMC Microbiology* 20: 84. https://doi.org/10.1186/s12866-020-01784-w.

5 Dorn, E.S., Tress, B., Suchodolski, J.S. et al. (2017). Bacterial microbiome in the nose of healthy cats and in cats with nasal disease. *PLoS One* 12 (6): e0180299. https://doi.org/10.1371/journal.pone.0180299.

6 Fillion-Bertrand, G., Dickson, R.P., Boivin, R. et al. (2018). Lung microbiome is influenced by the environment and asthmatic status in an equine model of asthma. *American Journal of Respiratory Cell and Molecular Biology* 60 (2): 189–197. 10.1165/rcmb.2017-0228OC.

7 Dickson, R.P., Erb-Downward, J.R., Falkowski, N.R. et al. (2018). The lung microbiota of healthy mice are highly variable, cluster by environment, and reflect variation in baseline lung innate immunity. *American Journal of Respiratory and Critical Care Medicine* 198 (4): 497–508. https://doi.org/10.1164/rccm.201711-2180OC.

8 Ericsson, A.C., Personett, A.R., Grobman, M.E. et al. (2016). Composition and predicted metabolic capacity of upper and lower airway microbiota of healthy dogs in relation to the fecal microbiota. *PLoS One* 11 (5): e0154646. https://doi.org/10.1371/journal.pone.0154646.

9 Aun, M.V., Bonamichi-Santos, R., Arantes-Costa, F.M. et al. (2016). Animal models of asthma: utility and limitations. *Journal of Asthma and Allergy* 10: 293–301. https://doi.org/10.2147/JAA.S121092.

10 Reinero, C.N., Mitchell, C.S., and Rabinowitz, P.M. (2010). Allergic conditions. In: *Human-Animal Medicine* (ed. P.M. Rabinowitz and L.A. Conti), 43–49. W.B. Saunders.

**11** Dear, J.D. (2019). Bacterial pneumonia in dogs and cats: an update. *Veterinary Clinics: Small Animal Practice* 50 (2): 447–465. https://doi.org/10.1016/j.cvsm.2019.10.007.

**12** Vientós-Plotts, A.I., Ericsson, A.C., Rindt, H. et al. (2019). Respiratory dysbiosis in canine bacterial pneumonia: standard culture vs. microbiome sequencing. *Frontiers in Veterinary Science* 6: 354. https://doi.org/10.3389/fvets.2019.00354.

**13** Lappin, M.R., Blondeau, J., Boothe, D. et al. (2017). Antimicrobial use guidelines for treatment of respiratory tract disease in dogs and cats: antimicrobial guidelines working group of the International Society for Companion Animal Infectious Diseases. *Journal of Veterinary Internal Medicine* 31 (2): 279–294. https://doi.org/10.1111/jvim.14627.

**14** Vientós-Plotts, A.I., Ericsson, A.C., Rindt, H. et al. (2017). Oral probiotics alter healthy feline respiratory microbiota. *Frontiers in Microbiology* 8: 1287. https://doi.org/10.3389/fmicb.2017.01287.

**15** Harper J. (2001). Feline immunocompetence, aging and the role of antioxidants; world small animal Veterinary Association World Congress Proceedings. https://www.vin.com/apputil/content/defaultadv1.aspx?id=3843820&pid=8708&print=1 (accessed 14 May 2022).

**16** Lappin, M.R., Veir, J.K., Satyaraj, E. et al. (2009). Pilot study to evaluate the effect of oral supplementation of *enterococcus faecium* SF68 on cats with latent feline herpesvirus 1. *Journal of Feline Medicine and Surgery* 11 (8): 650–654. https://doi.org/10.1016/j.jfms.2008.12.006.

**17** Rahman, I. (2006). Antioxidant therapies in COPD. *International Journal of Chronic Obstructive Pulmonary Disease* 1 (1): 15–29. 10.2147/copd.2006.1.1.15.

**18** Hand, M.S., Thatcher, C.D., Remillard, R.L. et al. (2010). Antioxidants. In: *Small Animal Clinical Nutrition*, 5e (ed. M.S. Hand et al.), 152–154. Mark Morris Institute.

**19** Leemans, J., Cambier, C., Chandler, T. et al. (2010). Prophylactic effects of omega-3 polyunsaturated fatty acids and luteolin on airway hyperresponsiveness and inflammation in cats with experimentally-induced asthma. *Veterinary Journal* 184 (1): 111–114. https://doi.org/10.1016/j.tvjl.2009.01.008.

# 11

# Oral Microbiomes

The oral cavity has many important functions for the body. It is the beginning of the respiratory and digestive systems; aids in the formation of sounds; it has protective, secretory, and sensory functions; and is the indicative source for taste [1]. Additionally, the mouth functions in communication and social interactions, grooming, protection, and heat regulation. Primarily, the function of the mouth is to obtain and prepare food for the digestive tract [2]. The actions required by the mouth for this function include bringing the food into the oral cavity, mastication of food, and swallowing, which require the use of muscles of the jaw and upper throat, the tongue, and teeth [2]. Dysfunction in any of these areas may result in malnutrition and dehydration [2].

## 11.1   The Oral Microbiome

The development of individual microbiomes is thought to be affected by the presentation of birth, neonatal feeding method, age of the host, diet, and health status [3]. The initial acquisition and type of early colonizing bacteria established may affect the lifelong health of the host [3]. The development of the resident oral microbiome is now believed to start in utero with human studies showing amniotic fluid containing microbiota that is similar to the oral microbiome of the mother [3]. The mode of birth, vaginal versus cesarian section, has been shown to affect the microbial diversity in neonates [3]. Post-birth environmental factors play a large role in the type of microbiota the neonatal is exposed to; this includes the air, mode of feeding (breastfed versus bottle-fed), type of food (breast milk versus formula), and physical contact with individuals [3]. Key differences have been noted between human and pet oral microbiomes, so research may not be transferable between these species in this area of research [3].

The oral microbiome covers all mucosal and dental surfaces in a biofilm. The biofilm is approximately 1 μm thick, is specific to each surface, and consists of the resident bacterial community combined with the extracellular matrix (ECM) [1]. The ECM contains specific cell-secreted proteins and polysaccharides that provide structure and biochemical support to the specific environment [3, 4]. The ability of the ECM to attach to various surfaces is an important mechanism of adhesion, along with the ability of microorganisms to aggregate and adhere to each other [1]. Like other areas in the body, the microbiome in the biofilm exists symbiotically with the host without evoking an inflammatory response, and they play a crucial role in the exclusion of pathogens in the biofilm [3, 4]. The continuous accumulation of the biofilm, particularly subgingival, can lead to dysbiosis and predispose the host to disease.

## 11.2 Factors Affecting Diversity and Density

In an established oral microbiome there are physical, chemical, and immunohistochemical factors that influence the diversity and density of microbes in the oral cavity, including the temperature, availability, and type of nutrients, colonization of microbiota or ability to exclude, pH of saliva, conditions of bacterial adhesion to plaque redox potential (ability to change of oxidation state of atoms), and the concentration of hydrogen ions. These conditions change when food is introduced as it lowers the pH in the oral cavity [1].

Variations in resident oral microbiomes are observed in different locations of the oral cavity. These areas or niches can be placed into groups: hard tissue surface (supragingival plaque), soft tissue surfaces (buccal and tongue dorsum mucosa), subgingival, and fluid or saliva [5]. The surface with the greatest diversity is the supragingival plaque, see Figure 11.1 [5]. Subgingival plaques between dogs and humans are

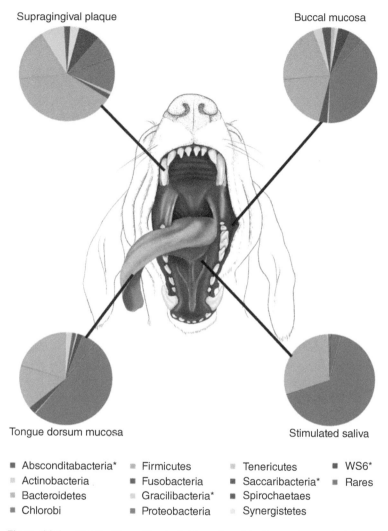

Supragingival plaque

Buccal mucosa

Tongue dorsum mucosa

Stimulated saliva

- Absconditabacteria*
- Actinobacteria
- Bacteroidetes
- Chlorobi
- Firmicutes
- Fusobacteria
- Gracilibacteria*
- Proteobacteria
- Tenericutes
- Saccaribacteria*
- Spirochaetaes
- Synergistetes
- WS6*
- Rares

**Figure 11.1** Distribution of bacterial taxa found in the canine oral niches. *Source:* Ruparell et al. [5] / Springer Nature / Public Domain CC BY 4.0.

quite different, with one study showing only 16.4% of taxa being similar [5]. Saliva pH in dogs ranges from 7.3 to 7.8 and 7.5 in cats and both lack salivary amylase, which initiates the digestion of carbohydrates [3]. Dogs and cats also do not normally have *Streptococcus mutans* in their oral microbiomes [3]. This specific bacteria is key in the formation of dental caries or tooth decay resulting in damage to the tooth when decay-causing bacteria produce acids that break down the enamel [3, 6]. Comparatively, dental caries are common in 92% of adult humans, less than 5% of dogs, and almost nonexistent in cats [3]. Cat oral communities are similar to communities found on their skin with an increase in *Bacteroides* [7]. Not all diseases associated with gum disease involve plaque; bacterial, viral, or fungal infections, genetic conditions, systemic diseases, and traumatic injury are conditions that do not arise due to the accumulation of the biofilm microbiota [1].

## 11.3 Diseases Associated with Dysbiosis and Inflammation

### 11.3.1 Periodontal Disease

The accumulation of the biofilm is one of the main factors in the pathogenesis of periodontal disease and may influence inflammatory processes (Table 11.1) [1]. When the balance between the resident microbiome and the host's immune balance is disturbed, immune tolerance shifts to a proinflammatory response [4]. Like other microbiomes, it is the proportion of more virulent species, along with damage to the barrier function that induce dysbiosis [4]. The variety in the microbial colonization in the oral cavity depends on the availability of individual nutrients and the level of the host's natural nonspecific immunity [1]. Adjuvants of the inflammatory process are the type of microbes, the type of toxin produced (endotoxins, exotoxins, and leukotoxins), the microbial enzymes, and their products of metabolism (butyric acid, propionic acid, ammonia, indole, amines, and volatile sulfur compounds), which when produced

Table 11.1 Common diseases of the oral cavity and the niches affected.

| Disease | Oral niche |
| --- | --- |
| Periodontitis | Chronic inflammation of alveolar and periodontium bones |
| Stomatitis | Inflammation of oral mucous membranes |
| Glossitis | Inflammation of the tongue |

in large amounts destroy the mucosa permeability and are reducers of collagen synthesis [1]. Simply, it is the pathogenic microbiota located in the subgingival plaque that degrades nitrogenous substrates (nutrients) into cytotoxic compounds such as short-chain fatty acids, ammonia, sulfur compounds, and indoles, which induce tissue inflammation and promote cell death, decreasing barrier functionality.

As indicated above, the composition of the supragingival and subgingival plaque is due to environmental differences and the ability of nutrients to flow into the gingival groove allowing the anaerobic bacteria to colonize and flourish. This is a step in the parthenogenesis of gingivitis, where the metabolites of the microbiota (endotoxins and protease) along the gum line and in the subgingival groove penetrate the epithelium [1]. This initiates inflammation with the dilation of blood vessels, increased vascular permeability, introduction of neutrophils into tissues, and damage to the collagen fibers that surround the blood vessels. Inflammatory lesions are confined to the supragingival tissues and can be modified by the endocrine system, blood diseases, and some pharmaceuticals (anticonvulsants and immunosuppressants) [1]. The pathogenesis for periodontitis occurs when the alveolar and periodontium bones experience chronic inflammation, which destroys the alveolar and periodontium bones resulting in periodontal pickers, gingival recessions, tooth mobility, and alterations in the consistency, shape, and resilience of the supragingival tissues [1]. The inflammatory lesions in periodontitis leak bacterial products that are absorbed by exposed cement becoming soft and necrotic [1]. While inflammation from gingivitis can be reversed with proper oral hygiene, severe periodontitis bone loss is permanent [3]. In humans, psychological stress that induces increased cortisol levels correlates positively with an increased risk of periodontal disease [1].

Both dogs and cats are susceptible to periodontal disease with gingivitis affecting 95–100% of pets and periodontitis affecting 50–70% [3]. Both cats and dogs have an increased risk of periodontal disease as they age. In cats, the upper and lower premolars are the most affected teeth. Multiple disease states are associated with gingivitis and periodontal disease in dogs and cats including, renal disease, endocarditis, systemic infection, and parenchymal liver disease [3].

In a study by Dewhirst, et al. approximately 89% of the 171 feline oral taxa analyzed were assigned to Firmicutes, Proteobacteria, Bacteroidetes, or Spirochaetes [3].

### 11.3.1.1 Stomatitis

Stomatitis is deep inflammation of oral mucous membranes. Commonly seen in specific dog breeds including Greyhounds, Maltese, Miniature Schnauzers, and Labrador Retrievers with symptoms including severe gum inflammation and recession, and oral sores on the inner surface of the lip most commonly by the upper canine and carnassial (4th premolar) teeth [2]. Cats have severe inflammation and sores that encompasses the entire oral cavity including the upper throat [8]. This disease is also associated with cats that have been diagnosed with calicivirus [8].

Fungal stomatitis occurs in both dogs and cats and is caused by an overgrowth of the fungus *Candida albicans* due to long-term antibiotic use, a suppressed immune system, or in conjunction with another oral condition. It is an uncommon cause of mouth inflammation in dogs and cats. Signs of fungal stomatitis differ slightly as in addition to inflammation and oral sores, creamy white plaques may be observed on the tongue of cats, and excessive drooling and bleeding may be observed in both dogs and cats [8, 9].

### 11.3.1.2 Glossitis

Inflammation of the tongue may be due to infection, or disease including renal disease or diabetes [8].

### 11.3.2 Systemic Antimicrobials

Systemic antimicrobials have been used preemptively and postoperatively for oral surgeries. According to a paper by Davis et al. [4], there is no evidence that adjunctive systemic antimicrobial treatment administered pre- or postoperatively is medically beneficial for canine or feline patients [4]. This also includes using antimicrobials alternatively for surgical treatment of periodontitis [4].

## 11.4 Key Nutritional Factors

Oral bacteria utilize nutrients in the mouth as a source of energy, with different species being able to thrive off these nutrients [1]. Some of these bacteria (*S. mutans, Streptococcus gordonii,* and *Lactobacillus*) can create a more acidic oral environment which in humans can promote the demineralization of enamel and dentin. Polypeptides also play a role with colonization by binding of bacteria cell walls with glycoproteins in saliva.

There is one published study looking at changes in the oral microbiomes (supragingival plaque) from birth through weaning onto commercial diets. The study began at birth with most oral bacteria being unclassified taxa. By 2 weeks of age, differences were noted in diversity between kittens born vaginally versus via C-section. The kittens were provided exclusively milk for the first 2 weeks and then were weaned onto a moisten extruded kibble and wet commercial diet starting at week 3 until 8 weeks of age where they were exclusively on the commercial diets. There were three main phyla found in all kittens (*Bacteroidetes, Firmicutes, and Proteobacteria*), which made up 76% of the total microbiota sequenced. *Porphyromonas* spp. and *Treponema* spp. were more abundant in kittens on the dry kibble, while cats consuming wet food had increased *Conchiformibius kuhniae* [3].

## 11.5 Chapter Summary

- The development of individual microbiomes is thought to be affected by the presentation of birth, neonatal feeding method, age of the host, diet, and health status.
- The oral microbiome covers all mucosal and dental surfaces in a biofilm. The biofilm is approximately 1 μm thick and is specific to each surface consisting of the resident bacterial community combined with the extracellular matrix (ECM).
- In an established oral microbiome there are physical, chemical, and immunohistochemical factors that influence the diversity and density of microbes in the oral cavity.
- Variations in resident oral microbiomes are observed in different locations of the oral cavity.
- It is the pathogenic microbiota located in the subgingival plaque that degrades nitrogenous substrates (nutrients) into cytotoxic compounds, which induce tissue inflammation and promote cell death.
- Polypeptides also play a role with colonization by binding of bacteria cell walls with glycoproteins in saliva.

# References

1 Rowińska, I., Szyperska-Ślaska, A., Zariczny, P. et al. (2021). The influence of diet on oxidative stress and inflammation induced by bacterial biofilms in the human oral cavity. *Materials (Basel)* 14 (6): 1444. 10.3390/ma14061444.

2 Disorders of the Mouth in Dogs (2022). Merck manual. https://www.merckvetmanual.com/dog-owners/digestive-disorders-of-dogs/disorders-of-the-mouth-in-dogs (accessed 12 June 2022).

3 Spears, J.K., Vester Boler, V., Gardner, C. et al. (2017). *Development of Oral Microbiome in Kittens*. The Campanion Animal Nutrition Summit Nestle, Research Center.

4 Davis, E.M. and Weese, J.S. (2022). Oral microbiome in dogs and cats: dysbiosis and the utility of antimicrobial therapy in the treatment of periodontal disease. *The Veterinary Clinics of North America. Small Animal Practice* 52 (1): 107–119. https://doi.org/10.1016/j.cvsm.2021.08.004.

5 Ruparell, A., Inui, T., Staunton, R. et al. (2020). The canine oral microbiome: variation in bacterial populations across different niches. *BMC Microbiology* 20: 42. 10.1186/s12866-020-1704-3.

6 Martins, K.S., de Assis Magalhães, L.T., de Almeida, J.G., and Pieri, F.A. (2017). Antagonism of bacteria from dog dental plaque against human cariogenic bacteria. *BioMed Research International* 2018: 10.1155/2018/2780948.

7 Older, C.E., Diesel, A.B., Lawhon, S.D. et al. (2019). The feline cutaneous and oral microbiota are influenced by breed and environment. *PLoS One* 14 (7): e0220463. https://doi.org/10.1371/journal.pone.0220463.

8 Disorders of the Mouth of Cats (2022ss). Merck Manual. https://www.merckvetmanual.com/cat-owners/digestive-disorders-of-cats/disorders-of-the-mouth-in-cats (accessed 12 June 2022).

9 Lee, D.B., Verstraete, J.M., and Arzi, B. (2020). An update on feline chronic gingivostomatitis. *The Veterinary Clinics of North America. Small Animal Practice* 50 (5): 973–982. https://doi.org/10.1016/j.cvsm.2020.04.002.

# 12

# Aural Microbiome

## 12.1 The Aural Microbiome

The anatomy of the canine and feline ear includes the pinna, the external ear canal (vertical and horizontal canals), the middle ear (an air-filled tympanic cavity, three auditory ossicles, and tympanic membrane), and the inner ear (bony labyrinth in the petrous portion of the temporal bone which is responsible for hearing and balance) [1].

While current research is limited in dogs and cats, there have been some trends found that are similar across body microbiomes, where healthy aural microbiomes tend to have greater species diversity. In trying to determine the normal flora, one study in dogs found *Cutibacterium acnes* (previously known as *Propionibacterium acnes*; 4.5%), *Staphylococcus pseudintermedius* (3.8%), and *Streptococcus* sp. (1.1%) to be the top three most abundant bacteria with *M. pachydermatis* (6.1%), *Capnodiales* (3.7%), and *Pleosporales* (1.0%) as the top three most abundant fungal taxa [2].

Multiple diseases are associated with aural conditions such as autoimmune disorders, allergic disease, and hypothyroidism though while ear infections have been identified as being a preliminary sign of hypothyroidism in dogs, there is no credible evidence to suggest that otitis externa, especially as the sole clinical sign, is a feature of hypothyroidism in dogs [3].

*Small Animal Microbiomes and Nutrition*, First Edition. Robin Saar and Sarah Dodd.
© 2024 John Wiley & Sons, Inc. Published 2024 by John Wiley & Sons, Inc.
Companion website: www.wiley.com/go/saar/1e

## 12.2   Factors Affecting Diversity and Density

As with most other trends, dogs, and cats with clinically affected aural microbiomes are characterized by a general lack of bacterial and fungal diversity and are often dominated by only one or two species [2].

### 12.2.1   Influencing Factors

Changes in a healthy microbiome are caused by three main factors:

1) Primary factors directly induce inflammation in the external ear. Examples of primary factors are hypersensitivity disorders such as allergies, parasites, masses, endocrine, and autoimmune diseases [4].
2) Predisposing factors are introduced factors that increase the risk of dysbiosis. Examples of predisposing factors are environmental changes such as humidity or water in the aural structure [4].
3) Perpetuating factors are those that maintain the problem once it has become established. For example, otitis media developing into post otitis externa. Secondary causes could be classified in this group though secondary causes require a predisposing factor(s) to lead to pathology. An example of this concept was described in a 2018 study by Paterson et al. in dogs. It was observed that dogs whose primary cause of infection was *Pseudomonas* were also affected with allergies, masses, endocrine disease, and autoimmune disease [5]. In cases where there was a mass or autoimmune disease, they perpetuated *Pseudomonas* infections to develop more quickly, compared to dogs with allergies and endocrinopathies [5] (Figure 12.1).

### 12.2.2   Biofilms

Like biofilms in other areas in the body, biofilms can exist in aural microbiomes. Bacteria exist in two forms in growth, and proliferation phases. The first form is referred to as planktonic where bacteria exist as single and independent cells. This is the most common form of bacteria in acute disease. If the condition is allowed to become chronic, the bacteria become more organized, in fixed groups known as biofilms [6]. These complex three-dimensional communities allow bacteria to communicate

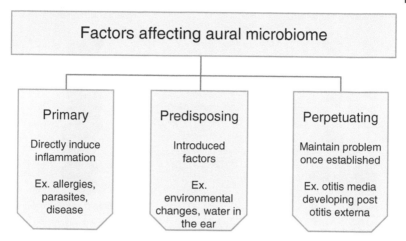

**Figure 12.1** Factors that can cause change in the microbiota diversity found in the aural cavity.

with each other by signaling molecules modulating gene expression, deliver nutrients, dispose of waste, and have many other advantages [7]. Bacteria in a biofilm produce extracellular polymeric substances composed of proteins, polysaccharides, and nucleic acids, and exhibit an altered phenotype which affects their growth, by slowing the rate of growth, and gene transcription; planktonic organisms are unable to develop this function [6, 7]. Bacteria have improved defense skills in biofilms including protection from environmental changes (temperature, moisture, pH), evading the host's immune system, and have an increased resistance to antibiotics [6, 7] (Figure 12.2).

The aural biofilm aids in antibiotic resistance by (i) decreasing cell growth making them less susceptible to antimicrobial agents and (ii) the utilization of the complex functions in the extracellular polymeric matrix. This diffusional barrier may protect bacteria from the penetration of antimicrobials. While high concentrations may still result in bacteria death, the biofilm increases the minimum inhibitory concentration allowing low concentrations of antimicrobials to be blocked by the matrix protecting bacteria in the biofilm [4, 6]. In cases where an intermediate concentration of antimicrobial may penetrate the barrier, some bacteria may be able to mutate and survive, leading to a more resistant population [4, 6].

Planktonic bacteria

Bacteria biofilm

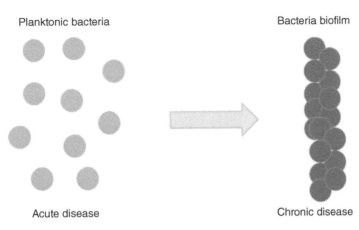

Acute disease

Chronic disease

**Figure 12.2** Disease progression from acute, with planktonic bacteria, to chronic, with the development of a biofilm. *Source:* George Andrew Abernathy, https://orcid.org/0000-0002-1336-3631, last accessed 8 December 2022 / Licensed under CC0 license.

Biofilms are a common occurrence in otitis. Pathogenic bacteria and yeast can form biofilms such as *Staphylococcus pseudintermedius, Malassezia pachydermatis,* and *Pseudomonas aeruginosa* [6].

## 12.3 Diseases Associated with Dysbiosis

Otitis is a commonly observed aural dysbiosis disease with 7.5–16.5% of canine cases seen in general practice being presented for otitis externa [2]. Otitis externa includes inflammation in the pinna, the vertical and horizontal ear canals to the tympanum, and may be acute or chronic, where the same condition persists or recurs for 3 months or longer [8]. The external ear may be physically altered in response to chronic inflammation. Some of these changes are glandular hyperplasia, glandular dilation, epithelial hyperplasia, and hyperkeratosis, which can contribute to an increase in humidity, and pH, predisposing the ear to secondary infections [8]. Secondary infections with bacterial pathogens (*P. aeruginosa, S. pseudintermedius, Escherichia coli, Klebsiella* spp., and *P. aeruginosa*), or fungus (*Malassezia pachydermatis*) occur in many instances of otitis externa. *Pseudomonas aeruginosa* is a gram-negative bacillus that is not considered to be a resident inhabitant in canine aural microbiomes, and once it has colonized, it can be difficult to manage [2] (Figures 12.3 and 12.4).

Another component of otitis externa is yeast with some dogs developing an allergic response to *Malassezia* spp., which can cause pruritus

**Figure 12.3** Beginning stages of otitis externa. Note increased debris soon to be followed by inflammation if not treated.

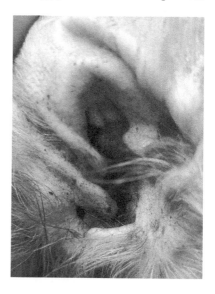

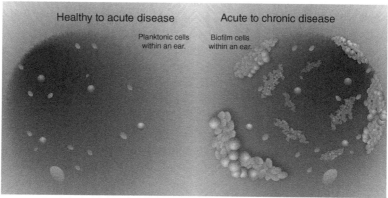

**Figure 12.4** Aural microbiome diversity is decreased when the patient becomes clinically affected. In some cases, a single bacteria or fungal microbiota can constitute more than 90% of the sample. *Source:* George Andrew Abernathy, https://orcid.org/0000-0002-1336-3631, last accessed 8 December 2022 / Licensed under CC0 license".

and pain [8]. A report that looked at *Malassezia* in both dogs and cats found some interesting differences between the species. This yeast species was found more frequently in animals under 5 years of age and was identified in cats more frequently in the winter wherein in dogs it was more common in the fall. In dogs, the type of ears affects the level of incidence, with pendulous ears having a higher level of occurrence when compared to erect ears. Finally, higher levels of Malassezia were identified in animals with otitis versus pets with healthy aural structures [9].

A recent study looked at samples from 257 dogs' aural microbiomes. Using next-generation sequencing (NGS), they were able to identify 7846 bacterial and fungal species from healthy and clinically affected dogs. Cases, where the dog was clinically affected, were characterized by an overall loss of microbial diversity, and an increase in microbial biomass. The overgrowth was in specific microbiota (69.8% bacterial, 16.3% fungal, and 7.0% both bacterial and fungal overgrowth) in 78.3% of clinically affected cases [2]. In 21% of the clinically affected cases, either a single bacteria or fungal microbiota (*M. pachydermatis* and *Staphylococcus pseudintermedius*) constituted more than 90% of the sample [2]. While many microbes were found in the healthy dog samples and there was a tendency to have a significantly higher density when the dog was clinically affected, *Enterococcus faecalis, Finegoldia magna, Arcanobacterium phocae, Streptococcus halichoeri, Peptoniphilus harei, Proteus mirabilis, Bacteroides pyogenes, Trueperella* sp., and *Pasteurella dagmatis* were rarely found in healthy ear samples. This study also identified *Malassezia pachydermatis, S. pseudintermedius, Staphylococcus schleiferi,* and a few anaerobic bacteria such *as Finegoldia magna, Peptostreptococcus canis,* and *Porphyromonas cangingivalis* as the most important microbial taxa found in clinically affected ears [2].

In cats, one study found higher fungal populations in both allergic and diseased cats along with higher bacterial populations in the allergic cats. Fungal and bacterial overgrowth was associated with the severity of otitis [10]. A 2017 study that compared skin microbiomes in healthy and allergic cats found healthy cats had more *Oxalobacteraceae* and *Porphyromonadaceae*, and allergic cats had increased *Staphylococcus* [11].

## 12.4    Key Nutritional Factors

Ensuring a complete and balanced diet is important to support pets with chronic otitis. Some nutrients may benefit the health of a pet experiencing aural dysbiosis.

The goal is to support the epithelium and decrease reactive oxygen species.

- Protein is the building block for skin cells and ensuring the pet is on a highly digestible source of protein can help improve the health of the epithelium of the aural canal.
- Omega 3 fatty acids improve skin barrier function and may reduce inflammation associated with aural disease.
- Manage allergic components by offering a hydrolyzed protein or limited ingredient diet. Ensuring that the diet is highly digestible and complete and balanced will additionally play a role in creating a homeostatic environment.
- Antioxidants such as carotenoids, tocopherols, polyphenols, and flavonoids have been frequently researched for their antioxidant effect on skin health.
- Probiotics may aid in improving skin health.

## 12.5    Chapter Summary

- As with most other trends, dogs, and cats with clinically affected aural microbiomes are characterized by a general lack of bacterial and fungal diversity and are often dominated by only one or two species.
- The changes in the healthy microbiome are caused by primary, predisposing, or perpetuating factors.
- Biofilms are complex three-dimensional communities: allow bacteria to communicate with each other by signaling molecules modulating gene expression, deliver nutrients, dispose of waste, and have many other advantages.
- The aural biofilm aids in antibiotic resistance.
- Nutrition can be used supportively to help ensure good skin barrier.

# References

1 Cole, L.K. (2010). Anatomy and physiology of the canine ear. *Veterinary Dermatology* 21 (2): 221–231. https://doi.org/10.1111/j.1365-3164.2010.00885.x.

2 Tang, S., Prem, A., Tjokrosurjo, J. et al. (2020). The canine skin and ear microbiome: a comprehensive survey of pathogens implicated in canine skin and ear infections using a novel next-generation-sequencing-based assay. *Veterinary Microbiology* 247: https://doi.org/10.1016/j.vetmic.2020.108764.

3 Graves, T.K. (2008). Canine hypothyroidism: fact or fiction. *DVM 360 Proceedings*. https://www.dvm360.com/view/canine-hypothyroidism-fact-or-fiction-proceedings (accessed 14 May 2022).

4 Pye, C. (2018). *Pseudomonas* otitis externa in dogs. *The Canadian Veterinary Journal* 59 (11): 1231–1234.

5 Paterson, S. and Matyskiewicz, W. (2018). A study to evaluate the primary causes associated with *Pseudomonas* otitis in 60 dogs. *The Journal of Small Animal Practice* 59 (4): 238–242. https://doi.org/10.1111/jsap.12813.

6 The role of biofilms in otitis (2017). Dermatology. http://fs-1.5mpublishing.com/vet/issues/2017/02/vp_2017_02_derm.pdf (accessed 8 May 2022).

7 Akyıldız, I., Take, G., Uygur, K. et al. (2012). Bacterial biofilm formation in the middle-ear mucosa of chronic otitis media patients. *Indian Journal of Otolaryngology and Head & Neck Surgery* 65 (Suppl 3): 557–561. https://doi.org/10.1007/s12070-012-0513-x.

8 Bajwa, J. (2019). Canine otitis externa – treatment and complications. *The Canadian Veterinary Journal* 60 (1): 97–99.

9 Cafarchia, C., Gallo, S., Capelli, G. et al. (2005). Occurrence and population size of *Malassezia* spp. in the external ear canal of dogs and cats both healthy and with otitis. *Mycopathologia* 160 (2): 143–149. https://doi.org/10.1007/s11046-005-0151-x.

10 Pressanti, C., Drouet, C., and Cadiergues, M.C. (2014). Comparative study of aural microflora in healthy cats, allergic cats and cats with systemic disease. *Journal of Feline Medicine and Surgery* 16 (12): 992–996. https://doi.org/10.1177/1098612X14522051.

11 Older, C.E., Diesel, A., Patterson, A.P. et al. (2017). The feline skin microbiota: the bacteria inhabiting the skin of healthy and allergic cats. *PLoS One* 12 (6): e0178555. 10.1371/journal.pone.0178555.

# 13

# Integumentary Microbiomes

## 13.1   The Cutaneous Microbiome

While the bulk of microbe research has been focused on residents of the gastrointestinal (GI) tract, more is being discovered about the micro-communities that inhabit the skin of dogs and cats. Normal cutaneous microbiota facilitates functions such as modulating the innate immune response and preventing the colonization of pathobionts [1]. The skin acts as a protective boundary between the ambient environment and the body of the animal [2]. It is a highly metabolic organ, containing hair, skin, and subcutis – adipose-rich tissue beneath the dermis responsible for attachment to the underlying muscle, fascia, or periosteum. Much like the intestine, the skin consists of epithelial cells, immune cells, and microbes offering multiple layers of protection, covering a large surface area, and is constantly exposed to possible allergens, toxins, and pathogens [3]. Pioneer microbes initiating colonization of the skin aid in the development of the immune response system, educating the immune cells to microbes considered commensal versus pathogenic through the release of signaling molecules and antimicrobial peptides [4–6].

In contrast to the gut microbiome, there are relatively few studies investigating normal core cutaneous microbes for both dogs and cats. Two corresponding studies by Hoffman et al. [1] and Older et al. [7] described the cutaneous microbiome of healthy versus allergic dogs and cats [1, 7], respectively, using modern sequencing techniques. In both

*Small Animal Microbiomes and Nutrition*, First Edition. Robin Saar and Sarah Dodd.
© 2024 John Wiley & Sons, Inc. Published 2024 by John Wiley & Sons, Inc.
Companion website: www.wiley.com/go/saar/1e

species, individual variability was high, more so for dogs than cats. Similar to the gut, which offers different microenvironments travelling from oral to aboral, the microenvironment of dog and cat skin differs between different regions of the body. Microbial diversity and density appear to be affected by sampling location, with higher richness and diversity in haired skin as opposed to hairless mucocutaneous junctions or mucosal surfaces. In agreement with older, culture-based studies, Proteobacteria predominated regardless of skin region, followed by Actinobacteria, Firmicutes, Bacteroidetes, and Fusobacteria [1, 8]. In cats, the core bacteria were similar to that of dogs, also dominated by Proteobacteria, though followed in a different order by Bacteroidetes, Firmicutes, and Actinobacteria. The higher prevalence of Bacteroidetes was suspected to result from feline grooming behavior, as members of this phyla are typically associated with the oral microbiome and may thus be deposited on the skin [7]. Skin-associated fungi have also been described in dogs and cats [9, 10]. In comparison to bacteria, there was less variability in fungal communities between body sites, but still reduced richness noted in mucosal sites. In both dogs and cats, *Alternaria* and *Cladosporium* were the most abundant fungal genera (Figure 13.1).

## 13.2 Factors Affecting Diversity and Density

### 13.2.1 Environment

Geographic location and habitat can exert influence on the microclimate of the skin surface, with environmental factors such as humidity, temperature and pH influencing the composition of the cutaneous microbiome [1, 2]. While the environment plays a role in some skin conditions, particularly allergy-associated conditions such as canine atopic dermatitis, this is not always a determining factor. One study in cats found that the genetics, or, more specifically, the breed of the cat, was a more influential factor compared to environment [11]. A study by Cuscó et al. [12], looked at a 35 Golden Retrievers that were genetically related and raised in the same environment. They found differences in diversity, based on the area of sampling, temporality (season, time spent in confinement), and sex to be the main factors of influence [12]. Individuality was a strong conclusion for both of these studies [11, 12].

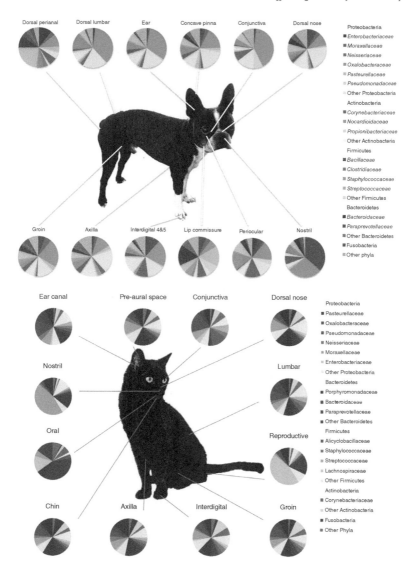

**Figure 13.1** The normal core skin microbes found on dogs and cats. *Source:* Adapted from [1, 6].

### 13.2.2 Diet and the Gut Microbiome

Though the epithelium lining the gut may seem distant and separate from that lining the external surface of the body, the two are intrinsically linked and interact extensively [6]. Nutrition can have an influence on the cutaneous microbiome by aiding in maintaining gut barrier health and the gut microbiome [13]. Disruption of the gut mucosal barrier can allow for antigen presentation and formulation of immune complexes against dietary components, resulting in systemic inflammation and manifesting dermatoses [14, 15]. Nutrition can also directly impact the external skin barrier. The epidermal barrier is composed of skin cells (corneocytes) and intracellular lipids (ceramides, sterols, and fatty acids), the health of which may be influenced by nutrient intake [13]. In turn, the cutaneous microbiome can both impact, and be impacted by, the health of the epidermal barrier.

### 13.2.3 Pharmaceuticals

Antimicrobials, both systemic and topical, impact the diversity and density of cutaneous microbiomes. Antimicrobials may be applied as a therapy to target pyoderma, which may reduce density of offending microbes and allow balance of the cutaneous microbiota to reestablish [16, 17]. However, risks of antimicrobial therapy include selection for drug-resistant organisms and suppression of core microbiome commensals. Furthermore, systemic antimicrobials may also disrupt the gut microbiome, with potential impacts on the skin and associated microbiome (Figure 13.2).

## 13.3 Diseases Associated with Dysbiosis

### 13.3.1 Dysfunctional Barrier Syndrome

To maintain a healthy protective barrier, microbial, immune, biochemical, and physical barriers are all required simultaneously [4, 6, 19]. All barrier system functions must work together for effective barrier function to occur [19]. When there is a disruption in one or more of these protective functions, there is an increased risk of pathogenic skin conditions, such as infections, inflammation, allergy, or neoplasia [20].

(a)

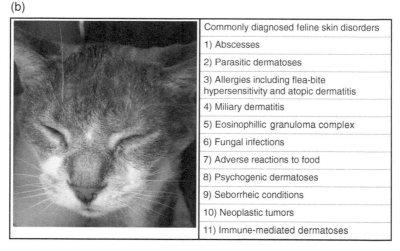

| | Commonly diagnosed canine skin disorders |
|---|---|
| | 1) Allergic including flea-bite hypersensitivity and atopic dermatitis |
| | 2) Cancer (neoplasia) |
| | 3) Bacterial pyoderma |
| | 4) Seborrhea |
| | 5) Parasitic dermatoses |
| | 6) Adverse reactions to food including food hypersensitivity or food intolerance |
| | 7) Immune-mediated dermatoses |
| | 8) Endocrine dermatoses |

(b)

| | Commonly diagnosed feline skin disorders |
|---|---|
| | 1) Abscesses |
| | 2) Parasitic dermatoses |
| | 3) Allergies including flea-bite hypersensitivity and atopic dermatitis |
| | 4) Miliary dermatitis |
| | 5) Eosinophillic granuloma complex |
| | 6) Fungal infections |
| | 7) Adverse reactions to food |
| | 8) Psychogenic dermatoses |
| | 9) Seborrheic conditions |
| | 10) Neoplastic tumors |
| | 11) Immune-mediated dermatoses |

**Figure 13.2** Figure (a) lists the most commonly diagnosed skin diseases in canines. *Source:* Marsella (2021)/MDPI/CC BY 4.0. (b) Lists the most commonly diagnosed skin diseases in felines. *Source:* Marsella (2021)/MDPI/CC BY 4.0. *Source:* Adapted from [1, 5, 18].

**Microbial barrier:** Similar to the GI microbiome, a healthy cutaneous microbiome can aid in preventing the colonization of pathogenic type bacteria [1, 7, 9, 16]. Commensals may compete with and inhibit the growth of pathogenic organisms.

**Immune barrier:** In human skin, a xenobiotic receptor has been implicated in epidermal differentiation, critical for epidermal stratification and formation of a protective stratum corneum [4, 20]. Immune functions utilize innate and adaptive immune cells to mount memory responses to protect against pathogens without reacting to benign commensals [6].

**Biochemical barrier:** A biochemical barrier functions work to inhibit the growth of bacterial pathogens by maintaining moisture and acid mantle – a thin film on the skin's surface composed of lipids from the oil glands mixed with amino acids from sweat of the skin [19]. In animals such as dogs and cats with reduced sweat glands, this function may not be comparable to that described in human skin.

**Physical barrier:** Physically, the skin consists of structured keratinocytes and tight junctions to create a cement-type barrier holding in moisture and prevent pathogens or toxins from crossing into the tissue [3]. The stratum corneum, the layer of cornified epidermal cells at the outermost surface of the skin, comprises of a complex system of tight junctions, adhesion complexes, and cytoskeletal networks. This barrier works to mediate cell–cell adhesion, creating a strong mechanical barrier between the environment and underlying tissue. The stratum corneum is constantly shedding dead cells from the keratin squames outermost layer which aids in the removal of surface pathogens [3] (Figure 13.3).

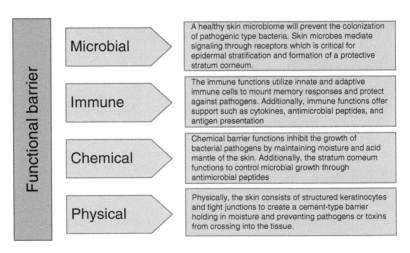

**Figure 13.3** Functions of a normal skin barrier. If any one of these is disrupted, there is an increased risk of pathogenic skin conditions, such as infections, inflammation, allergy, or neoplasia.

Dysfunctional barrier syndrome of the epidermis is pathologically similar to barrier dysfunctions discussed in Chapters 8, 15, and 16. Dysregulation in the immune system, deficiencies of antimicrobial compounds, impaired structural integrity, along with gut dysbiosis, may all contribute to skin barrier defects. Malfunction of epidermal barrier mechanisms can lead to primary dermatoses and allow for secondary infection with opportunistic pathogenic species [1].

### 13.3.2 Atopic Dermatitis

Atopic dermatitis describes a genetic predisposition to exaggerated immune response against diverse antigens leading to an overproduction of immunoglobulin E (IgE) resulting in inflammatory dermatosis [17]. The clinical consequence is an increased propensity to hypersensitivity reactions to common environmental antigens. Atopic dermatitis is a chronic inflammatory disease that may be complicated by a secondary bacterial and fungal infection [21]. The pathogenesis of atopic dermatitis is discussed in Chapter 15, but briefly: impaired mucosal barrier function can allow translocation of ingested environmental components and presentation of antigens to the gut-associated lymphoid tissue (GALT), resulting in hypersensitivity and inflammation [17, 22]. The gut microbiota play a role in maintaining the integrity of the mucosal barrier, as well as in modulating gut inflammation [14, 23]. Gastrointestinal dysbiosis may alter the balance of specific immune cells, called T helper cells, resulting in reduced tolerance and a predisposition to hypersensitivity, in conjunction with reduced production of anti-inflammatory microbial metabolites like SCFA. The resulting outcome is exaggerated inflammatory responses to ingested food and environmental substances. Atopic dogs may or may not show GI signs, as the disease condition is a systemic disease, not localized exclusively to the skin.

The cutaneous microbiome may also impact, and/or be impacted by, atopic dermatitis. In atopic dogs, cutaneous fungal and microbial richness were reduced in comparison to healthy dogs [1, 9]. This may allow for colonization with pathobionts and secondary infection, a common comorbidity associated with atopic dermatitis [17, 24] (Figure 13.4).

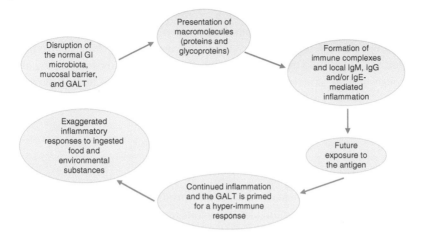

**Figure 13.4** Atopy pathway showing how disruption in the gut can lead to hypersensitivity and exaggerated inflammation.

## 13.4 Key Nutritional Factors

Nutrition plays a significant role in skin health with multiple dermatoses being associated with nutrient deficiencies or excesses or genetic impairment of nutrient absorption or use.

Commonly associated nutrients of concern are protein, fat, essential fatty acids, zinc, vitamin A, and vitamin E [13]. Several B-complex vitamins are also associated with some skin conditions as they function as cofactors in essential fatty acid (EFA) metabolism. Additionally, given the link between gut microbial dysbiosis and some dermatoses, dietary support for a balanced microbiome may also be required (see Chapter 15).

### 13.4.1 Protein

Skin cells contain a comparatively large amount of the proteins keratin and collagen, as well as elastin, which aids in normal barrier function, while hair is composed almost entirely of protein [3, 13]. It has been estimated that 25–30% of daily protein requirements are utilized for normal daily hair growth in dogs [13]. Meeting protein needs is thus essential for normal hair growth, skin keratinization and barrier function [25].

### 13.4.2 Essential Fatty Acids

Essential fatty acids (EFAs) play a structural role in cell membranes and are required to maintain normal cutaneous integrity and barrier function [13]. Deficiencies of the omega-6 polyunsaturated fatty acid (PUFA) linoleic acid is associated with reduced skin surface lipid production resulting in a dry, dull coat and can progress to greasy skin, hair loss and barrier dysfunction [13]. Both omega-6 and omega-3 PUFA are incorporated into and alter the composition and function of cellular membranes. Omega-3 PUFA, particularly eicosapentaenoic acid (EPA), and docosahexaenoic acid (DHA) are well studied for having anti-inflammatory properties by competing with the metabolism of the omega-6 PUFA arachidonic acid into pro-inflammatory eicosanoids, prostaglandins, and leukotriene [26]. The consumption of omega-3 fatty acids results in the production of fewer eicosanoids derived from arachidonic acid (omega-6) and an increase in eicosanoids derived from alpha-linolenic acid (omega-3), thereby reducing the inflammatory response. Thus, both adequate intake and balance of omega-6 and omega-3 fatty acids are required to maintain skin health.

### 13.4.3 Fiber

Indigestible carbohydrates such as oligosaccharides, sometimes referred to as prebiotics, may be beneficial in supporting the growth of microbes that produce SCFA and may aid in decreasing inflammation [27]. Oligosaccharides are rapidly fermented to SCFA through microbial fermentation. Dietary inclusion of fructooligosaccharides (FOS) may help to modulate the intestinal environment to favor the production of secretory IgA and are a preferred substrate for *Lactobacillus spp.* and *Bifidobacterium spp.*, both responsible for lactic acid, SCFA, and IgA production [28]. Mannooligosaccharide (MOS) may be able to influence the immune humoral response by increasing the activity of lysozymes, antibodies, and T cells and act as a physical blockade, preventing non-resident bacteria from binding to the gut mucosa [28].

### 13.4.4 Vitamins

Vitamin A is required for regulation of cellular replication and differentiation and plays an essential role in epithelial integrity and keratinization [13]. Both deficiency and excess of vitamin A can result in keratinization defects resulting in seborrhea and secondary infection [13, 18]. B-vitamins are cofactors in a wide variety of metabolic reactions, particularly in energy and anabolic pathways. As such, deficiencies of B vitamins can result in slow skin cell turnover, flaky, dry skin, alopecia, and impaired barrier function [13, 29]. Vitamin E is a critical antioxidant involved in maintenance of cell membrane stability [30, 31]. Deficiency of vitamin E may result in cutaneous lipid disorders such as steatitis [32].

### 13.4.5 Minerals

Zinc is a key component of a number of enzymes, particularly those associated with DNA replication, making it an essential requirement for rapidly dividing cells – including skin cells [13]. It is also required for biosynthesis of fatty acids and normal inflammatory and immune function. Zinc deficiency, either as a result of dietary insufficiency or genetic abnormality in zinc metabolism, often results in dermatoses [33–36]. Secondary skin infections are common in cases of zinc-deficient dermatoses [13].

## 13.5 Chapter Summary

- Normal skin microbiota facilitates functions such as modulating the innate immune response and preventing the colonization of pathobionts
- The skin consists of epithelial cells, immune cells, and microbes offering multiple layers of protection, covering a large surface area, and is constantly exposed to possible allergens, toxins, and pathogens
- Multiple factors influence the skin microbiome including genetics, environment, microbial imbalances or dysbiosis in the gut microbiome, and the status of both gut and skin barrier function
- Dysregulation in the immune system, nutritional deficiencies and gut dysbiosis may all contribute to skin barrier defects

- Atopic dermatitis is the result of a genetic tendency or predisposition to develop an exaggerated immune response against diverse antigens
- Multiple dietary factors can help support skin healthy, including nutritional support of the gut microbiome
- Further research is needed in the relationship between cutaneous microbiomes and skin health

## References

**1** Hoffmann, A., Patterson, A.P., Diesel, A. et al. (2014). The skin microbiome in healthy and allergic dogs. *PLoS One* 9 (1): e83197.

**2** Ross, A., Müller, K.M., Weese, J.S. et al. (2018). Comprehensive skin microbiome analysis reveals the uniqueness of human skin and evidence for phylosymbiosis within the class mammalia. *Proceedings of the National Academy of Sciences of the United States of America* 115 (25): E5786–E5795.

**3** Mauldin, E. and Peters-Kennedy, J. (2016). Integumentary system. In: *Jubb, Kennedy, and Palmer's Pathology of Domestic Animals* (ed. M. Maxie), 509–736. St Louis, Missouri: Elsevier.

**4** Uberoi, A., Bartow-McKenney, C., Zheng, Q. et al. (2021). Commensal microbiota regulates skin barrier function and repair via signaling through the aryl hydrocarbon receptor. *Cell Host & Microbe* 29: 1235–1248.

**5** Chen, Y., Fischbach, M., and Belkaid, Y. (2018). Skin microbiota-host interactions. *Nature* 553: 427–436.

**6** Tizard, I. and Jones, S. (2018). The microbiota regulates immunity and immunologic diseases in dogs and cats. *Veterinary Clinics of North America: Small Animal Practice* 48: 307–322.

**7** Older, C., Diesel, A., Patterson, A.P. et al. (2017). The feline skin microbiota: the bacteria inhabiting the skin of healthy and allergic cats. *PLoS One* 12 (6): e0178555.

**8** Saijonmaa-Koulumies, L. and Lloyd, D. (1996). Colonization of the canine skin with bacteria. *Veterinary Dermatology* 7: 153–162.

**9** Meason-Smith, C., Diesel, A., Patterson, A.P. et al. (2015). What is living on your dog's skin? Characterization of the canine cutaneous mycobiota and fungal dysbiosis in canine allergic dermatitis. *FEMS Microbiology Ecology* 91: fiv139.

**10** Meason-Smith, C., Diesel, A., Patterson, A.P. et al. (2017). Characterization of the cutaneous mycobiota in healthy and allergic cats using next generation sequencing. *Veterinary Dermatology* 28: 71–83.

**11** Older, C., Diesel, A.B., Lawhon, S.D. et al. (2019). The feline cutaneous and oral microbiota are influenced by breed and environment. *PLoS One* 14 (7): e0220463.

**12** Cuscó, A., Belanger, J.M., Gershony, L. et al. (2017). Individual signatures and environmental factors shape skin microbiota in healthy dogs. *Microbiome* 5: 139.

**13** Watson, T. (1998). Diet and skin disease in dogs and cats. *Journal of Nutrition* 128: 2783S–2789S.

**14** Jergens, A. (2002). Understanding gastrointestinal inflammation — implications for therapy. *Journal of Feline Medicine and Surgery* 4: 179–182.

**15** Verlinden, A., Hesta, M., Millet, S. et al. (2006). Food allergy in dogs and cats: a review. *Critical Reviews in Food Science and Nutrition* 46: 259–273.

**16** Weese, J. (2013). The canine and feline skin microbiome in health and disease. *Advances in Veterinary Dermatology* 24 (1): 137–e31.

**17** Olivry, T., DeBoer, D.J., Favrot, C. et al. (2010). Treatment of canine atopic dermatitis: 2010 clinical practice guidelines from the international task force on canine atopic dermatitis. *Veterinary Dermatology* 21: 233–248.

**18** Polizopoulou, Z., Kazakos, G., Patsikas, M.N. et al. (2005). Hypervitaminosis a in the cat: a case report and review of the literature. *Journal of Feline Medicine and Surgery* 7: 363–368.

**19** Eyerich, S., Eyerich, K., Traidi-Hoffman, C. et al. (2018). Cutaneous barriers and skin immunity: differentiating a connected network. *Trends in Immunology* 39 (4): 315–327.

**20** Gutowska-Owsiak, D., Podobas, E.I., Eggeling, C. et al. (2020). Addressing differentiation in live human keratinocytes by assessment of membrane packing order. *Frontiers in Cell and Development Biology* 8: 573230.

**21** Chermprapai, S., Podobas, E.I., Eggeling, C. et al. (2019). The bacterial and fungal microbiome of the skin of healthy dogs and dogs with atopic dermatitis and the impact of topical antimicrobial therapy, an exploratory study. *Veterinary Microbiology* 229: 90–99.

**22** Craig, J. (2016). Atopic dermatitis and the intestinal microbiota in humans and dogs. *Veterinary Medicine and Science* 2: 95–105.

**23** Barko, P., McMichael, M.A., Swanson, K.S. et al. (2018). The gastrointestinal microbiome: a review. *Journal of Veterinary Internal Medicine* 32: 9–25.

**24** Bradley, C., Morris, D.O., Rankin, S.C. et al. (2016). Longitudinal evaluation of the skin microbiome and association with microenvironment and treatment in canine atopic dermatitis. *Journal of Investigative Dermatology* 136: 1182–1190.

**25** NRC (2006). *Nutrient Requirements of Dogs and Cats*. Washington, DC: National Research Council.

**26** Bauer, J. (2011). Therapeutic use of fish oils in companion animals. *Journal of the American Veterinary Medical Association* 239 (11): 1441–1451.

**27** Propst, E., Flickinger, E.A., Bauer, L.L. et al. (2003). A dose-response experiment evaluating the effects of oligofructose and inulin on nutrient digestibility, stool quality, and fecal protein catabolites in healthy adult dogs. *Journal of Animal Science* 81 (12): 3057–3066.

**28** Perini, M., Rentas, M.F., Pedreira, R. et al. (2020). Duration of prebiotic intake is a key-factor for diet-induced modulation of immunity and fecal fermentation products in dogs. *Microorganisms* 8: 1916.

**29** Blanchard, P., Bai, S.C., Rogers, Q.R. et al. (1991). Pathology associated with vitamin b-6 deficiency in growing kittens. *Journal of Nutrition* 121: S77–S78.

**30** Van Vleet, J. (1975). Experimentally induced vitamin e-selenium deficiency in the growing dog. *Journal of the American Veterinary Medical Association* 166 (8): 769–774.

**31** Piercy, R., Hinchcliff, K.W., Morley, P.S. et al. (2001). Vitamin e and exertional rhabdomyolysis during endurance sled dog racing. *Neuromuscular Disorders* 11: 278–286.

**32** Niza, M., Vilela, C., and Ferreira, L. (2003). Feline pansteatitis revisited: hazards of unbalanced home-made diets. *Journal of Feline Medicine and Surgery* 5: 271–277.

**33** White, S., Bourdeau, P., Rosychuk, R.A.W. et al. (2001). Zinc-responsive dermatosis in dogs: 41 cases and literature review. *Veterinary Dermatology* 12: 101–109.

**34** Cummings, J. and Kovacic, J. (2009). The ubiquitous role of zinc in health and disease. *Journal of Veterinary Emergency and Critical Care* 19 (3): 215–240.

**35** Rolles, B., Maywald, M., and Rink, L. (2018). Influence of zinc deficiency and supplementation on nk cell cytotoxicity. *Journal of Functional Foods* 48: 322–328.

**36** Usama, U., Khan, M., and Fatima, S. (2018). Role of zinc in shaping the gut microbiome; proposed mechanisms and evidence from the literature. *Journal of Gastrointestinal & Digestive System* 8 (1): https://doi.org/10.4172/2161-069X.1000548.

# 14

# Hepatic Circulation and Bile Acid Involvement with Microbiomes

Bile has been historically acknowledged as playing a major role in health status. In approximately 400 BCE, Hippocrates developed the concept of humorism that had four pillars of health known as "humors" (blood, yellow bile, black bile, and phlegm) [1]. In this concept, balanced pillars are equated to health while imbalances in any of the pillars would reveal illness [1]. Bile is a complex aqueous secretion consisting of ~95% water and bile salts, bilirubin, phospholipid, cholesterol, amino acids, steroids, enzymes, porphyrins, vitamins, and heavy metals, along with exogenous drugs, xenobiotics (foreign substances), and environmental toxins [2]. The GI microbiota's role in bile acid metabolism has been known for decades though we are continuing to discover how this relationship is able to manipulate health status [3]. Research is revealing that GI microbiota are a major mediator of bile acid chemistry, with diseases such as diabetes, cirrhosis, inflammatory bowel disease, and cancer being linked to alterations in the normal chemistry of secondary bile acids [1].

## 14.1 Hepatic Circulation and Bile Acid Metabolism

While the hepatic circulation and bile acid recycling system are complex, in its simplest form we can summarize bile, consisting of a variety of organic and inorganic solutes [2], is created in the liver, stored in the gallbladder, and released into the intestines with multiple chemical

*Small Animal Microbiomes and Nutrition*, First Edition. Robin Saar and Sarah Dodd.
© 2024 John Wiley & Sons, Inc. Published 2024 by John Wiley & Sons, Inc.
Companion website: www.wiley.com/go/saar/1e

reactions occurring, followed by the metabolites of these reactions being absorbed through the intestinal epithelium to be utilized by the body, or flowing into the portosystemic system, recycling the chemically altered components back to the liver.

## 14.1.1 Primary Bile Acids

A well-known primary function of this system involves cholesterol being degraded in the liver into primary bile acids [4, 5]. Primary bile acids may differ between species. The two major primary bile acids in humans, dogs, and cats are cholic acid (CA) and chenodeoxycholic acid (CDCA) [6, 7]. In mice, muricholic acid and in pigs, hyocholic acid are the primary bile acids. Primary bile acids are also involved in energy metabolism due to their interaction with G-protein-coupled bile acid receptor (TGR-5) activation and release of glucagon-like peptide-1 (GLP-1) [8].

### 14.1.1.1 Conjugation of Primary Bile Acids

Within the hepatocyte, primary bile acids may be conjugated with an amino acid: glycine, taurine, glucuronic acid, and sulfates, with bile acids bound to glycine and taurine being referred to as bile salts [1, 5, 9]. Conjugated primary bile acids are excreted into the biliary canaliculi which set up an osmotic gradient, pulling water into bile and driving bile flow through a series of ducts (biliary tree) where it is released into the lumen or directed into the gallbladder [9]. The result of conjugation is the development of bile salts becoming a stronger acid, limiting their passive reabsorption as they pass through the biliary tree in the liver [2]. Additionally, the conjugated bile salts become water-soluble, enabling them to emulsify fats [9].

## 14.1.2 The Function of the Gallbladder and Micelles

The gallbladder allows for the storage and concentration of bile to be later secreted into the duodenum upon the ingestion of nutrients [5, 10, 11]. There, they interact with fat to form micellar structures and facilitate absorption of fat into enterocytes [12]. The formation of micelles greatly reduces the toxic detergent effects the bile salts have on the epithelium, while the detergent properties facilitate lipid absorption in the intestines [2].

### 14.1.3    Recycling of Bile Acids

The enterohepatic circulation of bile acids is very efficient with primary conjugated bile acids being absorbed by active transport in the ileum at >90% absorption [1, 5]. The intestinal bile acid transporter is the receptor that drives this uptake, and in dogs, it is primarily expressed in the ileum, cecum, and colon [5]. Once absorbed, bile acids move into the portal blood system circulating back to the liver with >95% being extracted by the hepatocyte for re-conjugation and re-secretion into the bile [1, 5, 10]. The relative amounts of bile-salt-dependent and bile-salt-independent canalicular flow and cholangiocyte secretion are very species-specific and are highly regulated by hormones, second messengers, and signal transduction pathways, with many determinants of bile secretion now characterized at the molecular level in animal models [11]. Being the primary pathway for cholesterol catabolism, bile acids account for approximately 50% of the daily volume of cholesterol [10]. Once synthesized in the liver, humans produce and secrete approximately 0.5 g of bile acids per day. The total amount of bile acids cycling through the body (bile acid pool) consists of primary and secondary bile acids approximately 3 g of bile acids [10] (Figure 14.1).

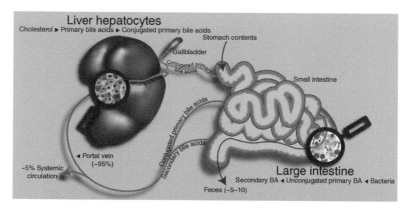

**Figure 14.1**    Recycling of bile acids. *Source:* George Andrew Abernathy, https://orcid.org/0000-0002-1336-3631, last accessed 8 December 2022 / Licensed under CC0 license.

### 14.1.4 Secondary Bile Acids

The remaining 5–10% of primary conjugated bile acids, which have not been absorbed in the small intestine, undergo a variety of microbial-mediated transformations in the large intestine into more hydrophobic molecules that enable them to be reabsorbed by passive diffusion across cell membranes [13]. This is completed by bile salt hydrolases (hydrolyze the amide bond), followed by transforming the now primary deconjugated bile acids into secondary bile acids, lithocholic acid (dehydroxylated chenodeoxycholic acid), and deoxycholic acid (dehydroxylated cholic acid) [1] mainly by 7α-dehydroxylation. While deconjugation reactions are completed by a broad spectrum of colonic bacteria, the 7α-dehydroxylation process is only completed by a limited number of intestinal bacteria [3]. In the recycling process, the remaining 5–10% of bile acids are either absorbed passively in the colon or excreted in the feces [1].

## 14.2 Microbiota's Role in Bile Acid Metabolism

There have been four distinct pathways related to microbial transformations of bile acids deconjugation, dehydroxylation, oxidation, and epimerization [1]. Re-conjugation is another pathway that has been more recently identified [1]. These pathways alter the molecules at different junctions with some pathways requiring multiple chemicals reducing actions [1].

### 14.2.1 Deconjugation

Deconjugation is the hydrolysis of bile salts into primary bile acid and amino acid, usually glycine or taurine [9]. This reaction dramatically alters the physicochemical properties of the bile acids, resulting in them being more lipophilic and partially protonated. This enables the products to be further metabolized by dehydroxylases and epimerases [13].

Bile salt hydrolases encoding genes have been listed in GI microbes including species belonging to the genera *Bacteroides*, *Clostridium*, *Lactobacillus*, and *Bifidobacterium*, with the most diversity found in the phylum *Firmicutes* [3]. The ability for enzymes to be capable of catalyzing this reaction across all major phyla suggests that the encoding genes are horizontally transferable [1]. Bile salt hydrolysis is completed by both gram-positive (*Bifidobacterium*, *Lactobacillus*, *Clostridium*, *Enterococcus*, and *Listeria*) and gram-negative (*Stenotrophomonas*, *Bacteroides*, and *Brucella*) bacteria in the GI tract [1]. In humans, approximately 26% of identified strains of GI microbiota are capable of bile salt hydrolysis [1].

Bile activity deconjugation may provide carbon, nitrogen, and sulfur to GI microbes, though some of the possible compounds (hydrogen sulfide) may have lasting health consequences as it increases colonocyte turnover and has been associated with inflammation and cancer [3]. Joyce et al. [14] proposed that bile salt hydrolysis has the capacity to profoundly alter host functions, particularly local (gastrointestinal) and systemic (hepatic) systems based on studies completed in mice [14]. A neutral to slightly acidic GI pH of 5–7 results in optimal bile salt hydrolysis activity [1].

### 14.2.2 Dehydroxylation

Dehydroxylation is the conversion of primary bile acid cholic acid to secondary deoxycholic acid or primary chenodeoxycholic acid to secondary lithocholic acid by 7α-dehydroxylases. This requires seven enzymes to complete eight catalytic reactions and is completed by species from the genera *Eubacterium* and *Clostridium* [3]. *One* enzyme capable of dehydroxylation, BaiE, is highly conserved (has remained relatively unchanged) structurally between *Clostridium scindens*, *Clostridium hylemonae*, and *Clostridium hiranonis* [1]. *Clostridium hiranonis* is a main microbiota that converts primary bile acids into secondary bile acids. When this microbiota is depleted, there is an increase in primary bile acids. This low level of fecal secondary bile acids is a common finding in many chronic inflammatory enteropathies [12].

### 14.2.3 Oxidation and Epimerization

Epimerization of bile acids is carried out by gut microbes and occurs in two distinct steps: oxidation of the hydroxyl group, followed by reduction, with reactions carried out by the same organism or cocultures of microbes [1]. Some microbes are able to complete oxidation at multiple (1–3) hydroxyl positions. When bile acids are oxidized, their ability to be amphipathic (a molecule that possesses both hydrophobic and hydrophilic elements) is decreased, which decreases their ability to act as a detergent. This prevents bile acids from being able to damage cell membranes [1].

### 14.2.4 Re-Conjugation

A 2021 study by Quinn et al. revealed that gut microbiota are also involved in the re-conjugation of amino acids with bile acids [15]. Unlike compounds conjugated within the hepatocyte, microbiota-conjugated compounds are bound with the amino acids phenylalanine, leucine, and tyrosine on a cholic acid backbone. *Enterocloster bolteae,* formerly *Clostridium bolteae,* was the identified species that are able to create microbially conjugated bile acids. The primary function of these compounds is to dissolve fat in the diet, which may result in a change in the bile acids' emulsifying properties [1] (Figure 14.2).

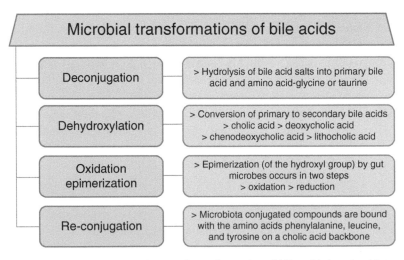

**Figure 14.2** Four main pathways of transformation of bile acids by microbiota.

## 14.3 Bile and Bile Acids Fundamental Roles in the Regulation of Various Physiological Systems

### 14.3.1 Digestion

Bile acids act as emulsifiers and create micelles [9, 10]. By acting as a functional biological detergent they allow water and fat to mix creating micelles [9]. This action promotes the intestinal absorption of nutrients including lipids and fat-soluble vitamins [9, 10]. Lipids are normally water-insoluble; once emulsified, lipase enzymes can be functional in digesting lipids and bringing them close to the intestine's brush border, augmenting lipid and fat-soluble vitamin absorption [3, 6, 9].

### 14.3.2 Metabolism

Bile salts aid in the metabolism of cholesterol, lipid, and glucose [1, 3]. They are active in gut metabolism by powering bile flow to remove various metabolites like bilirubin [1, 9].

### 14.3.3 Cell Signaling

Hormonally, bile salts act on the farnesoid X receptor (FXR) and G-protein-coupled bile acid receptor Gpbar1 (TGR5) receptors [9]. FXR-mediated pathways signal molecules regulating hepatic-glucose metabolism [8]. Additionally, many hormones and pheromones are excreted in bile and contribute to the growth and development of the intestine in some species [2].

### 14.3.4 Microbiome Composition

Bile acids are toxic for bacterial cells and thus they are able to influence the GI microbial density and diversity [3].

### 14.3.5 Immune Homeostasis

The host is protected from enteric infections by excreting immune globulin A (IgA), inflammatory cytokines, and stimulating the innate immune system in the intestine [2]. Leukotrienes, their metabolites, along with other inflammatory cytokines, appear in bile [2]. For example, tumor necrosis factor (TNF)-α is synthesized in bile duct epithelial cells [2].

### 14.3.6 Exogenous and Endogenous Substrate Disposal

This action aids in the removal of foreign or toxic substances, lipophilic substances (cholesterol), and bilirubin and bile salts that are not excreted by the kidney [2, 6].

### 14.3.7 Circulatory System Support

Bile is an essential component of the cholehepatic and enterohepatic circulation [2].

## 14.4 Nutrients in Bile

### 14.4.1 Fats (Cholesterol)

Cholesterol is the predominant sterol and phosphatidylcholine is a major phospholipid found in bile and is the major route of elimination for cholesterol from the body [2]. Neutral lipids (diglycerides, triglycerides) or acidic lipids (fatty acids) are not normally found in bile in large quantities [2].

### 14.4.2 Proteins

Many proteins, peptides, and amino acids are found in bile [2]. Individual amino acids are partially recovered from the bile by specific amino acid transporters that line the luminal membrane of the bile duct epithelium (46, 388) [2]. A study in humans revealed that an animal-based diet rapidly altered the GM, increasing the number of bile-tolerant anaerobes such as *Bacteroides*, *Alistipes,* and *Bilophila* along with decreasing the number of Firmicutes [16].

Proteomic analysis is still being developed with multiple barriers making the analysis of the bile proteome very difficult [2].

### 14.4.3 Vitamins

Bile also delivers vitamins to the intestine. The vitamin D metabolite, 25-hydroxyvitamin D, is first formed in the hepatocytes. In newborns, these metabolites may function in intestinal growth and development, and in adults they function in calcium homeostasis [2]. Folic acid, pyridoxine, and cobalamin also enter the intestine via the bile.

### 14.4.4 Other

Some solutes have the bile component absorbed by the bile duct epithelium prior to being released into the intestine. This can be seen with both glucose and phosphate solutes [2]. Steroid hormones, estrogens, prolactin, and insulin are other important substances that are excreted in bile. Bile also provides the pathway for the excretion of pheromones [2].

## 14.5 Liver–Gut–Brain Axis

There is a complex and bidirectional relationship between host to microbiota interactions and bile acids impact on intestinal physiology [8, 13]. Communication between the gut and liver are through the portal vein, biliary tract, and systemic circulation. Alterations in GI microbiota composition affect the diversity of microbiota that create intestinal products; this results in an alteration in the type and volume of metabolites and signaling molecules, resulting in changes in pathways affecting neurological, hepatic, and GI systems [3, 17]. Disruptions in the bile acid – microbial crosstalk have been associated with several gastrointestinal, metabolic, and inflammatory disorders; this also includes some diseases that have been associated with age-related decline [3]. A diseased liver is unable to effectively inhibit the overgrowth of bacteria and remove any harmful microbial by-products, with liver damage being closely related to the severity of gut dysbiosis. Knowing the role that the gut–brain axis has the role of the liver in the gut–brain axis cannot be ignored, especially in liver diseases where the microbiota–gut–liver–brain axis is considered to be a typical model, such as in hepatic encephalopathy [17].

GI microbiota can produce bioactive peptides, including neurotransmitters, secondary bile acid conversion, short-chain fatty acids (SCFAs), branched-chain amino acids, and intestinal hormones, which are signals for the gut–brain axis [2]. For example, SCFAs enter the circulatory system and send signals to the brain via the gut–brain axis [2]. Bile acids can affect multiple pathways by inducing cellular responses through recruiting "non-bile acid" receptors, in addition to binding and activating normal bile-acid-associated receptors [11]. A couple of examples of influential responses are TGR5's ability to transactivate epidermal growth factor receptor influencing pathways to regulate cell growth including hepatocytes, enterocytes, and pancreatic epithelial cells, and the ability to control the movement of proteins on and off cell surfaces by regulating endocytosis [11]. This bidirectional communication influences the immunological system. IgA is a major protein in bile that contributes to immunological surveillance within the biliary system [2].

The occurrence and development of many diseases are mediated by the microbiota–gut–liver–brain axis. Alterations in the microbiota and their ability to participate in physiological functions of the GI and hepatic systems result in diseases associated with inflammation such as irritable bowel syndrome, inflammatory bowel disease, functional dyspepsia, cirrhosis, and hepatic encephalopathy [17]. Mental illness is also associated with many GI- and hepatic-related disorders in humans with psychotherapy and psychotropic medications being associated with a multifocal treatment in human patients [17] (Figure 14.3).

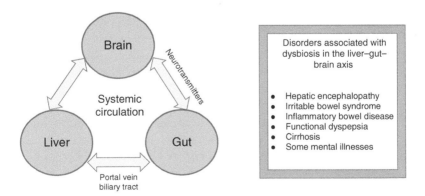

**Figure 14.3** Liver–gut–brain axis (simplified) and associated disorders when there is dysbiosis of the microbiota.

Various chronic liver diseases at the end stage are generally classified as cirrhosis [17]. Clinically human patients will experience portal hypertension, decreased liver function, with a measurable correlation between changes in the microbiome and disease progression [17]. Bacterial translocation is observed in hepatic encephalopathy, spontaneous bacterial peritonitis, and other infections [17]. Changes in the microbiota–gut–liver–brain axis are closely related to the progression of cirrhosis with specific gut microbes being associated with changes in neurons and synaptic functions that cause brain dysfunction associated with cirrhosis [17].

Hepatic encephalopathy is well known in dogs and cats and can manifest as a wide range of neurological abnormalities [17, 18]. Previous studies have indicated its development is due to increases in harmful microbial by-products such as ammonia, indole, oxindole, and endotoxin, with the diseased liver unable to clear the increased level of toxic metabolites [17, 18]. Pathogenesis of hepatic encephalopathy also includes inflammation (systemic or local), leaky gut, bacterial translocation, and overgrowth of small intestinal bacteria [17, 18].

## 14.6 Bile Acid Dysmetabolism

Disruptions in the efficiency of the bile acid recycling system can affect multiple physiological systems. Both the excretion of bile acids into the canaliculi and movement of bile acids from the portal blood involve energy-dependent pumps, which can be disrupted in a variety of conditions including cholestasis from obstruction or inflammation (cytokine-mediated) [5]. Malabsorption of bile acids leads to a disruption of the enterohepatic loop, resulting in a change in the production and excretion of more primary bile acids into the lumen where they can have secretory effects [12]. In humans with inflammatory bowel disease, the apical sodium-bile-acid transporter in the ileum is destroyed, which leads to decreased reabsorption of bile acids in the small intestine. Increases in primary bile acids in the colon cause secretory or a type of watery diarrhea. Glucocorticoids can potentially reduce this type of bile acid malabsorption as they induce the expression of ASBT in the small intestine [12]. In dogs with chronic intestinal inflammation, the intestinal bile acid transporter is downregulated, which leads to an increased loss of primary bile acids in the feces [5].

Microbiome composition may be altered through multiple means including diet, antibiotic therapy, and bile acid antimicrobial action where GI microbiota cell membranes are destroyed by the detergent properties of the primary bile acids. This function in normal function prevents bacterial overgrowth in the GI tract [16]. Fluctuations in the volume of primary bile acids will alter the density of the microbiome. This change in microbiome composition can have a domino effect on the bile recycling system [8].

1) These changes in the microbiome composition led to changes in bile acid metabolism and may affect the level of different bile acids in the colon [13]. Some liver-related disorders have been related to different intestinal microbial patterns where altered liver–microbiota–bile acid crosstalk has been identified. This may result in higher ratios between primary and secondary bile acids in feces and conjugated and unconjugated bile acids in serum in disease-affected patients [3]. Early studies are suggesting that the dysbiosis observed in chronic enteropathies also leads to a decrease in bacterial species with 7α-dehydroxylation activity [12].

2) Changes in metabolite production, which disrupt normal physiological functions. For example, changes in the fermentation resulting in a change in the production of lactate may lead to bile acid diarrhea [12]. A recent study in cats with various gastrointestinal disorders showed an increased serum D-lactate concentration, where normally, this form of lactic acid is not found in any appreciable quantities in serum from mammals [16]. GI microbial dysbiosis may lead to increased bacterial production of D-lactate with increased risks to health as D-lactate has been shown to lead to neurological signs in some cats [12]. There are more recent studies utilizing metabolomics where several hundred metabolites are measured in serum or feces of dogs with GI disease. In one study, the serum metabolite profile of dogs with idiopathic inflammatory bowel disease was analyzed with serum concentrations of metabolites associated with the pentose phosphate pathway were significantly more abundant in dogs with IBD. These indicate the presence of oxidative stress in dogs with IBD. More, importantly, the metabolic profiles did not normalize after 3 weeks of therapy, suggesting the persistence of intestinal inflammation despite improved clinical symptoms. Another recent study found significant

alterations in various metabolic pathways such as altered SCFA metabolism (decreased propionate), altered bile acid metabolism, altered glycolysis pathways, and altered tryptophan-indole pathways in dogs with inflammatory bowel disease. However, more in-depth studies evaluating additional metabolites are needed [12].

3) Alterations to the hydrophobicity to/hydrophilicity (ability to repel or attract water) ratio of the colonic bile acid pool [13].

4) A reduction in bile metabolizing microbiota will impair bile acid metabolism, affecting host metabolic pathways [3]. This results in altered bile acid signaling events through activation of receptors FXR and TGR5 in metabolically active tissues [8]. This may alter hepatic glucose and lipid metabolism, and cause metabolic dysregulation [3, 8]. Changes in bile acid metabolism have been observed in humans with diabetes, which may affect the ability to control blood glucose levels [8].

5) Alterations in nutrient absorption may be affected when transport systems are impaired during bile duct injury or when excessive amounts of the bile are released into the intestine [2].

6) Microbial contributions to disease pathogenesis through other mechanisms such as increased intestinal permeability, contributing to a chronic pro-inflammatory state, and increase energy intake [3].

7) An increase in the presence of unconjugated bile acids which are toxic to epithelial cells. This may result in increased intestinal permeability (Figure 14.4).

## 14.6.1 Diseases Associated with Bile Acid Dysmetabolism

### 14.6.1.1 Aging

While not a disease, aging may cause microbial shifts resulting in alterations in bile acid metabolism [3]. For example, old mice with an increase in fecal deconjugated bile acids have been associated with a shift toward a pro-inflammatory state in the GI microbiome. In mice models looking at Alzheimer's disease, a decrease in cholic acid with an increase in secondary bile acids through 7α-dehydroxylase is observed along with an increase in microbiota in the *Clostridium* group who are able of completing this type of dehydroxylation [3]. Similarly, fasting serum in obese humans contains decreased primary bile acids and increased secondary bile acid concentrations [8].

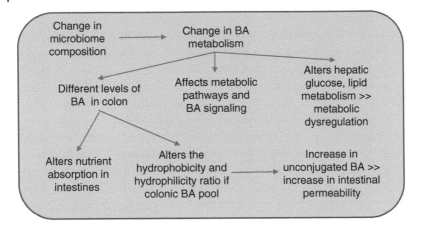

**Figure 14.4** Domino effect on the bile recycling system that occurs when there are changes in the GI microbiome.

### 14.6.1.2 Diabetes Mellitus

Diabetes mellitus is also associated with dysbiosis and bile acid dysmetabolism. An increase in Gram-negative bacteria increases lipopolysaccharide absorption, which may modulate inflammatory activity in the host [8]. High-fat diets in dogs where 75% of the total energy is coming from dietary fat sources has resulted in changes in fecal bile acid concentrations [8]. In a 7-week study with dogs fed a high-fat/low-fiber diet, there was an increased fecal concentration of both secondary bile acids deoxycholic acid (DCA), and ursodeoxycholic acid (UDCA), along with a significant increase in the *Clostridiaceae* family, who are adept in converting primary bile acids to secondary bile acids [8].

Secondary bile acids (deoxycholic acid and lithocholic acid) have both pro and anticancer activity [19]. In humans, bile acids are associated with colorectal cancer through four mechanisms:

1) High concentrations of bile acids cause epithelial cell destruction, initiating inflammatory reactions, which could transition into a precancerous state.
2) The induction of reactive oxygen species and reactive nitrogen species results in damaged DNA and repairs pathway disruptions.
3) Chronic exposure to bile acids, colonocytes become resistant to normal death cycles allowing for mutation of cells into cancer cells.
4) Bile acids regulate gene expression toward tumor development [19, 20].

#### 14.6.1.3 Bile Acid Diarrhea

Bile acid diarrhea is becoming recognized as a frequent cause of diarrhea in humans. This class of diarrhea has been described to have four possible causes [12].

1) Type 1 – Bile Acid Malabsorption. Observed post ileal resection or with GI inflammatory disorders resulting in bile acid malabsorption, and diarrhea [12].
2) Type 2 – Idiopathic Bile Acid Malabsorption. This dysfunction may be associated with an ileal hormone fibroblast growth factor 19, which causes a disruption in the feedback system for hepatic bile synthesis [12].
3) Type 3 – Disease-Associated Bile Acid Diarrhea. This disorder occurs secondary to various GI diseases. Examples include small intestinal dysbiosis, celiac disease, chronic pancreatitis, and radiation enteropathy [12].
4) Dysbiosis – Dysbiosis that leads to a decrease in bacterial species that complete 7α-dehydroxylation activity results in a change in bile acid metabolism [12]. There is a significant increase in fecal primary bile acids and a significant decrease in secondary bile acids compared to healthy controls in studies [12]. Preliminary data from dogs with chronic enteropathy suggest there is impaired bacterial conversion from primary to secondary bile acids [12]. A correlation has been observed between an increase in the dysbiosis index and bile acid dysmetabolism, with bile acid malabsorption being clinically relevant in dogs with chronic diarrhea [12].

## 14.7 Key Nutritional Factors

Diet plays a vital role in regulating the intestinal environment, which has been shown to alter hepatic function. While further research is needed there may be some nutritional approaches that could benefit pets with hepatic disease and associated disorders.

### 14.7.1 Water

The consumption of water has been shown to induce gallbladder contraction and emptying [21].

### 14.7.2 Fat

Dietary fat increases the synthesis and the volume of bile acids that reach the colon, which may result in an increase in the synthesis of secondary bile acids which may be proinflammatory, increasing the pathogenesis of several gastrointestinal diseases [3]. Fat tends to cause a decrease in diversity in the microbiome influencing metabolite production. High-fat diets should be avoided in pets with diarrhea and GI dysbiosis.

### 14.7.3 Protein

The source of protein offered may alter the variety of microbes in the GI tract. A study in humans showed that an animal-based diet rapidly altered the GI microbiome, increasing the number of bile-tolerant microorganisms (*Bilophila wadsworthia* and *Bacteroides*) while decreasing the number of *Firmicutes* [16]. Protein catabolism increases ammonia levels, and recommendations in pets with hepatic encephalopathy have been to limit protein intake. New studies have shown that normal protein intake is well tolerated by humans with hepatic encephalopathy [18]. The source of protein may play a role in the volume the pet can tolerate with a high-protein, high-calorie diet based on casein-vegetable significantly reducing blood ammonia level and mental status of humans with hepatic encephalopathy [22]. Hydrolyzed diets may prove to be beneficial for pets with hepatic encephalopathy as oral supplementation of branched-chain amino acids produces a nutritional effect on cirrhosis and reduces the risk of recurrence of hepatic encephalopathy [23].

### 14.7.4 Carbohydrates

Nonabsorbable disaccharides (lactulose and lactol) can treat and prevent overt hepatic encephalopathy and significantly improve the recovery rate of minimal hepatic encephalopathy [17]. While it is commonly known to have a laxative effect, a reduction in ammonia production, having a prebiotic effect regulating GI microbiota and improving cognitive function by enhancing neuroplasticity are other mechanisms of nonabsorbable disaccharides [17].

## 14.7.5 Fiber

Fiber is a well-known source of nutrition for some generally considered beneficial GI microbial species. Oligosaccharides are fast fermenters that enhance the growth rate of bacteria. *Bifidobacteria* produce SCFA during fermentation that decreases intestinal pH, which may improve the ability for deconjugation to occur, along with inhibiting the growth of pathogenic bacteria. Fructooligosaccharides (FOS) in particular are known to reduce fasting blood glucose, cholesterol, and low-density lipoprotein levels in people with diabetes [24].

## 14.7.6 Probiotics

Probiotics can provide some benefit to patients experiencing hepatic disease and secondary disorders as they inhibit the excessive growth of pathogenic bacteria; competitively exclude pathogens; strengthen the intestinal barrier; enhance host immunity; increase the production of IgA; regulate the production of cytokines, produce, or secrete SCFAs; and promote the absorption of ions and trace elements [17]. The specific strain is important in creating the desired effect. In one study, the probiotic *Lactobacillus rhamnosus GG* (LGG) increases beneficial bacteria in the distal small intestine, restores the intestinal barrier function, reduces liver inflammation and steatosis, and exerts protective effects on mice with fatty liver caused by a high-fructose diet [25]. However, another study found that dietary supplementation of *Lactococcus lactis* subspecies *cremoris* was more effective than dietary supplementation of LGG in reducing liver fat and inflammation development in female mice on a high-fat, high-carbohydrate diet [17, 26]. Probiotics that focus on improving mental health or anxiety should also be considered in these cases [17]. Fecal microbial transplant material may additionally be able to provide benefits in this type of dysbiosis. More studies in dogs and cats are needed to validate this form of treatment in bile acid dysmetabolism.

In humans with bile acid diarrhea, the treatment of choice is bile acid sequestrants. The frequency of bowel movements decreased in 38% of human patients with bile acid diarrhea when bile acid sequestrants were administered [12].

## 14.8 Chapter Summary

- Bile is a complex aqueous secretion consisting of ~95% water and bile salts, bilirubin, phospholipid, cholesterol, amino acids, steroids, enzymes, porphyrins, vitamins, and heavy metals, along with exogenous drugs, xenobiotics (foreign substances), and environmental toxins.

- GI microbiota are a major mediator of bile acid chemistry, with diseases such as diabetes, cirrhosis, inflammatory bowel disease, and cancer being linked to alterations in the normal chemistry of secondary bile acids.

- The two major primary bile acids in humans, dogs, and cats are cholic acid (CA) and chenodeoxycholic acid (CDCA).

- The result of conjugation is the development of bile salts becoming a stronger acid, limiting their passive reabsorption as they pass through the biliary tree in the liver.

- Once absorbed, bile acids move into the portal blood system circulating back to the liver with >95% being extracted by the hepatocyte for re-conjugation and re-secretion into the bile.

- There have been four distinct pathways related to microbial transformations of bile acids deconjugation, dehydroxylation, oxidation, and epimerization.

- Re-conjugation is another pathway that has been more recently identified.

- Bile and bile acids fundamental roles in the regulation of various physiological systems.

- Communication between the gut and liver are through the portal vein, biliary tract, and systemic circulation.

- GI microbiota can produce bioactive peptides, including neurotransmitters, secondary bile acid conversion, short-chain fatty acids (SCFAs), branched-chain amino acids, and intestinal hormones, which are signals for the gut–brain axis.

- Microbiome composition may be altered through multiple means including diet, antibiotic therapy, and bile acid antimicrobial action where GI microbiota cell membranes are destroyed by the detergent properties of the primary bile acids.

- Diabetes mellitus is also associated with dysbiosis and bile acid dysmetabolism.
- Dietary fat increases the synthesis and the volume of bile acids that reach the colon, which may result in an increase in the synthesis of secondary bile acids which may be proinflammatory (*Bernstein* et al. *2011*), increasing the pathogenesis of several gastrointestinal diseases.

## References

1 Guzior, D.V. and Quinn, R.A. (2021). Review: microbial transformations of human bile acids. *Microbiome* 9: 140. https://doi.org/10.1186/s40168-021-01101-1.

2 Baloni, P., Funk, C.C., Yan, J. et al. (2020). Metabolic network analysis reveals altered bile acid synthesis and metabolism in Alzheimer's disease. *Cell Reports Medicine* 1 (8): 100138. https://doi.org/10.1016/j.xcrm.2020.100138.

3 Molinero, N., Ruiz, L., and Sánchez, B. (2019). Intestinal bacteria interplay with bile and cholesterol metabolism: implications on host physiology. *Frontiers in Physiology* 10: 185. https://doi.org/10.3389/fphys.2019.00185.

4 Engelking, L. (2015). Bile acids. In: *Textbook of Veterinary Physiological Chemistry*, 3e (ed. L. Engelking), 397–405. Academic Press https://doi.org/10.1016/B978-0-12-391909-0.50062-1.

5 Cheng, H.M., Mah, K.K., and Seluakumaran, K. (2020). Recycling of bile salts: enterohepatic circulation (EHC). In: *Defining Physiology: Principles, Themes, Concepts*, vol. 2. Cham: Springer https://doi.org/10.1007/978-3-030-62285-5_12.

6 Chiang, J.Y.L. (2013). Bile acid metabolism and signaling. *Comprehensive Physiology* 3 (3): 1191–1212. https://doi.org/10.1002/cphy.c120023.

7 Miyazaki, T., Sasaki, S.I., Toyoda, A. et al. (2020). Impaired bile acid metabolism with defectives of mitochondrial-tRNA taurine modification and bile acid taurine conjugation in the taurine depleted cats. *Scientific Reports* 10: 4915. https://doi.org/10.1038/s41598-020-61821-6.

8 Jergens, A.E., Guard, B.C., Redfern, A. et al. (2019). Microbiota-related changes in unconjugated fecal bile acids are associated with naturally occurring, insulin-dependent diabetes mellitus in dogs. *Frontiers in Veterinary Science* 6: 199. 10.3389/fvets.2019.00199.

**9** Staels, B. and Fonseca, V.A. (2009). Bile acids and metabolic regulation: mechanisms and clinical responses to bile acid sequestration. *Diabetes Care* 32 (Suppl 2): S237–S245. https://doi.org/10.2337/dc09-S355.

**10** Ramírez-Pérez, O., Cruz-Ramón, V., Chinchilla-López, P. et al. (2017). The role of the gut microbiota in bile acid metabolism. *Annals of Hepatology* 16 (Suppl 1): S21–S26. https://doi.org/10.5604/01.3001.0010.5672.

**11** Boyer, J.L. (2013). Bile formation and secretion. *Comprehensive Physiology* 3 (3): 1035–1078. https://doi.org/10.1002/cphy.c120027.

**12** Blake, A.B., Guard, B.C., Honneffer, J.B. et al. (2019). Altered microbiota, fecal lactate, and fecal bile acids in dogs with gastrointestinal disease. *PloS One* 14 (10): e0224454. https://doi.org/10.1371/journal.pone.0224454.

**13** Fiorucci, S. and Distrutti, E. (2015). Bile acid-activated receptors, intestinal microbiota, and the treatment of metabolic disorders. *Trends in Molecular Medicine* 21 (11): 702–714. https://doi.org/10.1016/j.molmed.2015.09.001.

**14** Joyce, S.A., MacSharry, J., Casey, P.G. et al. (2014). Regulation of host weight gain and lipid metabolism by bacterial bile acid modification in the gut. *Proceedings of the National Academy of Sciences* 111 (20): 7421–7426. https://doi.org/10.1073/pnas.1323599111.

**15** Quinn, R.A., Melnik, A.V., Vrbanac, A. et al. (2020). Global chemical effects of the microbiome include new bile-acid conjugations. *Nature* 579: 123–129. https://doi.org/10.1038/s41586-020-2047-9.

**16** Singh, R.K., Chang, H.W., Yan, D. et al. (2017). Influence of diet on the gut microbiome and implications for human health. *Journal of Translational Medicine* 15: 73. https://doi.org/10.1186/s12967-017-1175-y.

**17** Ding, J.H., Jin, Z., Yang, X.X. et al. (2020). Role of gut microbiota via the gut-liver-brain axis in digestive diseases. *World Journal of Gastroenterology* 26 (40): 6141–6162. https://doi.org/10.3748/wjg.v26.i40.6141.

**18** Campion, D., Giovo, I., Ponzo, P. et al. (2019). Dietary approach and gut microbiota modulation for chronic hepatic encephalopathy in cirrhosis. *World Journal of Hepatology* 11 (6): 489–512. 10.4254/wjh.v11.i6.489.

**19** Epiphanio, T.M.F. and Santos, A. (2021). Small animals gut microbiome and its relationship with cancer. In: *Canine Genetics, Health and*

*Medicine* (ed. C. Rutland). IntechOpen https://doi.org/10.5772/intechopen.95780.

20 Nguyen, T.T., Ung, T.T., Kim, N.H. et al. (2018). Role of bile acids in colon carcinogenesis. *World Journal of Clinical Cases* 6 (13): 577–588. https://doi.org/10.12998/wjcc.v6.i13.577.

21 Svenberg, T., Christofides, N.D., Fitzpatrick, M.L. et al. (1985). Oral water causes emptying of the human gallbladder through actions of vagal stimuli rather than motilin. *Scandinavian Journal of Gastroenterology* 20 (6): 775–778. https://doi.org/10.3109/00365528509089212.

22 Gheorghe, L., Iacob, R., Vădan, R. et al. (2005). Improvement of hepatic encephalopathy using a modified high-calorie high-protein diet. *Romanian Journal of Gastroenterology* 14 (3): 231–238. PMID 16200232.

23 Amodio, P., Canesso, F., and Montagnese, S. (2014). Dietary management of hepatic encephalopathy revisited. *Current Opinion in Clinical Nutrition and Metabolic Care* 17 (5): 448–452. 10.1097/MCO.0000000000000084.

24 Hand, M.S., Thatcher, C.D., Remillard, R.L. et al. (2010). Macronutrients. In: *Small Animal Clinical Nutrition*, 5e (ed. M.S. Hand et al.), 70. Mark Morris Institute.

25 Ritze, Y., Bárdos, G., Claus, A. et al. (2014). Lactobacillus rhamnosus GG protects against non-alcoholic fatty liver disease in mice. *PloS One* 9 (1): e80169. 10.1371/journal.pone.0080169.

26 Naudin, C.R., Maner-Smith, K., Owens, J.A. et al. (2020). Lactococcus lactis subspecies cremoris elicits protection against metabolic changes induced by a western-style diet. *Gastroenterology* 159 (2): 639–651. e5. 10.1053/j.gastro.2020.03.010.

# 15

# Gastrointestinal Microbiomes

## 15.1 The Gastrointestinal Microbiome

The gastrointestinal (GI) tract of dogs and cats includes the oral cavity, pharynx, esophagus, stomach, duodenum, jejunum, ileum, colon, and rectum. The oral microbiome is discussed in Chapter 11 and will not be included here. Thus, this chapter will cover the microbiome of the tract from the pharynx to the rectum. It bears mentioning that there is vast variation in microbiomes between individual animals, thus a description of a "normal" or "healthy" microbiome that has been determined based on one or more "normal" or "healthy" individuals does not necessarily indicate that a differing microbiome in a different individual is "abnormal" or "unhealthy." The microbiomes of the gastrointestinal tract of the dog and cat are vast and complex systems and we are only just beginning to scratch the surface with our limited understanding of their true nature.

### 15.1.1 The Pharyngeal Microbiome

The pharynx is a relatively unique component of the GI tract with a largely aerobic environment, thanks to the communication of the naso-pharynx, a component of the respiratory tract, and the oropharynx, a component of the GI tract. Indeed, the oropharynx links the mouth, nasopharynx, larynx, lower airways, and the GI tract. However, description of the pharyngeal microbiome is limited even in human research and barely exists for dogs and cats.

*Small Animal Microbiomes and Nutrition*, First Edition. Robin Saar and Sarah Dodd.
© 2024 John Wiley & Sons, Inc. Published 2024 by John Wiley & Sons, Inc.
Companion website: www.wiley.com/go/saar/1e

The shared space of the pharynx thus includes epithelium, mucosa, and microbiota characteristic of both body systems [1]. In humans, the pharyngeal microbiota appear to be comprised of predominantly the same microbial phyla as the respiratory tract – Firmicutes, Actinobacteria, Bacteroidetes, Proteobacteria, and Fusobacteria – though with greater richness and evenness than observed in the rest of the respiratory tract [1]. A high prevalence of *Streptococcus* spp. has been reported, along with *Veillonella, Fusobacterium, Gemella, Granulicatella,* and *Rothia* [2]. In dogs, Bacteroidetes, Firmicutes, Fusobacteria, Proteobacteria, and Pseudomonadota were the phyla most present in the oropharynx, characterized by Pasteurellaceae, Moraxellaceae, and Porphyromona families and genera *Cutibacterium, Streptococcus, Acinetobacter, Brevundimonas,* and *Pseudomonas* [3]. Similar to findings in humans, the oropharyngeal microbiota of dogs appears intermediary between the nasal cavity, with a very strong predominance of Proteobacteria, and the oral cavity, with a less dominant Proteobacteria abundance and more Bacteroidetes, Firmicutes, Actinobacteria, and Fusobacteria [3].

In humans, pathobionts are common in the oropharynx, such as *Streptococcus, Haemophilus,* and *Neisseria* spp., as well as pathogens including *Streptococcus pneumonia, Streptococcus pyogenes, Streptococcus agalactiae, Streptococcus dysgalactiae* subsp. *Equisimilis* [1]. These potential pathogenic organisms contribute to diseases ranging from self-limiting pharyngitis to sepsis and toxic shock syndrome in humans. In dogs, *Streptococcus, Pasteurella, Moraxella, Enterobacteriaceae,* and *Fusobacterium* spp. are common potential pathogens and have all been detected from oropharyngeal swabs [3]. Protection of the host against the potential pathogenic activity of these microbes may be attributable to interaction between microbes within the oropharynx, as well as a healthy and functional mucosal and epithelial barrier, preventing invasion of potentially pathogenic microbes.

## 15.1.2 The Esophageal Microbiome

There is very little research regarding the esophageal microbiome of dogs and cats – even less than for the pharynx. In humans, the esophageal microbiome has been studied largely in relation to esophageal cancer.

In the healthy human esophagus, the population of microbes is markedly reduced in number in comparison to the intestine, measuring at only $10-10^4$ cells/g/ml in the esophagus as compared to $10^{12}$ per g/ml in the large intestine [2]. The microbiota of the esophagus in humans appear to be distinct from that of both the oral cavity and the stomach, supporting the concept that this region of the GI tract harbors its own microbiome and not just a transient population acquired from swallowing microbe-laden ingesta. In humans, the main microbe genera repeatedly identified in the healthy esophagus include *Streptococcus*, *Fusobacterium*, *Prevotella*, and *Veillonella* [2]. Specifically, *Streptococcus* spp. appear to be the dominant genus, with lower proportions of *Prevotella*, *Fusobacterium*, and *Veillonella* [4].

In humans, the majority of esophageal diseases are predominantly attributable to gastroesophageal reflux (GER) [2]. Gastroesophageal reflux is relatively common in dogs [5], though less commonly reported in cats [6]. In humans, alterations in the esophageal microbiota resulting from GER may contribute to metaplasia and progression of chronic esophagitis to esophageal adenocarcinoma [2]. Esophageal dysbiosis associated with metaplasia and adenocarcinoma are characterized by a dysbiotic shift from predominantly Gram-positive taxa, namely Firmicutes, to Gram-negative taxa, including Bacteroidetes, Proteobacteria, and Fusobacteria [2, 4, 7]. Specifically, the presence of *Helicobacter pylori*, *Escherichia coli*, and *Campylobacter* appear to be characteristic of pathogenic changes in the human esophagus [4, 7].

### 15.1.3 The Gastric Microbiome

The acidity of the gastric milieu and presence of gastric pepsin render the stomach an inhospitable environment for many of the microbes inhabiting the rest of the GI tract, indeed the stomach was long considered sterile as a result. The microbial density of the stomach is comparatively low, similar to that of the esophagus, with only around $10^2-10^4$ cells per g [4, 8]. Description of the typical gastric microbiome is sparse, even human studies are mainly related to alterations in the microbiome associated with disease, particularly associations between *H. pylori* and gastric cancer [9]. In humans, infection with *H. pylori* has been strongly associated with reduced microbial diversity and development of gastric disease, including gastritis, gastric ulceration, adenocarcinoma, and lymphoma, though few individuals develop clinical signs, despite an infection prevalence greater than 50% worldwide [9, 10]. In *H. pylori* negative humans, the gastric microbiome appears to be characterized largely by Firmicutes, Actinobacteria, Bacteroidetes, Proteobacteria, and Fusobacteria, in decreasing order, as compared to the *H. pylori* positive gastric microbiome, where over 70% of the microbial population can be comprised by *H. pylori* exclusively.

In dogs and cats, the *Helicobacter* species are the center of some controversy, as infections with *H. pylori* and non-*H. pylori* helicobacters have been detected in dogs and cats both with and without gastric pathology [11, 12]. Indeed, *Helicobacter* spp. may be the most abundant organisms in the typical feline or canine stomach [8, 12]. It has been suggested that *Helicobacter* spp. may be involved in the etiology of gastrointestinal lymphoma in cats [13], while non-*H. pylori* helicobacters have been demonstrated in dogs with gastric inflammation, follicular hyperplasia, erosions, and ulcers [14, 15]. Clinically, in dogs, treatment to eradicate *Helicobacter* may result in improvement in clinical signs, though recurrence of infection is common. At present, the "normal" canine or feline gastric microbiome is not clearly described, and the significance of *Helicobacter* spp. is yet unknown.

### 15.1.4 The Intestinal Microbiome

The intestinal tract (gut), starting from the duodenum and terminating at the rectum, is likely the microbial habitat most investigated with respect to canine and feline microbiota. The intestinal microbiota plays a role in gastrointestinal motility, the development and function of the intestinal epithelium and the immune system, metabolism and defense against pathogens. Thanks to its immense surface area, the gut is the body's largest communication with the extra-corporeal environment. The dog's intestines are about 6 times the length of their body, while that of the cat is about 4 times the length, the surface area of which are greatly enhanced by villi, each also bearing microvilli to the density of about 23 villi per square mm [16]. Within this tract, microbial cells can outnumber host cells 10-fold, with $10^5$–$10^{11}$ cells/g [8, 17]. Microbial abundance and richness increases along the tract from oral to aboral [18]. Additionally, the microbial communities in different sections of the gut are representative of the different environmental niches, based on presence or absence of oxygen, which is relatively abundant in the duodenum and practically absent in the colon, and the nutrient composition of the luminal milieu [18].

Often, fecal microbiota and metabolites are used as a proxy of the intestinal microbiome, but this only reveals a portion of the greater picture. Fecal samples are easy and noninvasive to procure, whereas sampling directly from the intestine itself requires more invasive techniques, such as endoscopy or fistulation performed under general anesthesia, or post mortem collection [19, 20]. Though there is marked variation between individuals and under different conditions, it is generally observed that the canine and feline intestinal microbiota is predominantly composed of bacterial species from five phyla: *Firmicutes, Proteobacteria, Fusobacteria, Bacteroidetes* and *Actinobacteria* [20, 21]. Three dominant phyla: *Fusobacteria, Bacteroidetes*, and *Firmicutes*, account for the majority of microbes detected in canine fecal samples [21], while feline fecal samples appear to be characterized predominantly by *Firmicutes*, followed by smaller representation from *Actinobacteria* and *Proteobacteria* [22] (see Table 15.1). It may seem surprising that such different animals with differing nutritional physiology – the facultatively carnivorous or omnivorous dog in comparison to the obligatorily carnivorous cat – would share the same bacterial phyla, but it must be remember that firstly, each phylum contains multiple classes, orders, families, genus, and species of bacteria, allowing for great diversity at the lower levels, and secondly, even where species are shared, their genetic expression can be very different, allowing for adaptations to quite distinct environments. Though bacteria are the microbes enjoying the most research and discussion, fungi present a strong population within the gut as well. In dogs, *Ascomycota, Basidiomycota, Glomeromycota* and *Zygomycota* phyla have been identified, while in cats *Ascomycota* was the single dominant fungal phylum [25].

The character of the gut microbiome in each section of the tract can be partially explained by the composition of the luminal milieu, including oxygen and nutrient content, which acts to nourish not only the host, but their microbes as well [24]. This can be seen by alterations in the composition of the bacterial communities or in alterations in the genes those bacteria express, or both [26].

**Table 15.1** Common bacterial components of the gastrointestinal microbiome.

| Phylum | Class | Order | Family | Genus |
|---|---|---|---|---|
| Firmicutes | Clostridia | Clostridiales | Clostridiaceae<br>Ruminococcaceae<br><br>Eubacteraceae | Clostridium<br>Ruminococcus<br>Faecalibacterium<br>Eubacterium |
| | Bacilli | Lactobacilliales | Latobacillaceae<br>Streptococcaceae | Lactobacillus<br>Streptococcus<br>Enterococcus |
| | Erysiphelotrichia | Erisophelotrichales | Erysiphelotrichaceae | Turicibacter<br>Catenibacterium<br>Coprobacillus<br>Allobaculum |
| | Negativicutes | Selenomonadales<br>Vellonellales | Selenomonadaceae<br>Veillonellaceae | Megamonas<br>Dialister<br>Megasphera<br>Veillonella |
| Bacteroidetes | Bacteroidia | Bacteroidales | Prevotellaceae<br>Bacteroidaceae | Prevotella<br>Bacteroides |

*(Continued)*

**Table 15.1** (Continued)

| Phylum | Class | Order | Family | Genus |
|---|---|---|---|---|
| Actinobacteria | Coriobacteria | Coriobacteriales | Coriobacteriaceae | Collinsella |
| | | | Atopobiaceae | Olsenella |
| | | Eggerthellales | Eggerthellaceae | Slackia |
| | | | | Eggerthella |
| | Actinobacteria | Bifidobacteriales | Bifidobacteriaceae | Bifidobacterium |
| Fusobacteria | Fusobacteria | Fusobacteriales | Fusobacteriaceae | Fusobacterium |
| Proteobacteria | Gammaproteobacteria | Enterobacteriales | Enterobacteraceae | Escherichia |
| | | | | Shigella |
| | | Aeromonadales | Succinivibrionaceae | Succinivibrio |
| | | | | Anaerobiospirillum |

*Source:* Adapted from Ritchie et al. [20], Pilla et al. [21], Barko et al. [23] and Pilla et al. [24].

## 15.2 The GI Microbiome's Role in the Production of Vitamins

The microbes within the GI tract provide essential functions in metabolizing, altering, and producing nutrients of benefit to the host, including essential vitamins. Metagenomics have demonstrated around 4–5% of the functions of one of the most dominant phyla in the canine and feline genome, *Proteobacteria*, to be associated with vitamins, cofactors, prosthetic groups, and pigments [27]. Indeed, vitamins account for the function of around 5–6% of the entire canine and feline GI metagenomes [28–30]. This represented the second highest known functional classification for this phyla, second only to protein metabolism.

The *de novo* vitamin biosynthetic capacity of the human GI microbiome has been well studied [31] and has served as a comparative baseline for research into vitamin synthesis by microbes in the canine and feline gut, especially B vitamins and vitamin K [32]. Thiamine (B1), riboflavin (B2), nicotinic acid (B3), pyridoxin (B6), folic acid (B9), cobalamin (B12), and menaquinone (K2) may all be synthesized by gut microbes [29, 32, 33]. Not only may microbes be directly responsible for biosynthesis of vitamins, but alterations in microbial populations and metabolism may indirectly affect host vitamin metabolism, such as impacts on fat-soluble vitamin absorption with changes in microbial bile acid metabolism [34].

## 15.3 Conditions Affected by or Associated with the GI Microbiome

The microbiome of the gut is not a passive ecosystem where microbes simply coexist with their host, feeding from the nutrients in the host's ingesta. As discussed in Chapter 2, the functions of the gut microbiome are diverse, playing roles in host nutrient metabolism, structural integrity, immunomodulation, and communication with distant body systems. As such, numerous health conditions affecting both the GI system directly and system-wide can be affected by and associated with the GI microbiome.

The term dysbiosis refers to upset of the healthy or normal microbiome (normobiosis) of an individual animal and can be both a cause or symptom of GI disease. Dysbiosis can include shift in microbial populations and/or function. Dysbiosis can arise as a result of infection with enteropathogens, as a sequel to antimicrobial administration, acute and/or chronic GI inflammation, intestinal dysmotility, alterations in gastric acid secretion including therapeutic suppression, and exocrine pancreatic insufficiency [35].

Consequences of dysbiosis are diverse, including:

- Alteration in metabolism and conjugation of bile acids, potentially leading to chronic GI inflammation, altered fat absorption, and dysregulation of glycemic control [36, 37]
- Reduced fermentation of indigestible carbohydrates, resulting in reduced production of anti-inflammatory short-chain fatty acids (SCFAs) and reduced energy substrate for enterocytes [35]
- Reduced synthesis and absorption of vitamins, contributing to alterations in cobalamin and folate metabolism [35, 38]
- Malabsorption and diarrhea [38]
- Alteration in mucosal immunity and dysfunction of the mucosal barrier, potentially allowing increased intestinal permeability and bacterial translocation, enterotoxaemia, and aberrant intestinal immune responses including hypersensitivity [35, 38]
- Loss of competition with enteropathogens, potentially leading to enteritis [35]

As discussed in Chapter 2, a robust GI microbiome serves to stimulate mucosal barrier function, including maintenance of tight junctions between epithelial cells and stimulation of mucus production [39, 40]. Dysbiosis can thus contribute to breakdown of the integrity of this barrier. Dysfunction of the gut barrier, or a "leaky gut," has been proposed as a potential component of multiple health condition. The healthy gut serves as a barrier between the external environment, with all its potential pathogens and toxins, and the animal's internal bodily systems. There are multiple potential consequences of dysfunction in the gut barrier, including those obvious and well known, such as chronic enteropathy, inflammatory bowel disease [41, 42], dietary hypersensitivity, and atopy [43, 44], as well as those that may seem to be more obscure and distant. Extra-GI conditions associated with dysbiosis and intestinal barrier dysfunction, such as chronic kidney disease and myxomatous mitral valve disease, may be associated via translocation of gut bacteria and their metabolites [45, 46]. Dogs and cats with dysbiosis may show no obvious clinical signs or may show signs consistent with multiple associated conditions. In many cases, dysbiosis may be a marker of disease or be caused by a disease process and/or may actively contribute to etiopathogenesis and cause or effect are not always easily distinguished.

## 15.3.1 Chronic Enteropathies

Chronic enteropathies describe a number of conditions of chronic inflammation of the intestine that may generate consistent, progressive, or waxing-waning clinical signs. Common clinical signs include vomiting, diarrhea, excessive borborygmus, flatulence, inappetence and weight loss. Regardless of underlying etiology, chronic enteropathies have been associated with dysbiosis to some degree [21].

### 15.3.1.1 Antibiotic-Responsive Enteropathy

A primary potential outcome from small intestinal dysbiosis in dogs is the phenomenon termed antibiotic responsive diarrhea (ARE), also sometimes referred to as small intestinal bacterial overgrowth or SIBO. Truly, SIBO is a misnomer, as there is no recognized pathological number of bacteria in the small intestine [35, 38, 47], so bacterial "overgrowth" per se is not an appropriately descriptive term, yet this is still commonly heard in clinical practice. A common diagnostic criterion to determine ARE is a reduction in serum cobalamin with corresponding increase in serum folate due to imbalance in the microbiota causing increased bacterial utilization of cobalamin and increased production of folic acid, though this is neither highly sensitive nor highly specific [35, 47]. Recently, indices of dysbiosis have been proposed for dogs and cats, using relative abundances of *Bacteroidetes*, *Bifidobacterium*, *Clostridium hiranonis*, *Fecalibacterium*, *Turicibacter*, *E. coli*, and *Streptococcus* in cats, and *Fecalibacterium*, *Turicibacter*, *E. coli*, *Streptococcus*, *Blautia*, *Fusobacterium*, and *C. hiranonis* in dogs [48, 49]. The most commonly prescribed antimicrobial therapies effective in ameliorating ARE in dogs are tylosin and metronidazole, with some animals requiring recurrent or indefinite therapy [35, 47]. Cats appear to have less response to antimicrobial administration, and ARE appears to be exclusive to dogs [47, 50]. Given that the disease appears to be directly related to microbial populations in the gut, it has been theorized the administration of beneficial bacteria (probiotics) may be an alternative to antimicrobial therapy. However, treatment of dogs with tylosin-responsive diarrhea with a single-strain probiotic failed to prevent relapse [51]. Instead, it is possible that tylosin-resistant beneficial bacteria may flourish during administration of the antimicrobial, potentially contributing to clinical resolution [52].

#### 15.3.1.2 Food-Responsive Enteropathy

As the name suggests, food-responsive enteropathy (FRE) is primarily attributable to an aberrant immune response to dietary antigens, which can be ameliorated by removal of offending foodstuffs [53, 54]. Dogs and cats with FRE have demonstrated similar histologic inflammatory lesions as dogs with inflammatory bowel disease (IBD), with similar alterations in microbiota richness and diversity [53–55]. Improvement of dysbiosis has been detected in dogs and cats successfully treated for FRE with dietary change, though administration of probiotics to dogs undergoing therapy for FRE failed to alter treatment outcome [53–56]. Potentially dysbiosis is an outcome, not cause, of FRE.

#### 15.3.1.3 Inflammatory Bowel Disease

Inflammatory bowel disease, or steroid-responsive enteropathy, is an idiopathic immune-mediated condition. A diagnosis of IBD is arrived through a combination of exclusion – failure to respond to dietary or antimicrobial therapies – and characteristic, but not pathognomonic, histologic features of inflammatory cell infiltration [57].

Alterations in the microbial communities within the GI tract have been associated with development of IBD. Though it appears unlikely that dysbiosis alone is sufficient to induce IBD, it is a causal component of a multifactorial etiology including genetic predisposition, aberrant immune response, and environmental factors [53, 57]. In dogs and cats with IBD, dysbiosis has been characterized by increases in *Proteobacteria* and decreases in *Firmicutes* and *Bacteroidetes* [57, 58]. The bacteria families most affected have been reported to be *Bacteroidaceae, Preveotellaceae, Ruminococcaceae, Veillonellaceae,* and *Lachnospiraceae,* all producers of SCFAs [21]. The reduction in SCFA production negatively impacts the colonocytes, for which luminal SCFAs are a main energy source [59]. It bears mentioning that differentiation of IBD from alimentary small-cell lymphoma can be challenging, as the clinical signs, histologic appearance, and dysbiosis can be very similar [60]. Indeed, it has been postulated that IBD may be a preliminary form of lymphoma, or progress to lymphoma, in cats [61].

### 15.3.2 Dietary Hypersensitivity and Atopy

Dietary hypersensitivity, also referred to as dietary allergies, and atopy are both associated with the GI microbiome. Both dietary hypersensitivity and atopy are immunologic adverse reactions to ingested material. The GI tract functions to allow absorption of nonpathogenic nutrients and exclude potential pathogenic substances and respond to potential pathogen invasion. A component of this function is the extensive immune system throughout the gut, termed the gut-associated lymphoid tissue (GALT) [23, 44, 62]. Briefly, the GALT is composed of mesenteric lymph nodes, lymphoid nodules, Peyers's patches, lymphocytes and plasma cells within the lamina propria, and enterocytes with intraepithelial lymphocytes [23, 44, 62]. In healthy animals, penetration of the mucosal barrier by protein components (free amino acids, dipeptides, and degraded proteins) results in the presentation of the antigen by specialized cells in the Peyer's patches to lymphocytes, with recognition of non-offensive antigens suppressing any immune reaction [44]. This is referred to as antigen tolerance and is influenced by commensal bacteria and their metabolites [63]. When the mucosal barrier is disrupted, macromolecules, specifically proteins and glycoproteins, are presented resulting in the formation of immune complexes against these components and local IgM-, IgG- and/or IgE-mediated inflammation [44, 62]. Future exposure to the antigen results in continued inflammation and the GALT is primed for a hyper-immune response. As previously discussed, the microbiota play a role in maintaining the integrity of the mucosal barrier, as well as in modulating gut inflammation [23, 62]. Dysbiosis may alter the balance of specific immune cells called T helper cells, resulting in reduced tolerance and a predisposition to hypersensitivity, in conjunction with reduced production of anti-inflammatory microbial metabolites like SCFAs [63]. The resulting outcome is exaggerated inflammatory responses to ingested food and environmental substances.

Dietary hypersensitivity is a term referring to a collection of immune-mediated responses to ingestion of non-tolerated foods [44].

Clinical signs of hypersensitivity may include gastrointestinal signs, dermatological signs, or both. In contrast to food intolerance, a hypersensitivity requires pre-sensitization to a food – that is to say: dogs and cats can only develop hypersensitivity to foods to which they have been previously exposed. Presentation of proteins and glycoproteins from ingested food leads to hypersensitivity of the GALT and intolerance to specific food components [44]. Thus, protein-rich foods are most commonly associated with dietary hypersensitivity, with the most common dietary protein sources being the most commonly implicated in hypersensitive cases – beef and dairy most predominant in both dogs and cats, along with wheat and chicken in dogs and fish in cats [44]. Altering the diet to remove antigenic proteins may improve clinical signs transiently, but new hypersensitivities may develop as penetration of the leaky gut barrier by antigenic proteins may continue, potentially necessitating the use of hydrolyzed protein sources [64].

The primary signs of atopy are dermatitis, and atopic dogs may show no gastrointestinal signs, though the disease condition is a systemic disease, not localized exclusively to the skin [43]. In addition to the integumentary microbiota, as discussed in Chapter 13, the gut microbiota also play a critical role in the etiology of atopy, by way of influencing immune cell activity, inflammation, and bioactive metabolites [43, 65]. Impairment of the intestinal mucosal barrier may allow translocation of ingested environmental components, leading to immune intolerance to otherwise benign substances. Preliminary data suggest that dysbiotic changes in the atopic canine gut appear to share similarities with atopic humans, with lower alpha-diversity than non-atopic dogs [65]. In that study, four genera were demonstrated to have higher prevalence in the atopic canine gut: *Conchiformibius*, *Catenibacterium*, *Ruminococcus gnavus* group, and *Megamonas*, while *Lachnospira* and *Ruminococcus torques* group were reduced. It was hypothesized that the loss of these two families in particular may contribute to reduced gut epithelial barrier integrity and immune regulation, predominantly via reduced production of SCFA and increased mucin degradation. Indeed, it appears that atopic dogs may responded to probiotics containing *Lactobaccilus* spp., a SCFA producer, with reports of partial prevention, persistent effect even after discontinuation, and reduction in disease severity [66–68].

### 15.3.3 Obesity

Overweight and obesity represent the most common nutritionally associated impairments to canine and feline health and well-being around the world, with somewhere around half or more of companion dogs and cats adversely affected [69]. Given the role that the microbiota play in nutrient digestion and metabolism, it is not surprising that alterations in the microbiome have been associated with obesity in dogs, cats, and other animals including humans. Studies have demonstrated altered microbial populations in obese dogs with lower diversity indices and higher proportion of Proteobacteria, Actinobacteria, and/or Bifidobacteriaceae than lean dogs [34, 70, 71]. In cats, similar findings have been reported, with reduced microbial diversity, lower proportion of Firmicutes, and a decreased Firmicutes to Bacteroidetes ratio in comparison to nonobese cats [72]. In this study, metagenomics also demonstrated upregulated fatty acid synthetic pathways in the obese feline microbiome. Furthermore, rate and capacity for weight loss in obese dogs also appears to be associated with microbial composition. In one study, Megamonas and Ruminococcaceae spp. were negatively correlated with weight loss [73]. In a second study of obese dogs undergoing weight loss, members of Clostridia and Bacilli phyla decreased, while *Allobaculum* (a Baccilota genus) increased [74]. In both of these studies, a higher proportion of SCFA producers were present in obese animals before weight loss and may suggest a higher efficiency of energy harvesting, contributing to the obese condition. However, these findings must also be interpreted with consideration that both obesity and weight loss are comprised of many factors, including changes in energy intake, energy output, and dietary composition, all of which may alter the GI microbiome [75].

### 15.3.4 Diabetes Mellitus

Manifestation of diabetes mellitus in companion animals is similar to humans, with cats typically presenting with type II-like insulin-resistant diabetes mellitus most often associated with obesity, while dogs present with type I-like autoimmune destruction of the pancreatic beta cells [76–78]. In humans, research has demonstrated associations between dysbiosis and both development and treatment of diabetes mellitus, leading to investigations in companion animals [37, 79]. In dogs, alterations reported have included an increased abundance of *Enterobacteriacea* and reduced *Mogibacteriacea* and *Anaeroplamataceae* in diabetic dogs compared to nondiabetic dogs [37]. In diabetic cats, reduced diversity indices have been reported as compared to lean nondiabetic cats, with fewer *Anaerotruncus*, *Dialister*, and *Ruminococcaceae* spp. [80] Feline findings may be complicated by the microbial changes associated with obesity, as well as diabetes, due to the high prevalence of obesity in diabetic cats.

The rectal microbiome of diabetic dogs also appears to shift in response to therapy, with one study demonstrating increasing *Bacteroides*, a genus associated with glucose tolerance and insulin sensitivity in humans, upon initiation of insulin therapy in newly diagnosed diabetic dogs [79]. Furthermore, the study found *Enterococcus* and *Escherichia-Shigella* to be positively associated with serum fructosamine, an indicator of chronic hyperglycemia. In cats, *Enterobacteriacea* were found to also be positively correlated with serum fructosamine, while *Prevotellaceae* were correlated negatively [80].

### 15.3.5 Neoplasia

Cancer arises as a result of interactions between host genetics and environmental aspects (epigenetics) leading to dysregulation of normal cellular replications. In humans, microorganisms have been implicated in the development of specific neoplasia, such as *Helicobacter* and gastric carcinoma, as mentioned in Section 15.1.3. Chronic inflammation can lead to metaplasia, then eventually dysplasia and neoplasia, with the GI microbiome being intrinsically linked with local and systemic inflammation [81]. Furthermore, alterations in the gut microbiome has been associated with local GI lymphoma and epithelial tumors as well as multicentric lymphoma [82–84]. In all three studies, dysbiosis was detected, with lower *Faecalibacterium* spp. (Order *Eubacteriales*), and higher *Streptococcus* spp. consistent among affected dogs. One study looked at the fecal microbiome of cats with IBD or small cell alimentary lymphoma compared to healthy cats and found lower abundance of *Firmicutes*, *Actinobacteria*, and *Bacteroidetes*, and increased *Enterobacteriaceae* and *Streptococcaceae* in cats with both IBD and lymphoma [60]. No differences in microbiome were detectable between IBD and GI lymphoma, highlighting the association between chronic GI inflammation and neoplasia.

## 15.3.6 Congestive Heart Failure

In comparison to local inflammatory diseases or systemic conditions associated with energy metabolism, the association between cardiac disease and the GI microbiome may seem less obvious. However, dysbiosis has been demonstrated in dogs with myxomatous mitral valve disease and congestive heart failure, characterized by reduced *Clostridium hiranonis*, a bile acid metabolizer, and increased abundance of trimethylamine *N*-oxide (TMAO)-producing *E. coli* [45, 85]. Advanced stages of mitral valve disease in dogs are associated with greater levels of TMAO, while secondary bile acids, produced by microbial bile acid metabolism, may inhibit growth of pathogenic microbes. These studies highlight the potential for microbial metabolites to affect extra-GI body systems and contribute to development of diseases appearing otherwise unassociated with the gut.

## 15.3.7 Chronic Kidney Disease

As discussed in Chapter 17, there is a demonstrated relationship between the GI microbiome and the kidney, referred to as the GI-renal or gut-kidney axis. Dietary components, for example phosphorus, and end-products of microbial fermentation of dietary components, such as the uremic toxins indole sulfates and kynurenate are known to contribute to or correlate with progression of chronic kidney disease (CKD) in dogs and cats [86]. Cats with CKD have been shown to have reduced gut bacterial diversity and richness, with increased serum uremic toxins suggestive of increased proteolytic bacterial activity as has been demonstrated in humans with CKD [87]. In one study, the fecal microbiome of cats with CKD had lower *Bacteroidales* than cats without CKD, which was improved with fiber supplementation [88]. Although CKD is not as common in dogs as in cats, it is still quite a common condition, yet fewer studies investigating the microbiome and CKD in dogs appear to have been performed. One found no difference in the fecal microbiota of dogs with or without early (International Renal Interest Society Stage I) CKD, yet the fecal metabolomes differed, with greater markers of glutathione, lysine, sulfur amino acid, and phenylalanine metabolism, and lower indicators of fatty acid and genistein sulfate [89].

## 15.4   Chapter Summary

- The gastrointestinal microbiome is a complex and vast community of microbes that differs along the length of the tract
- Some organisms may be commensals or potentially pathogenic, likely depending on multiple other factors
- More than density of individual species, the balance of the species comprising the gut microbiome is likely a better indicator of gut health, leading to the development of dysbiosis indices for cats and dogs
- Alterations in the gut microbiome have been associated with a number of local (such as chronic enteropathies, alimentary lymphoma) and distant (such as heart and kidney disease) health conditions
- It is often unknown whether dysbiosis is a cause or consequence of disease states and whether interventions to correct dysbiosis are effective or ameliorate signs of adverse health conditions.

## References

**1** de Steenhuijsen Piters, W., Sanders, E., and Bogaert, D. (2015). The role of the local microbial ecosystem in respiratory health and disease. *Philosophical Transactions B* 370: 20140294.

**2** Di Pilato, V., Freschi, G., Fingressi, M. et al. (2016). The esophageal microbiome in health and disease. *Annals of the New York Academy of Sciences* 1381: 21–33.

**3** Pereira, A. and Clemente, A. (2021). Dogs' microbiome from tip to toe. *Topics in Companion Animal Medicine* 45: 100584.

**4** Hunt, R. and Yaghoobi, M. (2017). The esophageal and gastric microbiome in health and disease. *Gastroenterology Clinics of North America* 46: 121–141.

**5** Muenster, M., Hoerauf, A., and Vieth, M. (2017). Gastro-oesophageal reflux disease in 20 dogs (2012 to 2014). *Journal of Small Animal Practice* 58: 276–283.

**6** Frowde, P., Battersby, I., Whitley, N., and Elwood, C. (2011). Oesophageal disease in cats. *Journal of Feline Medicine and Surgery* 13: 564–569.

**7** Okereke, I., Hamilton, C., Wenholz, A. et al. (2019). Associations of the microbiome and esophageal disease. *Journal of Thoracic Disease* 11 (S12): S1588–S1593.

**8** Lee, D., Goh, T., Kang, M. et al. (2022). Perspectives and advances in probiotics and the gut microbiome in companion animals. *Journal of Animal Science and Technology* 64 (2): 197–217.

**9** Noto, J. and Peek, R. Jr. (2017). The gastric microbiome, its interaction with helicobacter pylori, and its potential role in the progression to stomach cancer. *PLoS Pathogens* 13 (10): e1006573.

**10** Taiilieu, E., Chiers, K., Amorim, I. et al. (2022). Gastric helicobacter species associated with dogs, cats and pigs: signifcance for public and animal health. *Veterinary Research* 53: 1–5.

**11** Haesebrouck, F., Pasmans, F., Flahou, B. et al. (2009). Gastric helicobacters in domestic animals and nonhuman primates and their significance for human health. *Clinical Microbiology Reviews* 22 (2): 202–223.

**12** Teixeira, S., Filipe, D., Cerqueira, M. et al. (2022). Helicobacter spp. in the stomach of cats: successful colonization and absence of relevant histopathological alterations reveals high adaptation to the host gastric niche. *Veterinary Sciences* 9: 228.

**13** Bridgeford, E., Marini, R., Feng, Y. et al. (2008). Gastric helicobacter species as a cause of feline gastric lymphoma: a viable hypothesis. *Veterinary Immunology and Immunopathology* 123 (1–2): 106–113.

**14** Husnik, R., Klimes, J., Kovarikova, S., and Kolorz, M. (2022). Helicobacter species and their association with gastric pathology in a cohort of dogs with chronic gastrointestinal signs. *Animals* 12: 1254.

**15** Kubota-Aizawa, S., Ohno, H., Fukushima, K. et al. (2017). Epidemiological study of gastric helicobacter spp. in dogs with gastrointestinal disease in Japan and diversity of helicobacter *heilmannii sensu stricto*. *The Veterinary Journal* 225: 56–62.

**16** Kararli, T. (1995). Comparison of the gastrointestinal anatomy, physiology, and biochemistry of humans and commonly used laboratory animals. *Biopharmaceutics & Drug Disposition* 16: 351–380.

**17** Suchodolski, J. (2011). Intestinal microbiota of dogs and cats: a bigger world than we thought. *Veterinary Clinics of North America: Small Animal Practice* 41: 261–272.

**18** Suchodolski, J., Camacho, J., and Steiner, J. (2008). Analysis of bacterial diversity in the canine duodenum, jejunum, ileum, and colon by comparative16s rrna gene analysis. *FEMS Microbiology Ecology* 66: 567–578.

**19** Suchodolski, J., Morris, E., Allenspach, K. et al. (2008). Prevalence and identification of fungal DNA in the small intestine of healthy dogs and dogs with chronic enteropathies. *Veterinary Microbiology* 132: 379–388.

**20** Ritchie, L., Steiner, J., and Suchodolski, J. (2008). Assessment of microbial diversity along the feline intestinal tract using16s rrna gene analysis. *FEMS Microbiology Ecology* 66: 590–598.

**21** Pilla, R. and Suchodolski, J. (2020). The role of the canine gut microbiome and metabolome in health and gastrointestinal disease. *Frontiers in Veterinary Science* 6: 498.

**22** Tal, M., Verbrugghe, A., Gomez, D. et al. (2017). The effect of storage at ambient temperature on the feline fecal microbiota. *BMC Veterinary Research* 13: 256.

**23** Barko, P., McMichael, M., Swanson, K., and Williams, D. (2018). The gastrointestinal microbiome: a review. *Journal of Veterinary Internal Medicine* 32: 9–25.

**24** Pilla, R. and Suchodolski, J. (2021). The gut microbiome of dogs and cats, and the influence of diet. *Veterinary Clinics of North America: Small Animal Practice* 51: 605–621.

**25** Handl, S., Dowd, S., Garcia-Mazcorro, J. et al. (2011). Massive parallel16s rrna gene pyrosequencing reveals highly diverse fecal bacterial and fungal communities in healthy dogs and cats. *FEMS Microbiology Ecology* 76: 301–310.

**26** Suchodolski, J. (2021). Analysis of the gut microbiome in dogs and cats. *Veterinary Clinical Pathology* 50 (Suppl. 1): 6–17.

**27** Moon, C., Young, W., Maclean, P. et al. (2018). Metagenomic insights into the roles of proteobacteria in the gastrointestinal microbiomes of healthy dogs and cats. *Microbiology Open* 7: e00677.

**28** Deng, P. and Swanson, K. (2015). Gut microbiota of humans, dogs and cats: current knowledge and future opportunities and challenges. *British Journal of Nutrition* 113: S6–S17.

**29** Swanson, K., Dowd, S., Suchodolski, J. et al. (2011). Phylogenetic and gene-centric metagenomics of canine intestinal microbiome reveals similarities with humans and mice. *The ISME Journal* 5: 639–649.

**30** Barry, K., Middelbos, I., Boler, B.V. et al. (2012). Effects of dietary fiber on the feline gastrointestinal metagenome. *Journal of Proteome Research* 11: 5924–5933.

**31** LeBlanc, J., Milani, C., de Giori, G. et al. (2013). Bacteria as vitamin suppliers to their host: a gut microbiota perspective. *Current Opinion in Biotechnology* 24: 160–168.

**32** Young, W., Moon, C., Thomas, D. et al. (2016). Pre- and post-weaning diet alters the faecal metagenome in the cat with differences in vitamin and carbohydrate metabolism gene abundances. *Scientific Reports* 6: 1–6.

**33** Pilla, R., Guard, B., Blake, A. et al. (2021). Long-term recovery of the fecal microbiome and metabolome of dogs with steroid-responsive enteropathy. *Animals* 11: 2498.

**34** Forster, G., Stockman, J., Noyes, N. et al. (2018). A comparative study of serum biochemistry, metabolome and microbiome parameters of clinically healthy, normal weight, overweight and obese companion dogs. *Topics in Companion Animal Medicine* 33: 126–135.

**35** Suchodolski, J. (2016). Diagnosis and interpretation of intestinal dysbiosis in dogs and cats. *The Veterinary Journal* 215: 30–37.

**36** Duboc, H., Rajca, S., Rainteau, D. et al. (2013). Connecting dysbiosis, bile-acid dysmetabolism and gut inflammation in inflammatory bowel diseases. *Gut* 62: 531–539.

**37** Jergens, A., Guard, B., Redfern, A. et al. (2019). Microbiota-related changes in unconjugated fecal bile acids are associated with naturally occurring, insulin-dependent diabetes mellitus in dogs. *Frontiers in Veterinary Science* 6: 199. https://doi.org/10.3389/fvets.2019.00199.

**38** Minamoto, Y., Hooda, S., Swanson, K., and Suchodolski, J. (2012). Feline gastrointestinal microbiota. *Animal Health Research Reviews* 13 (1): 64–77.

**39** Kleessen, B. and Blaut, M. (2005). Modulation of gut mucosal biofilms. *British Journal of Nutrition* 93 (Suppl. 1): S35–S40.

**40** Jandhyala, S., Talukdar, R., Subramanyam, C. et al. (2015). Role of the normal gut microbiota. *World Journal of Gastroenterology* 21 (29): 8787–8803.

**41** Jergens, A., Parvinroo, S., Kopper, J., and Wannemuehler, M. (2021). Rules of engagement: epithelial-microbe interactions and inflammatory bowel disease. *Frontiers in Medicine* 8: https://doi.org/10.3389/fmed.2021.669913.

**42** Atherly, T., Rossi, G., White, R. et al. (2019). Glucocorticoid and dietary effects on mucosal microbiota in canine inflammatory bowel disease. *PLoS One* 14 (12).

**43** Craig, J. (2016). Atopic dermatitis and the intestinal microbiota in humans and dogs. *Veterinary Medicine and Science* 2: 95–105.

**44** Verlinden, A., Hesta, M., Millet, S., and Janssens, G. (2006). Food allergy in dogs and cats: a review. *Critical Reviews in Food Science and Nutrition* 46: 259–273.

**45** Li, Q., Larouche-Lebel, E., Loughran, K. et al. (2021). Gut dysbiosis and its associations with gut microbiota-derived metabolites in dogs with myxomatous mitral valve disease. *mSystems* 6: e00111–e00121.

**46** Bartochowski, P., Gayrard, N., Bornes, S. et al. (2022). Gut–kidney axis investigations in animal models of chronic kidney disease. *Toxins* 14: 626.

**47** Hall, E. (2011). Antibiotic-responsive diarrhea in small animals. *Veterinary Clinics of North America: Small Animal Practice* 41 (2): 273–286.

**48** AlShawaqfeh, M., Wajid, B., Minamoto, Y. et al. (2017). A dysbiosis index to assess microbial changes in fecal samples of dogs with chronic inflammatory enteropathy. *FEMS Microbiology Ecology* 93: fix136.

**49** Sung, C.-H., Marsilio, S., Chow, B. et al. (2022). Dysbiosis index to evaluate the fecal microbiota in healthy cats and cats with chronic enteropathies. *Journal of Feline Medicine and Surgery* 24 (6): e1–e2.

**50** Jergens, A., Crandell, J., Evans, R. et al. (2010). A clinical index for disease activity in cats with chronic enteropathy. *Journal of Veterinary Internal Medicine* 24: 1027–1033.

**51** Westermarck, E., Skrzypczak, T., Harmoinen, J. et al. (2005). Tylosin-responsive chronic diarrhea in dogs. *Journal of Veterinary Internal Medicine* 19: 177–186.

**52** Kilpinen, S., Rantala, M., Spillmann, T. et al. (2015). Oral tylosin administration is associated with an increase of faecal enterococci and lactic acid bacteria in dogs with tylosin-responsive diarrhoea. *The Veterinary Journal* 205: 369–374.

**53** Kalenyak, K., Isaiah, A., Heilmann, R. et al. (2018). Comparison of the intestinal mucosal microbiota in dogs diagnosed with idiopathic inflammatory bowel disease and dogs with food-responsive diarrhea before and after treatment. *FEMS Microbiology Ecology* 94: fix173.

**54** Bresciani, F., Minamoto, T., Suchodolski, J. et al. (2018). Effect of an extruded animal protein-free diet on fecal microbiota of dogs with food-responsive enteropathy. *Journal of Veterinary Internal Medicine* 32: 1903–1910.

**55** Ramadan, Z., Laflamme, D., Czarnecki-Maulden, G. et al. (2014). Fecal microbiota of cats with naturally occurring chronic diarrhea assessed using 16s rrna gene 454-pyrosequencing before and after dietary treatment. *Journal of Veterinary Internal Medicine* 28: 59–65.

**56** Sauter, S., Benyacoub, J., Allenspach, K. et al. (2006). Effects of probiotic bacteria in dogs with food responsive diarrhoea treated with an elimination diet. *Journal of Animal Physiology and Animal Nutrition* 90: 269–277.

**57** Vázquez-Baeza, Y., Hyde, E., Suchodolski, J., and Knight, R. (2016). Dog and human inflammatory bowel disease rely on overlapping yet distinct dysbiosis networks. *Nature Microbiology* 1: 1–5.

**58** Honneffer, J., Minamoto, Y., and Suchodolski, J. (2014). Microbiota alterations in acute and chronic gastrointestinal inflammation of cats and dogs. *World Journal of Gastroenterology* 20 (44): 16489–16497.

**59** Minamoto, Y., Minamoto, T., Isaiah, A. et al. (2019). Fecal short-chain fatty acid concentrations and dysbiosis indogs with chronic enteropathy. *Journal of Veterinary Internal Medicine* 33: 1608–1618.

**60** Marsilio, S., Pilla, R., Sarawichitr, B. et al. (2019). Characterization of the fecal microbiome in cats with infammatory bowel disease or alimentary small cell lymphoma. *Scientific Reports* 9: 1.

**61** Moore, P., Woo, J., Vernau, W. et al. (2005). Characterization of feline t cell receptor gamma (tcrg) variable region genes for the molecular diagnosis of feline intestinal t cell lymphoma. *Veterinary Immunology and Immunopathology* 106: 167–178.

**62** Jergens, A. (2002). Understanding gastrointestinal inflammation – implications for therapy. *Journal of Feline Medicine and Surgery* 4: 179–182.

**63** Tizard, I. and Jones, S. (2018). The microbiota regulates immunity and immunologic diseases in dogs and cats. *Veterinary Clinics of North America: Small Animal Practice* 48: 307–322.

**64** Cave, N. (2006). Hydrolyzed protein diets for dogs and cats. *Veterinary Clinics of North America: Small Animal Practice* 36: 1251–1268.

**65** Rostaher, A., Morsy, Y., Favrot, C. et al. (2022). Comparison of the gut microbiome between atopic and healthy dogs – preliminary data. *Animals* 12: 2377.

**66** Marsella, R., Santoro, D., and Ahrens, K. (2012). Early exposure to probiotics in a canine model of atopic dermatitis has long-term clinical and immunological effects. *Veterinary Immunology and Immunopathology* 146: 185–189.

**67** Marsella, R. (2009). Evaluation of lactobacillus rhamnosus strain gg for the prevention of atopic dermatitis in dogs. *American Journal of Veterinary Research* 70 (6): 735–740.

**68** Kim, H., Rather, I., Kim, H. et al. (2015). A double-blind, placebo controlled-trial of a probiotic strain lactobacillus sakei probio-65 for the prevention of canine atopic dermatitis. *Journal of Microbiology and Biotechnology* 25 (11): 1966–1969.

**69** Hamper, B. (2016). Current topics in canine and feline obesity. *Veterinary Clinics of North America: Small Animal Practice* 46: 785–795.

**70** Handl, S., Ge rman, A., Holden, S. et al. (2012). Faecal microbiota in lean and obese dogs. *FEMS Microbiology Ecology* 84: 332–343.

**71** Park, H.-J., Lee, S.-E., Kim, H.-B. et al. (2015). Association of obesity with serum leptin, adiponectin, and serotonin and gut microflora in beagle dogs. *Journal of Veterinary Internal Medicine* 29: 43–50.

**72** Ma, X., Brinker, E., Graff, E. et al. (2022). Whole-genome shotgun metagenomic sequencing reveals distinct gut microbiome signatures of obese cats. *Microbiology Spectrum* 10 (3): e0083722.

**73** Kieler, I., Kamal, S., Vitger, A. et al. (2017). Gut microbiota compostiion may relate to weight loss rate in obese pet dogs. *Veterinary Medicine and Science* 3: 252–262.

**74** Salas-Mani, A., Jeusette, I., Castillo, I. et al. (2018). Fecal microbiota composition changes after a bw loss diet in beagle dogs. *Journal of Animal Science* 96: 3102–3111.

**75** Bartges, J. (2019). Gut microbiome and obesity. In: *Hill's Global Symposium*. Toronto, Ontario.

**76** Hoenig, M. (2012). The cat as a model for human obesity and diabetes. *Journal of Diabetes Science and Technology* 6 (3): 525–533.

**77** Hoenig, M. (2002). Comparative aspects of diabetes mellitus in dogs and cats. *Molecular and Cellular Endocrinology* 197: 221–229.

**78** Clark, M. and Hoenig, M. (2016). Metabolic effects of obesity and its interaction with endocrine diseases. *Veterinary Clinics of North America: Small Animal Practice* 46: 797–815.

**79** Laia, N., Barko, P., Sullivan, D. et al. (2022). Longitudinal analysis of the rectal microbiome in dogs with diabetes mellitus after initiation of insulin therapy. *PLoS One* 17 (9): e0273792.

**80** Kieler, I., Osto, M., Hugentobler, L. et al. (2019). Diabetic cats have decreased gut microbial diversity and a lack of butyrate producing bacteria. *Scientific Reports* 9: 1–3.

**81** Epiphanio, T. and Santos, A. (2021). Small animals gut microbiome and its relationship with cancer. In: *Canine Genetics, Health and Medicine* (ed. C. Rutland). IntechOpen. http://dx.doi.org/10.5772/intechopen. 95780.

**82** Gavazza, A., Rossi, G., Lubas, G. et al. (2017). Faecal microbiota in dogs with multicentric lymphoma. *Veterinary and Comparative Oncology* 16: E169–E175.

**83** Herstad, K., Moen, A., Gaby, J. et al. (2018). Characterization of the fecal and mucosa associated microbiota in dogs with colorectal epithelial tumors. *PLoS One* 13 (5): e0198342.

**84** Omori, M., Maeda, S., Igarashi, H. et al. (2017). Fecal microbiome in dogs with inflammatory bowel disease and intestinal lymphoma. *The Journal of Veterinary Medical Science* 79 (11): 1840–1847.

**85** Seo, J., Matthewman, L., Xia, D. et al. (2020). The gut microbiome in dogs with congestive heart failure: a pilot study. *Scientific Reports* 10: 1–9.

**86** Summers, S. (2020). Assessment of novel causes and investigation into the gut microbiome in cats with chronic kidney disease. In: *Clinical Sciences*. Fort Collins, CO: Colorado State University.

**87** Summers, S., Quimby, J., Isaiah, A. et al. (2019). The fecal microbiome and serum concentrations of indoxyl sulfate and p-cresol sulfate in cats with chronic kidney disease. *Journal of Veterinary Internal Medicine* 33: 662–669.

**88** Hall, J., Jackson, M., Jewell, D., and Ephraim, E. (2020). Chronic kidney disease in cats alters response of the plasma metabolome and fecal microbiome to dietary fiber. *PLoS One* 15 (7): e0235480.

**89** Ephraim, E. and Jewell, D. (2020). Effect of added dietary betaine and soluble fiber on metabolites and fecal microbiome in dogs with early renal disease. *Metabolites* 10: 370.

# 16

# Neurological Interactions with Microbiomes

The concept that microbial changes or state of microbial health of the GI tract could alter neurological functions has become well-established though, all the mechanisms involved are not always completely understood. Neurogastroenterology is the study of neurology in the gastrointestinal tract, liver, gallbladder, and pancreas involving interactions between, and the integration of the enteric nervous system and the central nervous system [1]. The GI microbiota impact brain development, the host immune system, emotion, and behavior [2]. Molecular interactions that occur between the GI microbiome and its metabolome with the host's central nervous system are recognized as complex, bidirectional, and may involve endocrine, neuronal, toll-like receptors, and metabolite-dependent pathways. This bidirectional communication is vital for maintaining normal brain function and gastrointestinal homeostasis. Crosstalk between the gut and brain when there is perturbation or disruption in the communication axis can result in psychological and neurological disorders. Additionally, bacterial translocation due to intestinal barrier dysfunction results in neuroactive metabolites and other microbiota components that induce a neuroinflammatory response in the brain [2].

## 16.1   The Nervous System

The nervous system is made up of the central nervous system (CNS), which includes the brain and the spinal cord, and the peripheral nervous system (PNS), which includes the connection of nerves from the rest of the body (muscles, sense organs, glands) to the brain and spinal cord.

The PNS is then divided into the somatic nervous system, which controls muscle movements and relays information from ears, eyes, and skin to the CNS, and the autonomic nervous system, which is further broken down into the sympathetic, parasympathetic, and enteric branches. These areas regulate glands and control involuntary bodily functions including heart rate, blood pressure, sexual arousal, respiration, and GI tract function [3]. The sympathetic branch manages acute changes in homeostasis. For example, the body prepares for an acute emergent response resulting in the inhibition of intestinal contractions. The parasympathetic branch returns body functions to normal after a sympathetic stimulation [4]. The enteric nervous system (ENS) is the largest division of the autonomic system [5]. The ENS is embedded within the walls of the digestive tract and is "protected" from the luminal content by the intestinal barrier [6]. The ENS extends between the esophagus and anus and contains thousands of ganglia, and approximately 400 million neurons that are more than any other peripheral organ and are very equivalent to the number of neurons in the spinal cord [6]. This system is capable of governing itself and controlling the digestive system's local physiological state [6]. Functions completed by the ENS include digestion, intestinal contractions, barrier permeability, secretion of bile, maintenance of epithelial fluid levels, luminal osmolality and permeability, mucus production, mechanisms of manipulation of the GI mucosa, and mucosal immune response through ganglionated plexuses (myenteric and submucosal plexus) [1, 2]. The ENS can work independently from CNS input and utilizes an intrinsic system of microcircuits [5]. It works with gut-associated lymphoid tissue (GALT) and thousands of enteroendocrine cells. As discussed in Chapter 15, GALT contains more than two-thirds (70%) of the body's immune cells while enteroendocrine cells contain more than 20 currently identified hormones [7]. Neurotransmitters, signaling pathways, neuronal connections, and the immune system, provide conduits that allow GI diseases to affect the brain and for pathophysiological processes that involve the CNS to often gastrointestinal symptoms [5]. Communication between the gut and brain occurs through (i) primary afferent neurons,

(ii) immune-system-mediated connections, and (iii) enteroendocrine cell-mediated connections [7]. The brain contains four predominant types of cells including neurons, glia, microglia, and astrocytes, which may be influenced by metabolites in the gut–brain axis [8]. In the autonomic system, ganglionic neurons work as neurotransmitters. These neurons consist of a set of nerve fibers in two branch types: preganglionic neurons (acetylcholine) that connect the CNS to the ganglia and postganglionic neurons (noradrenaline or norepinephrine) that connect the ganglion to the effector organ [9]. These neurotransmitters are involved in connecting and transferring signals through neuronal pathways; afferent neuron pathways bring signals to the CNS, while efferent neuron pathways carry signals out to the muscles and glands [4]. Neurotransmitters provide fast, short-term responses in the nervous system.

Neuroimmune connections exist between afferent nerve terminals and immune cells including plasma cells, eosinophils, and mast cells, within the GI mucosa [7]. Lymphocytes and mast cells can secrete neuroactive compounds such as histamine, 5-hydroxytryptamine (5-HT or serotonin), prostaglandins, and various cytokines, and can also contain neuropeptide receptors acting as signal transducers providing slow-acting, prolonged result [7]. Toll-like receptors are able to detect microbial antigens, helping mucosal immune cells distinguish the difference between commensal and pathogenic bacteria [7]. Toll-like receptors can also indirectly alter the activity of enteroendocrine and dendritic immune cells [7]. Communication also exists between the immune system through cytokines and the nervous system cytokines [6].

Hormones and the hypothalamic–pituitary–adrenal axis influence communication as part of the limbic system, which is the part of the brain that regulates emotional responses and memory. The hypothalamic–pituitary–adrenal axis regulates efferent neurons to coordinate adaptive responses of the host to stressors. Stress, environmental stress, or increased systemic pro-inflammatory cytokines activate the hypothalamus to secrete corticotropin-releasing factor that stimulates the pituitary gland to secrete adrenocorticotropic hormone (ACTH). This leads to the adrenal glands releasing cortisol, a major stress hormone. It is the combination of both neural and hormonal lines of communication that allow the brain to influence the activities of intestinal functional effector cells (immune cells, epithelial cells, enteric neurons, smooth muscle cells, interstitial cells of Cajal, and enterochromaffin cells) [1].

## 16.2    The Gut–Brain Communication Axis

A loss of GI microbiome composition and homeostasis from antibiotic usage, infection, or inappropriate dietary patterns in conjunction with a genetic predisposition have been implicated in the lack of communication in the gut–brain axis and pathogenesis of GI tract and neurological disorders [2]. The gut–brain communication axis is a link between the emotional and cognitive centers of the brain and the functions of the peripheral intestine [10]. This axis monitors and integrates GI function and oversees the effects of environmental influences like hunger, stress, and emotions on GI functions. For example, those experiencing a high-stress situation or emotion may have a physiological response resulting in symptoms in the GI tract (gastrocolic reflex) [1]. The GI microbiota is able to communicate with the host through multiple signaling mechanisms, and direct stimulation of the host's cells in the lamina propria (enterochromaffin cells, neurons, immune cells), releasing signaling molecules into the gut lumen. The brain can provide indirect influence by altering gastrointestinal motility, secretions, and intestinal permeability [10] (Figure 16.1).

### 16.2.1    Enteroendocrine and Neuroendocrine Cells

Enteroendocrine cells are the collection of specific epithelial cells in the gastrointestinal tract, and even though they make up less than 1% of total epithelial cells, they are a foundation of digestive physiology [7, 9]. There are 20+ different types of enteroendocrine cells and they are classified based on the type of regulatory peptide or bioactive molecule they secrete [7]. They regulate digestive functions through ENS circuits and communicate with the CNS, either directly through endocrine pathways or by assisting afferent terminals in the GI tract to sense luminal chemo-signals [7].

Neuroendocrine cells also make hormones but are more like nerve cells (neurons). They are found in the gastrointestinal tract, pancreas, thyroid, and lungs and have multiple body functions, including aiding digestion and respiration [9].

Enterochromaffin cells are a type of both enteroendocrine and neuroendocrine cells and are the most common type of neuroendocrine cells in the GI tract. They play a role in GI regulation especially, intestinal motility and secretion, with cells also being predominant in the jejunum,

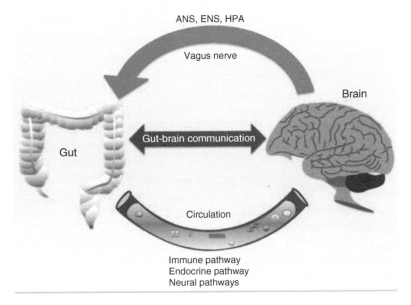

**Figure 16.1** The gut–brain axis. There is bidirectional communication between the brain and the gut that is affected by many pathways. These include the enteric nervous system (ENS), the autonomic nervous system (ANS), immune pathways, neural pathways, endocrine pathways, and hypothalamic–pituitary–adrenal (HPA) system [2]. Creative commons license: https://www.mdpi.com/openaccess.

ileum, colon, and appendix [10, 11]. These cells regulate the bidirectional communication between the GI lumen and the nervous system through vagal and afferent pathways which detect physiologic information from the viscera. Communication involving enterochromaffin cells can mediate pain and immune response and provide some influence on emotions and other homeostatic functions [10].

## 16.2.2 Microbial Metabolites

Microbial metabolites from the GI microbiome may affect neurological functions, and alterations in neurological functions may result in changes to the GI microbiome that initiates alterations in microbial metabolite production and functionality. Microbial metabolites have multiple functions in the body including the provision of energy and involvement in intrinsic and extrinsic communication including communication among the GI microbiota [2]. Microbial metabolites can alter barrier function through the autonomic nervous system gut synapses, which can affect mechanisms in the GI epithelium [2]. Changes in GI microbiome composition influence the type and concentration of the metabolome, alter barrier function, which may, in turn, result in intestinal permeability and the translocation of bacterial and/or their associated metabolites, with microbe-associated molecular patterns (MAMPs) into the mesenteric lymphoid tissues. This scenario has shown to result in the progression and development of various neurological diseases [2].

Metabolites and GI microbiota-derived cellular components with neuromodulatory properties can include gases (carbon monoxide, hydrogen sulfide, nitric oxide), short-chain fatty acids (SCFAs, propionate, butyrate, acetate), melatonin, gamma-aminobutyric acid (GABA), glutamine, histamine, branch-chained amino acids, lipopolysaccharides, secondary bile acids, acetylcholine, and catecholamines [1, 2, 7]. Additionally, microbiota can produce a wide range of molecules that mimic human hormones [1, 2, 7]. "Microbial endocrinology" includes neurochemicals (e.g. serotonin [5-Hydroxytryptamine], gamma-aminobutyric acid, glutamate) that are produced by both the host, multicellular organisms, and prokaryotes (bacteria and the archaea) that act as mechanisms for brain and behavior modification within the gut–brain axis [7, 12]. Some examples are muramyl dipeptide which is similar to serotonin, and indole is similar to melatonin; both are able to induce drowsiness. Lipopolysaccharides from Gram-negative bacteria can directly act on thyroid cells, via type 4 toll-like receptors [7]. These transmitters modulate important processes that occur during neurogenesis, myelination, synaptic pruning, glial cell function, and blood–brain barrier function [1]. Microbial metabolites are produced by specific phylum, family, genus, species, or strain of bacteria: SCFAs are produced by *Lactobacillus* and *Bifidobacterium species*; norepinephrine is produced by *Escherichia, Bacillus,* and *Saccharomyces* spp.; dopamine is a metabolite of *Bacillus*; Lactobacillus can produce acetylcholine; serotonin is produced from spore-forming microbes [13].

### 16.2.2.1 Gastrotransmitter – Gas Metabolites

Hydrogen sulfide ($H_2S$) is obtained through plant sources, L-cysteine or taurine, and may influence the density and function of GI microbiota. Sulfur is metabolized by anaerobic GI microbiota for energy, creating

$H_2S$ metabolites [14]. $H_2S$ is an important regulator of physiology, and the level of exposure determines the type of influence it has on the host. In lower provisions, $H_2S$ provides a therapeutic effect by decreasing inflammation, stabilizing mucus layers, preventing biofilm adhesion to the epithelium, inhibiting the release of invasive pathobionts, and increasing tissue repair [14]. Conversely, when produced at excessive concentrations, $H_2S$ can have toxic effects including causing disruptions in mucus layers, increased inflammation, and increase the risk and development of neoplasia in the host [14].

Nitric oxide (NO) is reduced from food (L-arginine) [15] to nitrate and then into nitrite by bacteria in the oral cavity and upper GI tract. Nitrite is able to take numerous pathways to be further reduced into NO. [16] NO is able to influence various neurotransmitter systems through the modulation of neurotransmitters norepinephrine, serotonin, dopamine, and glutamate. In humans, NO has been shown to play a role in multiple neurological pathophysiologies [17]. Like $H_2S$, NO has been shown to have beneficial effects, acting as an antibacterial, antiparasitic, antiviral, and tumoricidal agent, along with being potentially neurotoxic by contributing to excitatory amino-acid-induced neuronal injury and DNA damage [15]. Additionally, NO synthesis is linked to circulation, blood pressure, and cognition [18].

Carbon monoxide (CO) is commonly known to be an environmental pollutant, but it has the ability to provide some benefits. CO is a major neurotransmitter, acts as a vasodilator, functions in circadian rhythms, and is important for multiple neurologic functions including neuroprotection. It is involved in preventing platelet aggregation, as well as being a conditional anti-inflammatory agent [19, 20]. Like $H_2S$ and NO, CO can diffuse into any cell along a concentration gradient and has unique cell signaling (which involves the transmission of molecular signals from a cell's exterior to its interior) [20] (Figure 16.2).

### 16.2.2.2 Short-Chain Fatty Acids

Short-chain fatty acids (SCFAs) are probably the most researched metabolite having numerous benefits for the host [2]. SCFAs are a group of microbial metabolites resulting from the fermentation of nondigestible products, particularly dietary fiber and prebiotic classified sources, by mainly *Bacteroidetes* and *Firmicutes,* to produce acetate, propionate, and butyrate [2, 21], all of which have different metabolic and signaling

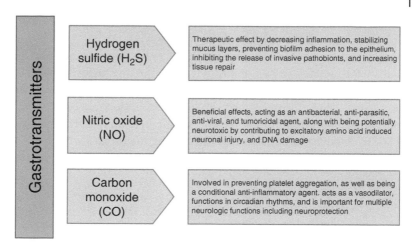

Figure 16.2 Benefits and actions of gastrotransmitters on the host.

capabilities [8]. These metabolites are rapidly absorbed into cells and the portal circulation where they travel to the brain and cross the blood–brain barrier. They play a crucial role in the regulation of hormones, GI motility, and neurological functions, including emerging evidence that SCFAs play a role in neuroimmune homeostasis, as well as influencing neurodegenerative diseases [2, 8, 21]. SCFAs are able to influence brain neurological functions through immune, vagal, endocrine, and humoral pathways. They are able to induce immune cells (microglia [8], regulatory T cells, endocrine cells, and vagal neuronal cells) to modulate brain functions by increasing the production of regulatory cytokines and GI-derived peptides [2]. SCFAs can stimulate mucosal serotonin release and are able to influence memory and learning capabilities [1]. Mice administered SCFA including oral butyrate resulted in improved responsiveness to stress and improved GI health [2].

Butyrate-producing bacteria *Clostridium*, *Eubacterium*, and *Butyrivibrio* genera are able to ferment nondigestible carbohydrates and fructooligosaccharides into the SCFA butyrate, which has multiple biological functions. This metabolite is the primary source of energy for colonocytes as they are able to utilize 70–90% of the butyrate pool [8]. Additionally, butyrate can act as a histone deacetylase inhibitor, preventing the accumulation of pro-inflammatory macrophages, and protecting the host from certain types of cancer, along with being able to activate

G-protein-coupled receptors (membrane proteins that convert extracellular signals into intracellular responses) [8, 22, 23]. The sodium form of butyrate (NAB) has also been shown to have a profound effect on enhancing memory and the ability to learn [22]. Mitochondrial dysfunction associated with acute and chronic neurological diseases may be due to a reduction of glucose metabolism in the brain. Butyrate could repair energy homeostasis through metabolic and mitochondrial influences [22]. In these ways, butyrate is an interesting microbial metabolite for countering neurological injury and disease.

### 16.2.2.3 Neurotransmitters

5-Hydroxytryptamine (5-HT), commonly known as serotonin, is a microbial metabolite that can be produced from tryptophan and enzymatic activity of tryptophan hydroxylase 1 (TH1). 5-HT is recognized as a neurotransmitter and plays a role in the regulation of GI contractions (peristalsis), vagal circuits (a main component of the parasympathetic system) that are associated with nausea, vomiting, and pain perception [7]. Enterochromaffin cells in the GI mucosa are the predominant site for the synthesis (90%) and storage of 5-HT in mammals, with microbial 5-HT production adding to the total GI tract pool [7, 8]. Its production is associated with *Clostridium perfringes* in humans and mice [2], though strains belonging to *Streptococcus* spp., *Escherichia* spp., and lactic acid bacteria are also known to synthesize 5-HT [7]. Chemical stimuli (presence of nutrients such as glutamate and glucose, or toxins in the intestinal lumen) cause the release of 5-HT. While serotonin is a well-known neurological influencer, it has also been utilized for the treatment of inflammatory bowel disease, irritable bowel syndrome, and idiopathic constipation [7]. When "germ-free" mice have increased production or supplementation of 5-HT, there is an increase in intestinal transit time and colonic motility [2].

Trace amines are neuroactive compounds that play a role as co-transmitters and neuromodulators. They are involved in mood control, appetite, and satiety circuits. Examples of trace amines are β-phenylethylamine, tyramine, tryptamine, and octopamine. Lactic acid bacteria strains are able to produce β-phenylethylamine, tyramine, and tryptamine; tyramine and β-phenylethylamine are produced by *Leuconostoc* and *Enterococcus species*, and *Lactobacillus bulgaricus* have been identified as being able to produce tryptamine. While there are fewer trace amines compared to 5-HT, they are physiologically present in the nervous system of mammals and play a significant role in neurological functions despite their low volume. Dysfunction with trace amine production and pathways are associated with attention/hyperactivity and some psychiatric disorders, Parkinson's disease, and hepatic encephalopathy in humans [7].

Histamine is produced when fish or shellfish products are contaminated by lactic acid bacteria or other types of bacteria. This interaction produces a large amount of histamine that has been indicated in allergy and anaphylaxis and plays a role as a neurotransmitter in both the CNS and ENS [7].

Glutamate is a main nutrient for enterocytes and is mostly oxidized into $CO_2$, or converted into other amino acids by microbial transformation; only 5–17% of glutamate is absorbed into the portal circulation [7]. Multiple bacterial strains are able to produce glutamate: *Corynebacterium glutamicum, Brevibacterium lactofermentum, Brevibacterium flavum,* and lactic acid bacteria *Lactobacillus plantarum, Lactobacillus paracasei,* and *Lactococcus lactis* [7]. Increasing glutamate intake does not necessarily result in increased concentrations in the plasma or brain tissue [7]. Glutamate is a major excitatory and inhibitory neurotransmitter found in the CNS and is part of a complex circuit that includes gamma-aminobutyric acid (GABA) and glutamine, which plays a role in recycling neurotransmitters in the brain [7].

GABA is a nonprotein amino acid from plants, animals, and microorganisms and can be synthesized from L-glutamate by α-decarboxylation. It is the principal inhibitory neurotransmitter in the brain playing a key role in CNS function in mammals [24]. GABA is involved in anxiety, depression, and aids in regulating blood pressure and heart rate, sleep cycles, appetite, mood, cognition, and plays a role in the perception of pain and anxiety [24]. There is also a genetic component with the ability of some genomes of bacteria being able to complete glutamate decarboxylation (gad genes); lactic acid bacteria (*Lactobacilli*), and *Bifidobacteria* are encoded with GABA production gad genes [24].

Substance P is a neuropeptide made up of 11 amino acids (an undeca-peptide) and functions as a neurotransmitter and a modulator of pain perception by altering cellular signaling pathways [25]. Additionally, substance P plays a role in gastrointestinal functioning, memory processing, angiogenesis, vasodilation, and cell growth and proliferation [25]. In mice, enhanced mucosal inflammation results in an increase in substance P expression in the ENS. This effect can be normalized by the administration of *L. paracasei*. In humans, it is hypothesized that patients with irritable bowel symptoms (IBS) have an abnormal microbiota that activates a mucosal innate immune response. This increases permeability, activates pathways that induce visceral pain, and dysregulates the ENS [1].

### 16.2.2.4 GI Microbiota-Derived Cellular Components

GI microbiota-derived cellular components can affect the function of both the CNS and ENS. Toll-like receptors in enteric neurons, sensory afferent neurons, and other cells in the brain are expressed by microglial cells and astrocytes and are activated by the GI microbiota-derived cellular components.

Lipopolysaccharides (LPS) are a main component of microbiota cell-wall structures and are known to induce neuroinflammation and neurodegenerative disease through toll-like receptor activation in brain cells. Signaling by LPS and toll-like receptors on microglial cells increases the expression of inflammatory cytokines in both the CNS and/or the GI tract [1, 21]. LPS may enter the brain under certain physiological conditions that induce neuroinflammation and cognitive impairment in mice [1]. Multiple studies reveal that when LPS travels from the GI tract to the brain via the circulatory system, it can induce neuroinflammation in the brain [2].

Microbial exocellular polysaccharides (EPSs) are extracellular metabolites that are similar to microbial biofilms. These metabolites are essential for protecting bacteria from the host immune response. Additionally, they interact with intestinal mucosal cells, including epithelial and enteroendocrine cells, modulating neural signaling or directly acting on primary afferent axons [7].

### 16.2.3 The Importance of Barrier Function

Changes in the normal function of the GI tract barrier result in alterations in permeability functions that can alter neurological behaviors. Alterations in barrier function can allow noxious substances from the lumen to cross the epithelium layer into the ENS. Changes in tight junction function can increase paracellular permeability. Signaling pathways that govern tight junction permeability are regulated by proinflammatory cytokines such as tumor necrosis factor-α and are associated with inflammation-induced intestinal permeability. A healthy and effective functioning GI tract barrier includes functional mucus layers, an effective glycocalyx (dense, gel-like meshwork consisting of polysaccharides, glycoproteins, and glycolipids that surround the cell or bacteria, creating a physical barrier) influence from secretory IgA and the mucosal immune response, antimicrobial peptides, chloride, and water secretions, along with a healthy functioning microbiome [6].

What are "germ-free" animal model studies showing us?

Utilizing "germ-free" mice, researchers can provide proof of how dysbiosis in GI microbiomes can result in neurological abnormalities [1]. These studies aim to be reproducible and predictable with results being altered by the addition or removal of species-specific microbes. Some frequently observed results in these studies are:

- Dysregulation of hormone signaling, including modulation of the serotoninergic system [1, 2].
- Varying expression of brain-derived neurotrophic factor [2].
- Differences in neurotransmission [1, 2].
- Changes in anxiety-like behaviors [1, 8].
- Changes in blood–brain barrier (BBB) expressions [1].
- Alterations in the release of corticosterone and adrenocorticotropin hormone (ACTH) [4].
- Change in the paracellular permeability of tight junction [1].
- Differences in amino acid metabolism [2].
- Alterations of gut sensory-motor functions (changes in gastric emptying and intestinal transit) [1].
- Neuromuscular abnormalities [1].
- Alterations in intrinsic sensory signaling [1].
- Modulation of afferent sensory nerves, which alter GI motility and pain perception [1].
- Alterations in memory function [1].

## 16.3 Anxiety

Stress is a state that is associated with a physiological response that aids the body in being able to defend or flee from the threat. A threat could be from a variety of sources such as infectious, psychological, traumatic, or toxic [26]. Stress is relieved by the removal of the stressor. Anxiety consists of a consistent state of worry or being in a constant state of preparation to defend or flee from a threat, even in the absence of the stressor or threat [27]. Stress and anxiety play a role in the modulation of the GI microbiome composition and total biomass, with up to 70% of behavioral disorders in dogs being attributed to some form of anxiety [1, 28]. The *"emotional motor system"* consists of the host's physiological response to stress. This system includes efferent neural pathways that are both directly and indirectly influenced by the host's GI microbiota signaling and are associated with the pain-modulator endogenous pathways, the activation of the hypothalamic–pituitary–adrenocortical axis, and the production of glucocorticoids [1, 29]. Initial colonization of the commensal GI microbiome plays a critical role in the development and must occur to ensure normal development of the hypothalamic–pituitary–adrenal (HPA) axis [4]. Stress can also affect the function of the GI tract with stress having been shown to induce a variation in the volume and quality of mucus secretion [1].

Different kinds of stress have different results on the GI tract, GI microbiomes, ENS, and CNS. Exposure to a social stressor for only 2 hours results in a reduction of the relative proportions of the main microbiota phyla [1]. Sound can be a stress trigger with acoustic stress altering gastric and postprandial motility in dogs, which slows gastric emptying [1]. In humans, psychological stress is associated with an increased occurrence of periodontal disease. Those experiencing high stress have twice the risk of experiencing a periodontal disease compared to people with minimal stress, which may be due to increased cortisol levels altering immune function in those experiencing high stress [26]. Mental stress has also been shown to increase the frequency of coeloconic spike-burst activity (three or more spikes with <8 ms interval in the hippocampus) [1]. Stress-associated alterations to the GI microbiome facilitate the expression of virulent bacteria. For example, during surgery, norepinephrine induces the expression of *Pseudomonas aeruginosa*, which may lead to GI sepsis. Additionally, norepinephrine can stimulate several other strains of enteric pathogens along with increasing the virulence of *Campylobacter jejuni* and allow for the overgrowth of pathogenic and non-pathogenic strains of *Escherichia coli* [1].

Aggression and phobia are both correlated to distress conditions and are expressions of anxiety disorders [29]. Aggressiveness includes both genetic and environmental influences and is displayed through physical attributes such as stance, vocalization, and attacking with or without biting. Phobia is a long-lasting and intense state of fear, which can be debilitating and are resulting from trauma. One study found a significantly lower relative abundance of *Oscillospira, Peptostreptococcus, Bacteroides, Sutterella,* and *Coprobacillus* in aggressive dogs when compared to a group of dogs with normal behavior and another group with phobic behaviors. The phobic group exhibited an enrichment of *Lactobacillus,* which are well-known GABA producers. In mice, this CNS inhibitory neurotransmitter is able to regulate emotional behavior via the vagus nerve [29]. *Lactobacillus rhamnosus* has been identified as having anxiolytic and anti-depressant-like effects that are mediated by GI-microbiota communication through the vagus nerve. What is unclear is whether the bacteria stimulate the vagus nerve with GABA it produces, or if it induces GABA production [7].

Enteropathogens may also be able to alter the behavior of infected animals. Mice inoculated with *C. jejuni* showed signs of increased anxiety (decreased exploratory type behaviors) despite any measurable activation of the immune system [30]. Infectious agents such as *Toxoplasma gondii,* influenza virus, and coronavirus have been hypothesized to be associated with an increased GI barrier permeability causing mood disorders [30].

Chronic gastrointestinal inflammation has been shown to induce anxiety-like behaviors. Studies looking to modify anxiety or emotion have been demonstrated with specific probiotic bacteria strains, *Bifidobacterium longum NCC3001 (BL999),* and *Lactiplantibacillus plantarum* (PS128) [28].

## 16.4 Cognitive Dysfunction

A decline in normal cognitive function over the course of aging is common in some mammals including humans and dogs, with cognitive dysfunction syndrome in dogs being similar to human dementia conditions including Alzheimer's disease [18]. Cognitive dysfunction syndrome is associated with irreversible loss of brain cells and synapses resulting in severe brain atrophy. Additionally, chronic low-grade inflammation is associated with this syndrome, which may result from altered bidirectional gut–brain communication [31]. Normal aging results in a

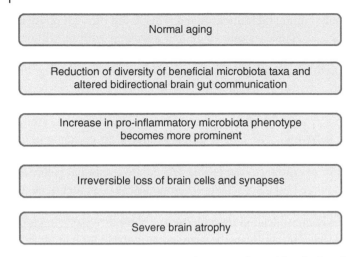

**Figure 16.3** Attributing factors and process of cognitive dysfunction syndrome in animals.

reduction of diversity and beneficial taxa with a pro-inflammatory phenotype being more prominent (see Figure 16.3). A precursor to the onset of neuroinflammation may be a microbial-derived neurotoxin metabolite that is able to cross the GI epithelial barrier and enter the systemic system, establishing pathogenic pathways of communication between the innate immune systems [31]. Microbial-derived polylipo-saccharides may be an important trigger for low-grade inflammation, neuroinflammation, and cognitive deficits due to GI permeability and its interaction with toll-like receptors on mononuclear cells, which can include immune cells such as lymphocytes [31].

Clinical signs of dogs and cats experiencing cognitive dysfunction include disorientation, alterations in social interactions, sleep–wake cycles, elimination habits, and activity, as well as an increase in generalized anxiety [32]. Additionally, deficits in learning and memory have been well documented [31]. Visuospatial learning and memory impairments are early markers for cognitive decline. Visuospatial function refers to cognitive processes necessary to "identify, integrate, and analyze space and visualize form, details, structure and spatial relations" in more than one dimension [33]. Visuospatial skills are needed for movement, depth and distance perception, and spatial navigation [33]. Aged dogs show a decline in visuospatial learning and memory deficits [34]. An example of visuospatial skills in dogs and cats could be changes in the ability to go up and down stairs or be able to jump up or down from furniture.

It is estimated that 28–29.5% dogs between 11 and 14 years of age experience cognitive dysfunction syndrome with a spike to 47.6–68% once a dog is 15+ years [18]. Like dementia in humans, once established, there is no known cure for cognitive dysfunction syndrome, though diet, supplements, and drugs are available to help slow progression, by reducing oxidative stress and inflammation, providing a viable energy source for neurons, or improving neuronal function [18, 32].

## 16.5 Psychobiotics

Psychobiotics is a term that is being used for probiotics that are able to influence CNS function [24]. Microbiota are able to produce a variety of neuroactive compounds such as orexant, anorexant, opioid, and opioid antagonists [7]. Understanding how each probiotic strain alters the proteome and metabolome will allow a better understanding of how to treat specific health conditions [7].

One-way psychobiotics benefit the host is by restoring the tight junction and improving intestinal barrier function. Animals administered a psychobiotic consisting of *Lactobacillus helveticus R0052* and *Bifidobacterium longum R0175* pre-stressor had restored tight junction barrier integrity, along with a reduced stress response [1]. The microbes in psychobiotics or their by-products can directly target intestinal sensory nerves, impacting the ENS. For example, a Cholera toxin can activate the mucosa to release 5-HT, which acts on sensory nerve receptors [6].

There are multiple studies that have identified the ability of psychobiotics to modulate mood and stress along with reducing anxiety and depression [7]. *Bifidobacteria* and lactic acid bacteria have been shown to increase the levels of melatonin in morning saliva [7]. *Lactobacillus helveticus R0052* and *B. longum R0175* taken together have been shown to reduce anxiety in rats [6]. Some microbial strains, *Escherichia* spp. and *Lactobacillus* spp. are able to produce GABA and modulate GABA receptors that impair anxiety-like symptoms in mice [2]. More studies are needed for both dogs and cats to verify what bacterial strains may act as effective psychobiotics (Figure 16.4).

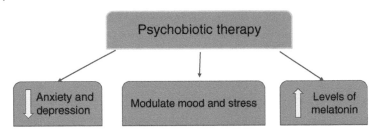

Figure 16.4   The benefits of psychobiotics on the central nervous system of the host.

## 16.6   Nutrients

Nutrients can modulate the growth of the microbiota in the GI tract, altering metabolite production and affecting cognition and behavior [30]. The GI microbiota are also able to influence nutrient availability through nutrient sensing (the cell's ability to recognize and respond to the concentration of energy substrates and produce only the molecules it needs at the time by regulating gene expression and modifying proteins) [1, 35]. Each type of energy source requires an alternative pathway and accessory molecules [35].

### 16.6.1   Simple Carbohydrates

The type of carbohydrate can influence changes at the genus and species level of GI microbiota. Mice fed resistant starch have shown to have more pronounced anxiety-like behaviors. In humans with autism, potential carbohydrate malabsorption has been identified in the small intestine; the long-term dysbiosis resulting in the formation of undesirable metabolites has been identified as the source of altered behavior in autistic children [30]. There are no studies at this time correlating this condition in dogs or cats with more research required.

### 16.6.2   Fat and Essential Fatty Acids

#### 16.6.2.1   Medium-Chain Triglycerides (MCT)
MCTs consist of glycerol esters that contain a carbon chain length between 7 and 12 compared to long-chain triglycerides that contain 13–21 carbon chains. MCT requires fewer steps to reach the mitochondria and

brain. During digestion, lipase hydrolyzes MCTs into medium-chain fatty acids that cross into the portal vein and are absorbed by the mitochondria of the liver and extrahepatic tissues, including the brain. Astrocytes in the brain metabolize the medium-chain triglyceride fatty acids, which is more efficient compared to long-chain fatty acids, where there is limited metabolism in the brain [35]. The ability of medium-chain fatty acids to cross the blood–brain barrier and be directly oxidized by the brain make this nutrient a key nutritional factor for pets with neurological disorders [36, 37]. Studies have shown that dietary supplementation with MCT improves brain and mitochondrial functions, alleviating the frequency of seizures and improving cognitive function in dogs [37, 38]. While not discussed in this book, some seizures can be triggered by impaired energy metabolism in the brain resulting in ion and neurotransmitter imbalances. By providing an alternative source of energy to the brain, we can avoid inducing perturbed metabolic processes [36]. Trials have shown improvement in cognitive function as early as 30 days with continuous improvement at 90 days. Additionally, 87% of dogs experienced a 33% reduction in seizure activity, while 50% had a 50% reduction in daily seizure activity [36–38].

### 16.6.2.2 Omega 3 Fatty Acids

Docosahexaenoic acid (DHA), a component of omega-3 fatty acids coming from marine sources, has been shown to provide anti-inflammatory benefits. Through multiple mechanisms, DHA has neuroprotective effects that include but are not limited to reducing pro-inflammatory metabolites from omega-6 fatty acids, enhanced antioxidant defenses, increased glucose transporters, and enhanced neurogenesis [18]. Additionally, when higher levels of DHA and eicosapentaenoic acid (EPA) (another component of omega 3 fatty acids) are provided, there is a decrease in inflammation due to effective levels of resolvins, protectins, and maresins that have been shown to be neuroprotective [18].

### 16.6.3 Vitamin and Mineral "Brain Blend"

It is sometimes not the supplementation of one nutrient but the addition of a complementary combination of a variety of vitamins and minerals serving to have an antioxidant and anti-inflammatory effect. Oxidative stress can be high in patients experiencing neural deficits including dementia and seizures and may require the addition of nutrients that aid in countering the effects of excessive oxidation and inflammation. A deficiency or low status of pyridoxine (B6), cobalamin (B12), and folate (B9) is associated with dementia in humans. Antioxidants can be used to protect against oxidative damage and damage associated with inflammation in both the brain tissues and blood vessels. A study on both cats and dogs looked at the benefits of supplementing omega-3 fatty acids, in the form of fish oil, arginine, B vitamins, and antioxidants vitamin E, C, and selenium to aging pets [18]. Both cats and dogs fed the supplement had improved cognition and memory [18, 39].

### 16.6.4 Fiber Sources – Oligosaccharides

*Morinda officinalis* How. (*M. officinalis*), is a Chinese traditional natural herbal medicine, that contains saccharides (49.79–58.25%), which are highly composed of oligosaccharides. Oligosaccharides from *M. officinalis* have been thought to inhibit oxidative stress, decrease neuronal cell death, restore normal energy metabolism, and significantly increase mitochondrial membrane and cell viability [13]. Hexasaccharide is an inulin-type of oligosaccharide that has shown to have antidepressant effects. Bajijiasu is another oligosaccharide from *M. officinalis* that improves D-galactose-induced cognitive deficits in mice along with improving blood flow by protecting against ischemia-induced neuronal damage and death [13]. Bajijiasu is also known to be a potential androgen-like drug that modulates hormone levels in male mice and humans [40]. Fructo-oligosaccharides (FOS) are known to be rapidly fermentable by beneficial microbiota in the GI tract resulting in a positive health effect for the host [13]. FOS from *M. officinalis* has shown to increase microbiota that are known to be beneficial similar to *Bifidobacteria* and *Lactobacilli* [13].

## 16.7 Chapter Summary

- Neurogastroenterology is the study of neurology in the gastrointestinal tract, liver, gallbladder, and pancreas involving interactions between, and the integration of the enteric nervous system and the central nervous system.

- The enteral nervous system (ENS) is embedded within the walls of the digestive tract and is "protected" from the luminal content by the intestinal barrier.
- The ENS works with gut-associated lymphoid tissue (GALT) and thousands of enteroendocrine cells.
- Enteroendocrine cells are the collection of specific epithelial cells in the gastrointestinal tract and even though they make up less than 1% of total epithelial cells, they are a foundation of digestive physiology.
- Neuroendocrine cells also make hormones but are more like nerve cells (neurons).
- Enterochromaffin cells play a role in GI regulation, especially in intestinal motility and secretion, with cells also being predominant in the jejunum, ileum, colon, and appendix.
- Microbial metabolites from the GI microbiome may affect neurological functions, and alterations in neurological functions may result in changes to the GI microbiome, which initiates alterations in microbial metabolite production and functionality.
- Metabolites and GI microbiota-derived cellular components with neuromodulatory properties can include gases (carbon monoxide, hydrogen sulfide, nitric oxide), SCFAs (propionate, butyrate, acetate), melatonin, gamma-aminobutyric acid (GABA), glutamine, histamine, branch-chained amino acids, lipopolysaccharides, secondary bile acids, acetylcholine, and catecholamines.
- *"Microbial endocrinology"* includes neurochemicals (e.g. serotonin [5-Hydroxytryptamine], gamma-aminobutyric acid, glutamate) that are produced bythe host, multicellular organisms, and prokaryotes (bacteria and the archaea) that act as mechanisms for brain and behavior modification within the gut–brain axis.
- Utilizing *"germ-free"* mice, researchers can provide proof of how dysbiosis in GI microbiomes can result in neurological abnormalities.
- Stress and anxiety play a role in the modulation of the GI microbiome composition and total biomass, with up to 70% of behavioral disorders in dogs being attributed to some form of anxiety.
- Cognitive dysfunction syndrome is associated with irreversible loss of brain cells and synapses resulting in severe brain atrophy.
- Clinical signs of pets experiencing cognitive dysfunction include disorientation, alterations in social interactions, sleep–wake cycles, elimination habits, and activity, as well as an increase in generalized anxiety.

- Psychobiotics is a term that is being used for probiotics that are able to influence CNS function. Microbiota are able to produce a variety of neuroactive compounds such as orexant, anorexant, opioid, and opioid antagonists.
- Nutrients like MCT, antioxidants, and SCFA are beneficial for pets with cognitive dysfunction.

## References

1 Chen, Z., Jalabi, W., Shpargel, K.B. et al. (2012). Lipopolysaccharide-induced microglial activation and neuroprotection against experimental brain injury is independent of hematogenous TLR4. *The Journal of Neuroscience* 32 (34): 11706–11715. https://doi.org/10.1523/JNEUROSCI.0730-12.2012.

2 Suganya, K. and Koo, B.S. (2020). Gut-brain axis: role of gut microbiota on neurological disorders and how probiotics/prebiotics beneficially modulate microbial and immune pathways to improve brain functions. *International Journal of Molecular Sciences* 21 (20): 7551. https://doi.org/10.3390/ijms21207551.

3 Waxenbaum, J.A., Reddy, V., and Varacallo, M. (2022). Anatomy, autonomic nervous system. In: *StatPearls*. Treasure Island (FL): StatPearls Publishing https://www.ncbi.nlm.nih.gov/books/NBK539845.

4 Carabotti, M., Scirocco, A., Maselli, M.A. et al. (2015). The gut-brain axis: interactions between enteric microbiota, central and enteric nervous systems. *Annals of Gastroenterology* 28 (2): 203–209.

5 Rao, M. and Gershon, M. (2016). The bowel and beyond: the enteric nervous system in neurological disorders. *Nature Reviews. Gastroenterology & Hepatology* 13: 517–528. 10.1038/nrgastro.2016.107.

6 Saulnier, D.M., Ringel, Y., Heyman, M.B. et al. (2013). The intestinal microbiome, probiotics and prebiotics in neurogastroenterology. *Gut Microbes* 4 (1): 17–27. https://doi.org/10.4161/gmic.22973.

7 Mazzoli, R. and Pessione, E. (2016). The neuro-endocrinological role of microbial glutamate and GABA signaling. *Frontiers in Microbiology* 7: 1934. https://doi.org/10.3389/fmicb.2016.01934.

8 Chambers, E.S., Preston, T., Frost, G. et al. (2018). Role of gut microbiota-generated short-chain fatty acids in metabolic and cardiovascular health. *Current Nutrition Reports* 7 (4): 198–206. https://doi.org/10.1007/s13668-018-0248-8.

**9** Gunawardene, A.R., Corfe, B.M., and Staton, C.A. (2011). Classification and functions of enteroendocrine cells of the lower gastrointestinal tract. *International Journal of Experimental Pathology* 92 (4): 219–231. https://doi.org/10.1111/j.1365-2613.2011.00767.x.

**10** Rhee, S.H., Pothoulakis, C., and Mayer, E.A. (2009). Principles and clinical implications of the brain-gut-enteric microbiota axis. *Nature Reviews. Gastroenterology & Hepatology* 6 (5): 306–314. https://doi.org/10.1038/nrgastro.2009.35.

**11** Bistoletti M, Bosi A, Banfi D, Giaroni C, Baj A. The microbiota-gut-brain axis: Focus on the fundamental communication pathways. *Progress in Molecular Biology and Translational Science* 2020;176:43–110. doi: https://doi.org/10.1016/bs.pmbts.2020.08.012.

**12** Lyte, M. (2014). Microbial endocrinology: host-microbiota neuroendocrine interactions influencing brain and behavior. *Gut Microbes* 5 (3): 381–389. https://doi.org/10.4161/gmic.28682.

**13** Chen, D., Yang, X., Yang, J. et al. (2017). Prebiotic effect of fructooligosaccharides from Morinda officinalis on Alzheimer's disease in rodent models by targeting the microbiota-gut-brain-axis. *Frontiers in Aging Neuroscience* 9: 403. https://doi.org/10.3389/fnagi.2017.00403.

**14** Buret, A.G., Allain, T., Motta, J.P. et al. (2022). Effects of hydrogen sulfide on the microbiome: from toxicity to therapy. *Antioxidants & Redox Signaling* 36: 4–6. https://doi.org/10.1089/ars.2021.0004.

**15** Danilov, A.I., Anderson, M., Bavand, N. et al. (2003). Nitric oxide metabolite determinations reveal continuous inflammation in multiple sclerosis. *Journal of Neuroimmunology* 136 (1–2): 112–118. https://doi.org/10.1016/S0165-5728(02)00464-2.

**16** Lundberg, J., Weitzberg, E., and Gladwin, M. (2008). The nitrate–nitrite–nitric oxide pathway in physiology and therapeutics. *Nature Reviews. Drug Discovery* 7: 156–167. https://doi.org/10.1038/nrd2466.

**17** Dhir, A. and Kulkarni, S.K. (2011). Nitric oxide and major depression. *Nitric Oxide* 24 (3): 125–131. https://doi.org/10.1016/j.niox.2011.02.002.

**18** Pan, Y., Kennedy, A.D., Jönsson, T.J. et al. (2018). Cognitive enhancement in old dogs from dietary supplementation with a nutrient blend containing arginine, antioxidants, B vitamins and fish oil. *The British Journal of Nutrition* 119 (3): 349–358. https://doi.org/10.1017/S0007114517003464.

**19** Mahan, V.L. (2015). Metabonomics, brain apoptosis, and carbon monoxide. *Journal of Translational Biomarkers & Diagnosis (JBR-TBD)* 1 (1): 1–8.

**20** Hanafy, K.A., Oh, J., and Otterbein, L.E. (2013). Carbon monoxide and the brain: time to rethink the dogma. *Current Pharmaceutical Design* 19 (15): 2771–2775. https://doi.org/10.2174/1381612811319150013.

**21** Panther, E.J., Dodd, W., Clark, A. et al. (2022). Gastrointestinal microbiome and neurologic injury. *Biomedicine* 10 (2): 500. https://doi.org/10.3390/biomedicines10020500.

**22** Bourassa, M.W., Alim, I., Bultman, S.J. et al. (2016). Butyrate, neuroepigenetics and the gut microbiome: can a high fiber diet improve brain health? *Neuroscience Letters* 625: 56–63. https://doi.org10.1016/j.neulet.2016.02.009.

**23** Zhao, J., Deng, Y., Jiang, Z. et al. (2016). G protein-coupled (GPCRs) in Alzheimer's disease: a focus on BACE1 related GPCRs. *Frontiers in Aging Neuroscience Cellular and Molecular Mechanisms of Brain-aging.* 8: 58. https://doi.org/10.3389/fnagi.2016.00058.

**24** Duranti, S., Ruiz, L., Lugli, G.A. et al. (2020). Bifidobacterium adolescentis as a key member of the human gut microbiota in the production of GABA. *Scientific Reports* 10: 14112. 10.1038/s41598-020-70986-z.

**25** Sharun, K., Jambagi, K., Arya, M. et al. (2021). Clinical applications of substance P (Neurokinin-1 receptor) antagonist in canine medicine. *Archives of Razi Institute* 76 (5): 1175–1182. https://doi.org/10.22092/ari.2021.356171.1797. PMID: 35355772; PMCID: PMC8934081.

**26** Rowińska, I., Szyperska-Ślaska, A., Zariczny, P. et al. (2021). The influence of diet on oxidative stress and inflammation induced by bacterial biofilms in the human oral cavity. *Materials* 14: 1444. https://doi.org/10.3390/ma14061444.

**27** Tynes, V.V. and Landsberg, G.M. (2021). Nutritional management of behavior and brain disorders in dogs and cats. *Veterinary Clinics of North America: Small Animal Practice* 51 (3): 711–727.

**28** Yeh, Y.-M., Lye, X.-Y., Lin, H.-Y. et al. (2022). Effects of *Lactiplantibacillus plantarum* PS128 on alleviating canine aggression and separation anxiety. *Applied Animal Behaviour Science* 247: 105569.

**29** Mondo, E., Barone, M., Soverini, M. et al. (2020). Gut microbiome structure and adrenocortical activity in dogs with aggressive and phobic behavioral disorders. *Heliyon* 6 (1): e03311. https://doi.org/10.1016/j.heliyon.2020.e03311.

**30** Suchodolski, J.S. (2018). Gut brain axis and its microbiota regulation in mammals and birds. *Veterinary Clinics: Exotic Animal Practice* 21 (1): 159–167. https://doi.org/10.1016/j.cvex.2017.08.007.

**31** Wu, M.L., Yang, X.Q., Xue, L. et al. (2021). Age-related cognitive decline is associated with microbiota-gut-brain axis disorders and neuroinflammation in mice. *Behavioural Brain Research* 402: 113125. https://doi.org/10.1016/j.bbr.2021.113125.

**32** Landsberg, G.M., Nichol, J., and Araujo, J.A. (2012). Cognitive dysfunction syndrome: a disease of canine and feline brain aging. *The Veterinary Clinics of North America. Small Animal Practice* 42 (4): 749–768. vii. https://doi.org/10.1016/j.cvsm.2012.04.003.

**33** Dickerson, B. and Atri, A. (2014). *Dementia Comprehensive Principles and Practices*, vol. 3 (19), 467–468. Oxford University Press.

**34** Studzinski, C.M., Christie, L.A., Araujo, J.A. et al. (2006). Visuospatial function in the beagle dog: an early marker of cognitive decline in a model of human aging and dementia. *Neurobiology of Learning and Memory* 86 (2): 197–204. https://doi.org/10.1016/j.nlm.2006.02.005.

**35** Duca, F.A., Waise, T.M.Z., Peppler, W.T. et al. (2021). The metabolic impact of small intestinal nutrient sensing. *Nature Communications* 12: 903. 10.1038/s41467-021-21235-y.

**36** Han, F.Y., Conboy-Schmidt, L., Rybachuk, G. et al. (2021). Dietary medium chain triglycerides for management of epilepsy: new data from human, dog, and rodent studies. *Epilepsia* 62 (8): 1790–1806. https://doi.org/10.1111/epi.16972.

**37** Molina, J., Jean-Philippe, C., Conboy, L. et al. (2020). Efficacy of medium chain triglyceride oil dietary supplementation in reducing seizure frequency in dogs with idiopathic epilepsy without cluster seizures: a non-blinded, prospective clinical trial. *The Veterinary Record* 187 (9): 356. https://doi.org/10.1136/vr.105410.

**38** Pan, Y., Larson, B., Araujo, J.A. et al. (2010). Dietary supplementation with medium-chain TAG has long-lasting cognition-enhancing effects in aged dogs. *The British Journal of Nutrition* 103 (12): 1746–1754. https://doi.org/10.1017/S0007114510000097.

**39** Pan, Y., Araujo, J.A., Burrows, J. et al. (2012). Cognitive enhancement in middle-aged and old cats with dietary supplementation with a nutrient blend containing fish oil, B vitamins, antioxidants and arginine. *The British Journal of Nutrition* 110 (1): 40–49. https://doi.org/10.1017/S0007114512004771.

**40** Wu, Z.Q., Chen, D.L., Lin, F.H. et al. (2015). Effect of bajijiasu isolated from Morinda officinalis F. C. How on sexual function in male mice and its antioxidant protection of human sperm. *Journal of Ethnopharmacology* 164: 283–292. https://doi.org/10.1016/j.jep.2015.02.016.

# 17

# Urinary System

The urinary system includes the kidneys, ureters, bladder, and urethra with a basic physiological role of extracting and removing waste products of metabolism and maintaining water and electrolyte balance within the cells. This system functions in the production of erythropoietin and renin hormones that maintain blood pressure, produce blood cells, and accurately absorb sodium. Additionally, this system processes vitamin D [1]. In the nephrons of the kidney, metabolic waste, excessive electrolytes, minerals, and water are filtered through the glomerulus and then moved through the tubule. Here, the viable substances are returned to the bloodstream and any waste products are moved through the ureters into the bladder for storage until the collection of urine products is released through the urethra and expelled outside the body. While this entire system has been historically considered to be sterile, there are findings of resident microbiomes, biofilms, and microbiota due to bacterial translocation in this system [1, 2].

## 17.1 GI–Renal Axis

Current research is minimal in this area and while it does not reflect a resident microbiome in the kidneys, it has shown that there is a gut–kidney/GI–renal axis (see Figure 17.1). Dysbiosis in the GI microbiome is showing to be associated with multiple renal conditions such as chronic kidney disease (CKD), nephrolithiasis, hypertension, and acute

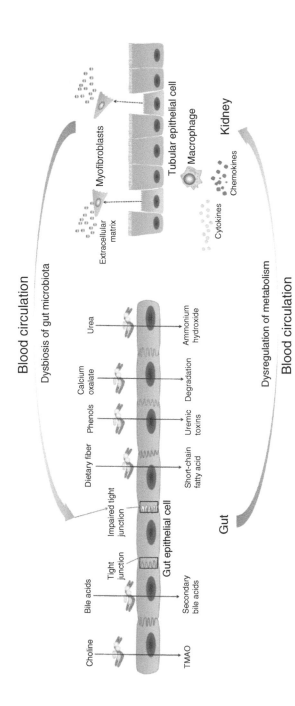

**Figure 17.1** The gut–kidney axis. Endogenous metabolites dysregulation and gut microbiota dysbiosis are contributing factors to renal injury. *Source:* Yuan-Yuan et al. [2] / Springer Nature / Public Domain CC BY 4.0.

renal injury. Intestinal dysbiosis may lead to intestinal barrier dysfunction allowing for bacterial translocation. The GI dysbiosis may also lead to excessive uremic toxin production such as indoxyl sulfate, *p*-cresyl sulfate, and trimethylamine-N-oxide. These products are all implicated in the development of renal diseases [2].

Interestingly, GI dysbiosis may be involved with the development of calcium oxalate uroliths in the kidneys. While nephrolithiasis may be caused by genetic and environmental factors, and some renal diseases are not directly correlated to dogs and cats, the GI microbiota may play a role in the formation of kidney stones. With 75% of kidney stones (uroliths) containing calcium oxalate, the concentration of calcium and oxalate can play a role in the development of uroliths. *Oxalobacter formigenes* is a bacterium that degrades oxalate in the intestinal tract that decreases the concentration of oxalate for intestinal absorption, which would lower the oxalate concentration for urinary excretion in humans. An inverse relationship has been noted between the recurrence of kidney uroliths and intestinal colonization of *O. formigenes,* meaning that when there is a high concentration of colonization, there is a low risk of urolith recurrence. One study found differences in the resident GI flora between healthy humans and those with nephrolithiasis with *Bacteroides* spp. being more abundant in patients that form kidney uroliths, and Prevotella spp. was more abundant in the healthy human patients [2]. Studies are required in dogs and cats to see if there is a similar correlation.

Melamine toxicity results in severe renal insult from the formation of kidney stones from the microbial metabolites of melamine, such as uric acid and cyanuric acid. It is possible that the type of microbiota in the GI tract plays a role in the level of toxicity the host experiences. In rats, when *Klebsiella* (*Klebsiella terrigena*) was colonized in the GI tract, melamine-induced renal nephrotoxicity was exacerbated. The effect of toxicity could be reduced through antibiotic suppression of this bacteria in the GI tract, which allowed an increased volume of melamine to be passed in the feces, unaffecting the health of the rat [3]. Further research in this area could see if this microbe plays a role in this toxicity in dogs and cats, explaining why some pets are more effected in cases of toxicity.

Key nutritional factors play a role in the maintenance and slowing of the progression of pathogenesis in pets with renal disease. The restriction of phosphorus, increased levels of antioxidants and omega 3 fatty acids, and moderate provision of proteins are known factors that influence the level of renal work and provide support to the kidneys. It should also be considered to address any concurrent GI conditions where there may be intestinal barrier dysfunction. Further information on supporting the health of the microbiome in the GI tract can be found in Chapter 15.

## 17.2   Urobiome

Urine in the bladder was once thought to be sterile and several studies on humans are now disproving that concept. Like other regions in the body, resident microbial communities play a role in the maintenance of the host health, with dysbiosis being associated with multiple urinary pathologies such as urinary tract infections (UTI) [1]. Studies have begun, using new tools, such as next-generation sequencing techniques, to identify common resident bacteria in the canine and feline urobiome [1, 4]. One study in dogs found that overall the four dominant taxa were *Pseudomonas* sp., *Acinetobacter* sp., *Sphingobium* sp., *and Bradyrhizobiaceae*. These taxa were substantially different from the rectal samples. *Pseudomonas* sp. was the most predominant bacteria genus for both male and female dogs [5]. Cats have multiple urinary tract-related conditions that may benefit from further research in this area. Currently, there is no evidence has been found to implicate the bladder microbiome in the pathogenesis of feline idiopathic cystitis [4]. Cats experiencing chronic kidney disease can have urobiome dysbiosis, which may favor *Escherichia-Shigella* colonization [4].

### 17.2.1   Urinary Tract Infections

Urinary tract infections (UTI) can be classified into simple uncomplicated and complicated (recurrent). Simple UTI occurs in a healthy pet with normal urinary tract anatomy and function, who suffers from a sporadic bacterial infection of the bladder. This can progress to a complicated UTI when there are three or more infections per year particularly when they are associated with the same bacteria culprit, along with the presence of relevant comorbidities [6].

Clinical signs may include dysuria (painful urination), pollakiuria (increased frequency), along with an increase in urgency to urinate.

The presence of bacteria in the urine should be identified though it requires the combination of clinical evaluation, gross, cytological, and cultured evaluation of the urine to determine the clinical significance of the UTI [6]. A subclinical infection or asymptomatic bacteriuria may not indicate antimicrobial treatment [6, 7]. The use of antimicrobials in these cases may increase the risk of clinical infection and can increase the development of antibiotic resistance [5, 6].

The identification of a UTI currently involves collecting a urine sample and identifying the components of the urine through the use of specifically treated paper or litmus paper, sediment analysis, and growing bacteria for identification. Collection of the sample can be easily contaminated through both invasive (catheterization or cystocentesis), and noninvasive (free catch) samples. These samples may be contaminated with epithelial cells or bacteria from the skin, urethral, or genital area. Microscopic detection includes either wet- or dry-mount analysis. Wet-mount detection of bacteria is not always an accurate way to assess urine samples. Using the modified Sternheimer-Malbin urinary stain (Sedi-Stain, Becton Dickinson) red blood cells, white blood cells and casts will be highlighted, and the stain will only be attached to dead bacteria. Dry-mount preparations with Gram and Wright-Giemsa staining have a higher specificity in both dogs and cats. Despite Wright-Giemsa and Gram staining of samples being more time-consuming to prepare, the use of these samples may reduce unnecessary culture and/or over-prescribing of antimicrobials in both dogs and cats (see Figure 17.2). One study identified that the wet-mount preparations of cat urine had a sensitivity of 76% and specificity of 57%, whereas Wright-stained dry-mount preparations had a sensitivity of 83% and a specificity of 99% [7]. Standard urine cultures are limited in the array of bacteria species they can detect, with mainly aerobic, fast-growing bacteria thriving on current culture media, such as *Escherichia coli*. Anaerobic microorganisms that grow slowly or bacteria with complex nutrient needs do not thrive in this environment [1].

The most common bacteria isolated from UTIs in dogs and cats is *Escherichia coli*. In dogs, *Staphylococcus* species, *Proteus*, *Klebsiella*, are seen along with *Enterococcus* as secondary species. *Enterococcus faecalis* and *S. felis* are the next most common microbiota in UTIs in cats [7] (Figure 17.3).

The health of the pet, the environment of the bladder, and the host immune response play a role in the development of a urinary tract infection [7].

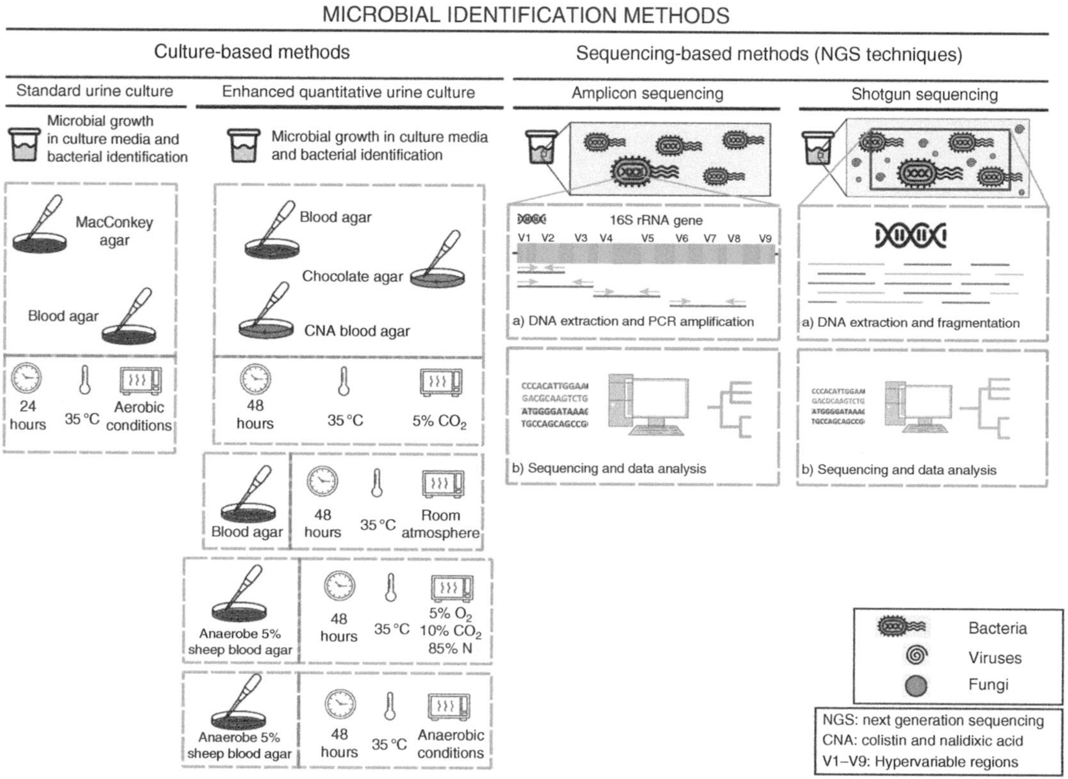

**Figure 17.2** Different methods of microbial identification in urine samples. *Source:* Perez-Carrasco et al. [1] / Frontiers Media S.A / Public Domain CC BY 4.0.

Risks of experiencing a UTI

- Age
- Sex
- Presence of a comorbidity
- Functional abnormalities
- Contamination from the microbiota in the rectum and urogenital area (vulva)
- Inability to completely empty bladder
- Presence of uroliths (urolithiasis)
- Urinary incontinence
- Immunosuppression
- Glucosuria (to emphysematous cystitis and not other UTIs)[5]

**Figure 17.3** Risk factors for contracting a urinary tract infection.

## 17.2.2 Biofilm in the Bladder

Similar to other areas in the body, bacteria in the lower urinary tract exist as planktonic (nonadhered, generally more susceptible to antimicrobials) or in a biofilm. Biofilms are structured communities of microorganisms. These microorganisms are able to secrete a gel-like polymer that aids in the creation of a stronger structure along with adhering to either the urothelium or on inert surfaces such as urinary catheters, ureteral stents, and subcutaneous ureteral bypass systems [7]. The biofilm may begin by creating a film using proteins and fibrinogen in the urine, which provide receptor sites for bacterial adhesions [7]. Once the biofilm structure is formed, the adhesion is irreversible. Urinary biofilms consist of 10–25% bacteria and 75–90% polysaccharides with water and nutrient transport channels [7]. Biofilms are able to provide protection to the bacteria in the structure from antimicrobials by:

1) Decreasing penetration of antimicrobials into the structure.
2) Slow the growth rate of bacteria, which decreases sensitivity to antimicrobials.
3) Alter gene expression to allow for resistance.
4) Binding and inactivating antibiotics using polysaccharides in the matrix [7].

Uropathogenic *E. coli* is the most widely studied bacterial biofilms in the urinary tract, and some uropathogenic *E. coli* are able to establish colonies in the bladder interstitium known as "quiescent intracellular reservoirs" where they can remain dormant for several months before reactivation. There are some bacteria, such as *Proteus* spp., that will create a crystalline biofilm structure. This is completed by producing urease and inducing struvite precipitation around the organism, as a protective barrier.

## 17.3  Defenses Against Urinary Tract Infections

### 17.3.1  Innate Immune System's Role

As part of the innate immune system, the urinary tract prevents ascending infection and mechanically removes bacteria. Urine is pulsated from the renal pelvis through the ureters into the bladder, and the strong flow of urine through the urethra when the bladder voids urine are two ways the innate system functions to remove planktonic bacteria from the body. There are also several antimicrobial peptides in the lower urinary tract that can prevent the colonization of bacteria in a variety of ways, along with the immune response, including the release of neutrophilic defenses [7] (Figure 17.4).

#### 17.3.1.1  Bacterial Interference

A novel therapy for recurrent UTI is the use of low-virulence nonpathogenic organisms like *E. coli* strains to decrease the risk of colonization with more pathogenic organisms. The beneficial bacteria strains are flushed directly into the bladder and have a "probiotic" effect. One study utilizing this technique found 44.4% of dogs achieve removal of the current UTI with 30% of those dogs having no recurrence of an infection [8].

**Figure 17.4**  Key elements in natural defenses against UTIs.

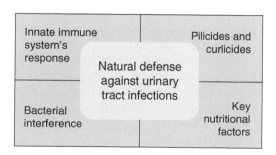

**17.3.1.2 Pilicides and Curlicides**

Bacterial adhesion pili are designed to bind and maintain the attachment of the bacteria to target cells [9]. Uropathogenic P-pili are able to resist the innate cleansing action of urine flow that removes most other bacteria [9]. Pilicides are able to effectively reduce motility and decrease the ability of P-pili to adhere to the bladder mucosa [8]. Curli are bacterial surface appendages that may facilitate biofilm formation. Curlicides are inhibitors that reduce the biofilm and virulence of uropathogenic *E. coli* [8].

## 17.4  Key Nutritional Factors

Proanthocyanidins from cranberry have been indicated in humans to be effective in inhibiting the ability of *E. coli* fimbriae to adhere to the uroepithelium. Studies do not align on the ability of cranberry to be effective in the treatment of UTIs though the antioxidant effects in higher concentration extracts of proanthocyanidins may aid in providing some protection with antiadhesion activity [6, 8].

Probiotics in humans have been utilized to aid in reducing recurrent UTIs in women. Several *Lactobacilli* strains are able to clear potential uropathogenic *E. coli*, stimulate the immune system, and alter vaginal flora [8]. Probiotic use to "normalize" vaginal flora has been successful in suppressing the recurrence of chronic UTI in women though this has not been as successful in dogs and cats. While the human vaginal microbiome may be different in those with or without a UTI, dogs' vaginal microbiomes remain unchanged regardless of the presence of a UTI [8].

### 17.4.1  Mannose (D-Mannose)

Uropathogenic *E. coli*'s ability to adhere to the uroepithelium can be blocked by D-mannosides as shown in both *in vivo* and *in vitro* studies in humans. D-mannose has been used to influence glyconutrient status, and it is able to bind proteins that ultimately block uropathogenic *E. coli*'s ability to adhere [8]. Studies in humans have shown promise in this area for dogs and cats [8].

## 17.5 Chapter Summary

- Dysbiosis in the GI microbiome is showing to be associated with multiple renal conditions such as chronic kidney disease (CKD), nephrolithiasis, hypertension, and acute renal injury.
- GI dysbiosis may be involved with the development of calcium oxalate uroliths in the kidneys.
- Dysbiosis in the urobiome is associated with multiple urinary pathologies such as urinary tract infections (UTI).
- The most common bacteria isolated from UTIs in dogs and cats is *Escherichia coli.*
- Bacteria in the lower urinary tract exist as planktonic (nonadhered, generally more susceptible to antimicrobials) or in a biofilm.
- Once the biofilm structure is formed the adhesion is irreversible.
- Some nutritional factors including the use of probiotics have been shown to be supportive to pets with urinary tract dysbiosis.

## References

1 Perez-Carrasco, V., Soriana-Lerma, A., Soriano, M. et al. (2021). Urinary microbiome: Yin and Yang of the urinary tract. *Frontiers in Cellular and Infection Microbiology* 11: 617002. 10.3389/fcimb.2021.617002.

2 Chen, Y.Y., Chen, D.Q., Chen, L. et al. (2019). Microbiome-metabolome reveals the contribution of gut-kidney axis on kidney disease. *Journal of Translational Medicine* 17: 5. https://doi.org/10.1186/s12967-018-1756-4.

3 Zheng, X., Zhao, A., Xie, G. et al. (2013). Melamine-induced renal toxicity is mediated by the gut microbiota. *Science Translational Medicine* 5: 172. https://doi.org/10.1126/scitranslmed.3005114.

4 Kim, Y., Carrai, M., Leung, M.H. et al. (2021). Dysbiosis of the urinary bladder microbiome in cats with chronic kidney disease. *Microbial Ecology* 6 (4): e00510–e00521. https://doi.org/10.1128/mSystems.00510-21.

5 Burton, E.N., Cohn, L.A., Reinero, C.N. et al. (2017). Characterization of the urinary microbiome in healthy dogs. *PLoS One* 12 (5): e0177783. https://doi.org/10.1371/journal.pone.0177783.

6 Weese, J.S., Blondeau, J.M., Boothe, D. et al. (2011). Antimicrobial use guidelines for treatment of urinary tract disease in dogs and cats: antimicrobial guidelines working group of the International Society for

Companion Animal Infectious Diseases. *Veterinary Medicine International* 2011: 263768. 10.4061/2011/263768.

**7** Byron, J.K. (2019). Urinary tract infection. *Veterinary Clinics of North America: Small Animal Practice* 49 (2): 211–221. https://doi.org/10.1016/j.cvsm.2018.11.005.

**8** Terlizzi, M.E., Gribaudo, G., and Maffei, M.E. (2017). UroPathogenic *Escherichia coli* (UPEC) infections: virulence factors, bladder responses, antibiotic, and non-antibiotic antimicrobial strategies. *Frontiers in Microbiology* 8: 1566. https://doi.org/10.3389/fmicb.2017.01566.

**9** Bullitt, E. and Makowski, L. (1995). Structural polymorphism of bacterial adhesion pili. *Nature* 373 (6510): 164–167. https://doi.org/10.1038/373164a0.

# Section III

# Emerging Ingredients and Alternative Diets

We have observed an evolution in the pet food industry over the last 10–15 years with a recognizable change in how pets are viewed in the family dynamic [1, 2]. We also have a greater understanding of the intrinsic involvement of the microbiome with the body's physiological functions, and the role nutrition plays beyond providing energy [3]. During this same time frame, the human diet culture evolved along with disease and fad-focus diets gaining public awareness, resulting in an increase in the number of diet-specific products in the market, such as keto, vegetarian, vegan, gluten-free, and raw diets. To meet pet parents' emotional needs when purchasing food, they consider to be better for their pets, there was an influx of "specialized" pet food diets in the market while scientifically there was very little or no indication that these diets resulted in better health for pets [4].

The world is experiencing and acknowledging the effects of climate change. With the pressing impact of global warming, environmental sustainability may require alternative protein sources in pet food [5]. Multiple factors are driving this necessity with the growth of the world population being the main component followed by numerous subsequent factors [6]. An increase in the number of people will result in an increased number of pets. Morgan Stanley Research strategists expect a 14% growth in pet ownership by the year 2030 [2]. Both of these factors will increase the competition for protein sources. Western diets have an increased demand for meat protein sources

*Small Animal Microbiomes and Nutrition*, First Edition. Robin Saar and Sarah Dodd.
© 2024 John Wiley & Sons, Inc. Published 2024 by John Wiley & Sons, Inc.
Companion website: www.wiley.com/go/saar/1e

with an expected increase in demand of 75% by the year 2050 [6]. There is less appropriate farmland to grow crops and raise protein sources, along with the effects of global warming such as changes in weather patterns resulting in weather extremes – droughts, flooding, heatwaves, and extreme cold such as a polar vortex, resulting in a decreased crop output [6]. These crops are utilized as a nutrient source for both humans and the animals being raised for consumption [6]. To help mediate these concerns, alternative protein sources are required to keep up with demand. To be successful, these new protein sources need to require fewer resources (water, land, feed) than what is currently being used to produce present-day protein sources [6].

The use of new alternative ingredients in pet food has many concerning factors that require further research such as digestibility, nutrient interactions, any possible associated toxicities, and the effects on the body's microbiomes [6]. Possible alterations in the body's microbiome, specifically the GI microbiome from feeding these new ingredients, may involve changes in diversity, the type of metabolites produced, and the effect of the metabolome on the host [7]. It can take years of research to understand any possible long-term health effects of using new ingredients in pet food, and with many of these emerging ingredients either having minimal or no current studies, the amount of information we have on their effects on the microbiome is minimal.

## References

**1** 2021 pet food trends Clarkson consulting. https://clarkstonconsulting. com/insights/2021-pet-food-trends/ (accessed 6 January 2022).

**2** 2021 ADM Unveils the next big consumer trends ADM news details. https://investors.adm.com/news/news-details/2021/ADM-Unveils-the-Next-Big-Consumer-Trends/default.aspx (accessed 6 January 2022).

**3** Kau, A.L., Aharn, P.P., Griffin, N.W. et al. (2011). Human nutrition, the gut microbiome, and immune system: envisioning the future. *Nature* 474 (7351): 327–336. 10.1038/nature10213.

**4** 2020 Alternative pet diets: Grain-free, raw, and other trends Today's veterinary nurse. https://todaysveterinarynurse.com/articles/alternative-pet-diets-grain-free-raw-and-other-trends/ (accessed 6 January 2022).

**5** 2021 Food for thought: The protein transformation BCG. https://www. bcg.com/publications/2021/the-benefits-of-plant-based-meats%20 (accessed 6 January 2022).

**6** van Huis, A. and Oonincx, D.G.A.B. (2017). The environmental sustainability of insects as food and feed. A review. *Agronomy for Sustainable Development* 37: 43. 10.1007/s13593-017-0452-8.

**7** Singh, R.K., Chang, H.W., Yan, D. et al. (2017). Influence of diet on the gut microbiome and implications for human health. *Journal of Translational Medicine* 15: 73. 10.1186/s12967-017-1175-y.

# 18

## Raw Ingredient Diets

The use of raw or uncooked ingredients, particularly uncooked meat products, as a source of pet nutrition has increased in popularity over the last few decades with pet parents looking for a diet that is considered to be more "natural" or "species-appropriate" [1, 2]. Pet parents like having some control over their pet's health by participating in making food from scratch or supplementing diets with ingredients they would feed their human family members or consist of ingredients they consider to be appropriate for their pet [3]. Presentation of raw diets has evolved in the commercial market to include fresh, frozen, freeze-dried, dehydrated, and high pressure pasteurized products [4]. Some diets have been identified as raw meat-based diets or "Biologically Appropriate Raw Food" [2] or BARF (Bones And Raw Food), which focus on a higher meat content (70–80%) coming from livestock or wild animals with less dietary ingredients coming from plant sources (20–30%) [2, 5]. Some countries (the United States and European Union [EU]) have increased guidelines and regulations on all commercial diets including raw to ensure that all food intended for animal consumption, meet nutrient requirements including more stringent regulations such as zero-tolerance for *Salmonella* and a defined acceptable level of *Enterobacteriaceae* [6]. With the increased use of raw products in pets' diets, it is important that we have a basic understanding of the differences, if any, between raw and cooked food sources regarding their effect on the body's microbiomes.

*Small Animal Microbiomes and Nutrition*, First Edition. Robin Saar and Sarah Dodd.
© 2024 John Wiley & Sons, Inc. Published 2024 by John Wiley & Sons, Inc.
Companion website: www.wiley.com/go/saar/1e

## 18.1 Raw vs Cooking

Raw food poses a substantial risk of infectious disease to the pet, the pet's environment, and the humans in the household, with raw pet food commonly exceeding hygiene thresholds for counts of *Enterobacteriaceae* [2, 3]. One claimed benefit of raw is the altered physiochemical properties to the nutrients from extreme heat used in cooked or commercial diets, which can result in a decrease or increase in the bioavailability of nutrients. While studies are limited in dogs and cats regarding raw versus cooked ingredients, there is some consideration that there has been some evolution of the gastrointestinal tract in pets [7]. Additionally, individual ingredients and the cooking method is showing to affect the composition and bioavailability of the nutrient for the host and the GI microbiota [8].

### 18.1.1 Starches and Vegetables

When cooked, starch is gelatinized which increases ileal digestibility. This leaves fewer nutrients for amylolytic (able to ferment starches) microbiota to ferment as an energy source. In a study of raw vs cooked tubers fed to mice, the diversity between the two groups' fecal microbiome was significantly different within only 24 hours of diet initiation [7]. The digestibility of the tubers was increased when cooked. The cooked tubers, in particular sweet potato and white potato, exhibited the greatest compositional shift and trended toward a reduced metabolite complexity [7]. There was an increased expression of genes for the metabolism of starch in the raw and less digestible tubers [7].

Vegetables provide a good source of vitamins including β-carotene (provitamin A), Vitamin C (ascorbic acid), Vitamin E (α-tocopherol), and Vitamin K [9]. Several epidemiological studies show a relationship between diets that are high in vegetables with a reduced risk of disease [9]. An abstract review of studies from 1994 to 2003 summarizing the relationship between cooked and raw vegetables and cancer found an inversely related relationship; the higher consumption of either raw or cooked vegetables resulted in a decreased risk of cancer [10].

A study in 2018 looked at changes in the retention of 10 vegetables (broccoli, chard, mallow, potato, sweet potato, carrot, crown daisy, pellia leaf, spinach, and zucchini) through 4 different cooking processes (boiling, blanching, steaming, and microwaving) [9]. Vitamin C (ascorbic acid) is water-soluble and temperature-sensitive and is easily degraded during the cooking process with higher temperatures and increase exposure times causing more severe loss. In this study, micro-waving and steaming showed the highest retention of vitamin C [9]. There were varied results on vitamin K with each type of vegetable through each cooking process. In some circumstances, vitamin K amounts were increased after cooking with the hypothesis that vitamin K is released when the plant proteins are broken down in the cooking process. Vitamin K is relatively stable when heated. Green leafy vegetables had higher retention of vitamin E ($\alpha$-tocopherol) compared to root vegetables though overall vitamin E (other tocopherol forms) was increased. Heat treatments could cause the breakdown of plant structure and possibly the loss of tocopherol oxidase allowing for the tocopherol varieties to be more available [9]. Carotenoids are precursors to vitamin A and were found to show lower and higher retention in the vegetables included in the study. This may be due to where the carotenoids are located; they may be released from chloroplasts of all green plant tissues, or the carotenes may be altered by heating resulting in lower retention [9].

Cooking vegetables causes an increase in the soluble dietary fiber content and decreases the insoluble fiber content [8]. Legumes can have the total dietary fiber increased by 1.2–8.2% when soaked in tap water at a 1 : 2 ratio for 12 hours at room temperature, with a considerable increase seen in soluble fibers [8]. It should be noted that cooking lentils can aid in removing anti-nutritional factors including tannins, phytic acid, and phenolic compounds, which can be a good source of nutrition for beneficial bacteria [11].

### 18.1.2 Meat (Protein)

The Association of American Feed Control Officials (AAFCO) defines meat in part as "the clean flesh derived from slaughtered mammals and is limited to that part of the striated muscle which is skeletal or that part which is found in the tongue, in the diaphragm, in the heart or in the esophagus; with or without the accompanying and overlying fat and portions of the skin, sinew, nerve, and blood vessels which normally accompany the flesh" [12]. Meat provides multiple nutrients such as protein, essential fatty acids, minerals, and vitamins [13]. While living muscle tissue in healthy animals contains little to no microorganisms, meat is easily perishable as it is a good medium for the growth.

Contamination with microorganisms may occur during slaughter and transport [13]. Sources of contamination during the slaughter process can come from processing tools, clothes, hands, and air [13].

Freezing is a widely accepted process for the inactivation of pathogens, and while the number of pathogens is reduced through the freezing process, certain pathogens can remain dormant, maintaining their pathogenicity, multiplying once the product is removed from storage and thawed [14]. Contamination and pathogen transfer from previously frozen raw products continue to pose a significant risk to the animals and the pet parents, which could be associated with potential health problems [14]. Commonly associated foodborne pathogens that are found in raw meat diets are *Escherichia coli, Salmonella* spp., *Clostridium* spp., *Campylobacter* spp., and *Listeria* spp. [14].

Colonic microbes are highly proteolytic (capable of fermenting protein) [15]. During digestion, proteins are hydrolyzed to polypeptides by peptidases and then into tripeptides, dipeptides, and single amino acids [15]. Bacterial proteases can then ferment smaller peptides and single amino acids to produce SCFAs, including acetate, propionate, and n-butyrate. Certain amino acids arginine, aspartic acid, glycine, phenylalanine, proline, serine, threonine, and tryptophan are more likely to undergo bacterial fermentation, rather than intestinal digestion [15]. In healthy humans, approximately 10% of protein reaches the large intestine and is available for bacterial fermentation [15]. The quality or digestibility of the protein source can alter the volume that reaches the gut microbiota, influencing intestinal microbiota diversity [16]. Raw meat advocates have promoted that raw meat has increased health benefits when compared to cooked meat, though current research does not reveal many differences between cooked and raw meat on the GI microbiome [8]. One recent study in cats compared a raw beef-based diet, cooked beef-based diet, and a commercial extruded diet. There were no significant differences between the cooked and the raw diet in digestibility or microbial [17]. A 2018 study looked at the true digestibility differences between raw, boiled, barbecued, grilled, roasted bovine meat, and/or milk proteins fed to rats for 3 weeks. The rats were divided into six groups with one group being fed only milk proteins. Each of the remaining five meat-fed groups was divided into a low-meat diet (5%) and a high-meat diet (15%) [18]. The findings between the meat-fed groups showed very similar digestibility except for boiled meat, which had a lower digestibility [18]. The mean true fecal

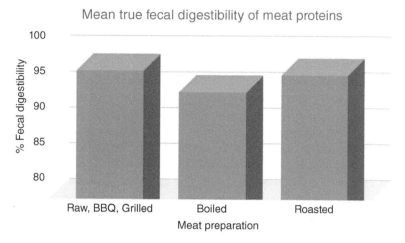

**Figure 18.1** The mean true fecal digestibility of meat proteins when prepared in different ways. The findings between the meat-fed groups showed very similar digestibility except for boiled meat that had a lower digestibility.

digestibility of meat proteins was 97.5% for raw, barbecued, and grilled meat, 94.5% for boiled meat, and 96.9% for roasted beef (see Figure 18.1). The SCFA concentrations did not differ between the diets though histologically, there were discrete signs of inflammation, and some excessive mucus secretion observed in all groups that ingested meat [18]. Interestingly, boiling hamburger meat has been commonly recommended by veterinary professionals as the ideal way to provide beef to pets with GI upset, and while it may lower the fat content, there could be an increase of undigested protein reaching the colon [18]. In a similar study in 2019, the gut microbiomes of mice fed raw and cooked meat were similar in composition and transcriptional profile [7]. More studies are needed in dogs and cats to better understand if raw meat ingredients have an effect on the gut microbiome.

## 18.2 Comparing Extruded, Canned, and Raw

There are very few studies in dogs and cats that compare extruded, and/or canned diets to raw meat-based diets. One very small more recent study by Kim et al. [19] compared the diversity of gut microbiota using fecal metagenomic DNA samples in 11 small breed dogs that were fed either a raw or kibble diet [19]. The findings revealed increased GI diversity in dogs fed the raw diet. At the phylum level, 8 different bacterial phyla in the 11 dog samples were identified [19]. The core microbiota in the natural diet group consisted of *Firmicutes, Bacteroidetes, Fusobacteria, Actinobacteria, and Proteobacteria,* and in the commercial feed group were *Firmicutes, Bacteroidetes, Proteobacteria*, and *Actinobacteria*. There are multiple limitations in the paper, including the nutrients of the diets on a dry matter basis, along with all the dogs being considered small or toy breeds [19].

In a comparison of the GI microbiota, 27 dogs were fed a BARF diet, and 19 were fed a conventional diet. The metabolomes from 10 BARF and 9 conventional diet dogs were analyzed via an untargeted metabolomics approach (see Figure 18.2) [5]. This study revealed changes in

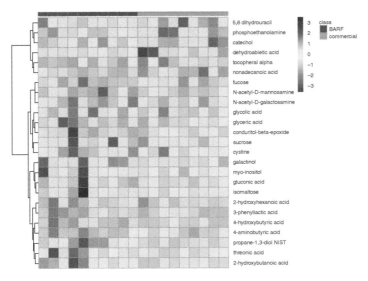

**Figure 18.2**   Heatmap showing the abundance of metabolites found in fecal samples of dogs fed a BARF diet (red columns) vs dogs fed a commercial diet (green columns). Red boxes show metabolites in a higher abundance and blue boxes show metabolites in lower abundance. Higher abundance of phosphoethanolamine, 5,6 dihydrouracil, dehydroabietic acid, and alpha-tocopherol were found in dogs fed the commercial diet. Conversely, dogs fed the BARF diet showed higher abundances of gluconic acid, myo-inositol, 4-aminobutyric acid, threonic acid, and 4-hydroxybutyric acid. *Source:* Schmidt et al. [5] / PLOS / Public Domain CC BY 4.0.

diversity with a significantly higher abundance of *Proteobacteria* and *Fusobacteria* with lower levels of *Firmicutes*, in dogs fed with the raw-based diet. The raw diet promoted a more balanced growth of bacterial communities and a positive change in the readouts of healthy gut functions in comparison to the commercial extruded diet [5]. This is also consistent with a study by Sandri et al., with the exception of not observing a significant change in *Firmicutes* [6].

In a study following kittens from birth, the oral microbiome became less variable once all the kittens were fed a commercial diet, though the type of commercial diet (kibble versus canned) reflected a difference in the populations of oral bacteria. Kittens fed the dry kibble had increased *Porphyromonas* spp. and *Treponema* spp., while kittens fed the wet-canned diets show an increase in C. kuhniae [20].

Inconsistencies in results, and limitations in the studies including varying amounts of macronutrients between diets, low subject and sample numbers, along with multiple studies being completed by home fed dogs that were not in a controlled environment, show the need for more research in this area until reproducible results can be obtained [2, 5].

## 18.3 Antimicrobial Resistance

Antimicrobial resistance awareness has become more common among veterinary practitioners. The evolution of antimicrobial-resistant bacteria is a concern in both human and veterinary medicine with the risk of pets developing, harboring, and possibly transmitting these strains to their human family members [21, 22]. Improper stewardships of antimicrobial agents has played a role along with some contributing factors including the increased administration of antimicrobial drugs, both by humans and animals, and improper prescribing of antimicrobial therapy, including the use of broad-spectrum antibiotics when they are either ineffective or unnecessary [23]. The World Health Organization published a list of antimicrobial-resistant bacteria in 2017, placing them in priority groups of "medium," "high," and "critical" [23] (Figure 18.3).

When bacterial cells are exposed to an antimicrobial agent, there are two possible scenarios: (i) some of the cells are resistant to the antimicrobial agent. The nonresistant cells are killed, leaving only resistant cells. When those resistant cells are regrown, all of the cells will be resistant.

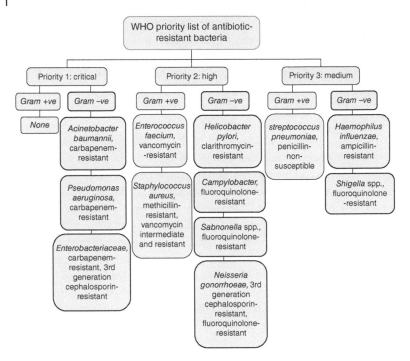

**Figure 18.3** WHO list of antibiotic-resistant pathogens listed in three categories of priority, critical, high, and medium, for the purpose of encouraging research and development of new antibiotics. *Source:* Brejyeh et al. [23] / MDPI / Public Domain CC BY 4.0.

(ii) The other possibility is the presence of dormant persister cells and not resistant cells. The non-persister cells are killed, leaving only persister cells. When these persister cells are regrown, they will not be in a dormant state and will still be susceptible to the antimicrobial agent [24].

Antimicrobial resistance can be defined as "a trait acquired by previously susceptible bacteria, on the basis of which can be attributed to the horizontal acquisition of new genes or the occurrence of spontaneous mutation" [25]. There are two ways that antimicrobial resistance is developed, intrinsic resistance or acquired resistance. Intrinsic resistance is where there is an innate ability for a bacteria species to resist the action of an antibiotic as a consequence of the bacteria's structural or functional characteristics [25]. An intrinsic resistance gene is involved in intrinsic resistance, and its presence in bacterial strains is independent of previous antibiotic exposure and is not caused by horizontal gene transfer [25]. Acquired resistance is where new resistance genes and DNA are horizontally transferred from one bacterium to another [23]. Bacteria can acquire resistant genes and easily transfer that information to related genera [26].

Gene transfer is the transfer of genes between organisms [27]. Unlike vertical gene transfer, where genes are transferred from parent to off-spring, horizontal genes (known as transposons) are transferred from the donor organism to the recipient organism through gene copying and insertion [27]. There are four types of horizontal gene transfer:

1) Transformation – the natural ability to take up exogenous DNA from the environment [28].
2) Transduction – the transfer of DNA from one cell to another by bacteriophage [28].
3) Conjugation – the contact-dependent, unidirectional transfer of DNA from a donor to a recipient via a conjugation (or mating) apparatus expressed in the donor [28].
4) Fusion – joining of two cells, and perhaps a fusion of cells with DNA-containing vesicles [28].

Another component of the development of resistant genes is the ability for the gene transfer elements to interact with each other as a large group [26]. This mass exchange of genetic information enhances their ability to transfer resistant genes more efficiently [26]. In addition, these elements can rapidly adapt to a new host, retaining memory of resistant genes even when they have not been exposed to the specific antibiotic [26].

The mechanisms that bacteria use to escape the effects of antibiotics are (i) limiting drug uptake, (ii) drug target modification, (iii) drug inactivation, and (iv) active drug efflux which transports the toxic compound out of the cell [23]. Intrinsic resistance may use limiting drug uptake, drug inactivation, and active drug efflux, while acquired resistance mechanisms may utilize drug target modification, drug inactivation, and active drug efflux [23].

Gram-negative bacteria are structurally more adept to protect themselves from antibiotics. The cell wall in Gram-negative bacteria consists of three structural layers [23]. Gram-positive bacteria do not have the outer or most inner layer making them more susceptible to antibiotics [23]. This can be observed when bacteria are stained with crystal

Table 18.1  Examples of gram negative bacteria and their actions.

| Disease | Oral niche |
| --- | --- |
| Periodontitis | Chronic inflammation of alveolar and periodontium bones |
| Stomatitis | Inflammation of oral mucous membranes |
| Glossitis | Inflammation of the tongue |

violet-iodine and a safranin counterstain. The violet stain can penetrate the cell wall of Gram-positive bacteria that appear purple under the microscope. The structure of the cell wall in Gram-negative bacteria does not allow the violet stain to transfer through these bacteria microscopically appearing pink [23].

Gram-negative bacteria make use of all four main mechanisms, whereas Gram-positive bacteria less commonly use limiting drug uptake, due to not having the outer membrane, and they do not have the capacity for certain types of drug efflux mechanisms [24] (Table 18.1).

When we discuss raw products in consideration of antimicrobial resistance, there are a few risk factors. The process may begin at the agricultural level where animal-based food sources may be inappropriately administered antimicrobials. These resistant strains of bacteria may contaminate the meat or by-products during slaughter and processing [26, 29]. Some risk factors for increased development and shedding of microbial-resistant bacteria are historical antibiotic treatment allowing for possible microbial evolution and feeding raw meat diets, which has shown to increase the rate at which bacterial contaminants are shed in the feces of pets [21]. Wedley et al. [21] reported that dogs eating raw poultry were 48 times more likely to shed ESBL *E. coli*, and 104 times as likely to shed *E. coli* that is resistant to fluoroquinolones [21].

## 18.4  Fermented Products

During fermentation, products are broken down by yeast, bacteria, or other microorganisms in a chemical reaction [30]. Fermented foods are defined as foods or beverages produced through controlled microbial growth and the conversion of food components through enzymatic action, with the use of variables such as the microorganisms, nutritional ingredients, and specific environmental conditions [30]. Historically, foods such as meat, fish, dairy, vegetables, soybeans, legumes, cereals, and fruits have undergone fermentation and were used as a form of preservation. Some foods require fermentation to become edible, for example fermentation removes the bitter phenolic compounds in olives [30]. Some probiotics are from lactic-acid-producing bacteria coming from fermented foods [31].

Highly fermented food diets have been shown to steadily increase microbial diversity [32]. This may be due to the potentially probiotic microorganisms in the fermented products. A fermented food effect on microbial diversity will depend on where the product came from, the age, and time the products are analyzed and consumed, with an average of 106 microbial cells per gram of fermented product [30]. The survival of the probiotic through the GI tract has the same risk as commercially available probiotics, though studies have indicated that these microbes do reach the large colon and have a transient presence in the GI tract [33].

Another possible benefit of fermented foods is health benefits from the fermentation-derived bioactive metabolites, which may have a direct health benefit on the host [33]. For example, lactic acid bacteria generate bioactive peptides and polyamines and can convert phenolic compounds (flavonoids) to biologically active metabolites, which may have positive effects on immune and metabolic health [30].

## 18.5 Chapter Summary

- The use of raw or uncooked ingredients, particularly uncooked meat products, as a source of pet nutrition has increased in popularity over the last couple of decades with pet parents looking for a diet that is considered to be more "natural" or "species-appropriate" [1, 2].
- Raw food poses a substantial risk of infectious disease to the pet, the pet's environment, and the humans in the household, with raw pet food commonly exceeding hygiene thresholds for counts of *Enterobacteriaceae* [2, 3].
- Studies are limited though a common conclusion of the evolution of the species GI tract [7], the individual ingredients, and the heating method will individually affect the composition and bioavailability of the nutrient for the host and the GI microbiota [8].

- When cooked, starch is gelatinized which increases ileal digestibility, which leaves fewer nutrients for amylolytic (able to ferment starches) microbiota to ferment as an energy source.
- The retention or increase in vitamins in vegetables depends on the type of vegetable and the cooking method.
- While muscle in healthy animals contains little to no microorganisms, meat is easily perishable as it is a good medium for the growth of various microorganisms that may contaminate the meat during slaughter and transport [13]. Sources of contamination during the slaughter process can come from processing tools, clothes, hands, and air [13].
- Colonic microbes are highly proteolytic (capable of fermenting protein) [15].
- Inconsistencies in results, and limitations in the studies including varying amounts of macronutrients between diets, low group, and sample numbers, along with multiple studies being completed by home-fed dogs that were not in a controlled environment, show the need for more research in this area until reproducible results can be obtained [2, 5].
- Gram-negative bacteria are structurally more adept to protect themselves from antibiotics due to their well-structured three-layered cell membrane.
- Pets that eat raw meat are more likely to shed pathogens at an increased rate compared to those fed a heat-processed diet.
- A fermented food product's microbial diversity will depend on where the product came from, the age, and time the products are analyzed and consumed, with an average of 106 microbial cells per gram of fermented product [30].

## References

1 Butowski, C.F., Moon, C.D., Thomas, D.G. et al. The effects of raw-meat diets on the gastrointestinal microbiota of the cat and dog: a review. *New Zealand Veterinary Journal* 70 (1): https://doi.org/10.1080/00480169.2021.1975586.

2 Davies, R.H., Lawes, J.R., and Wales, A.D. (2019). Raw diets for dogs and cats: a review, with particular reference to microbiological hazards. *The Journal of Small Animal Practice* 60 (6): 329–339. https://doi.org/10.1111/jsap.13000.

**3** Schlesinger, D.P. and Joffe, D.J. (2011). Raw food diets in companion animals: a critical review. *The Canadian Veterinary Journal* 52 (1): 50–54.

**4** Stogdale, L. (2019). One veterinarian's experience with owners who are feeding raw meat to their pets. *The Canadian Veterinary Journal* 60 (6): 655–658.

**5** Schmidt, M., Unterer, S., Suchodolski, J.S. et al. (2018). The fecal microbiome and metabolome differs between dogs fed bones and raw food (BARF) diets and dogs fed commercial diets. *PLoS One* 13 (8): e0201279. 10.1371/journal.pone.0201279.

**6** Sandri, M., Dal Monego, S., Conte, G. et al. (2017). Raw meat based diet influences faecal microbiome and end products of fermentation in healthy dogs. *BMC Veterinary Research* 13 (1): 65. 10.1186/s12917-017-0981-z.

**7** Carmody, R.N., Bisanz, J.E., Bowen, B.P. et al. (2019). Cooking shapes the structure and function of the gut microbiome. *Nature Microbiology* 4 (12): 2052–2063. https://doi.org/10.1038/s41564-019-0569-4.

**8** Dhingra, D., Michael, M., Rajput, H. et al. (2012). Dietary fibre in foods: a review. *Journal of Food Science and Technology* 49 (3): 255–266. https://doi.org/10.1007/s13197-011-0365-5.

**9** Lee, S., Choi, Y., Jeong, H.S. et al. Effect of different cooking methods on the content of vitamins and true retention in selected vegetables. *Food Science and Biotechnology* 27 (2): 333–342. https://doi.org/10.1007/s10068-017-0281-1.

**10** Link, L.B. and Potter, J.D. (2004). Raw versus cooked vegetables and cancer risk. *Cancer Epidemiology, Biomarkers & Prevention* 13 (9): 1422–1435.

**11** Joshi, M., Timilsena, Y., and Adhikari, B. (2017). Global production, processing and utilization of lentil: a review. *Journal of Integrative Agriculture* 16: 2898–2913. https://doi.org/10.1016/S2095-3119(17)61793-3.

**12** AAFCO (Association of Feed Control Officials) (2018). Chapter 6; 338:359. Association of Feed Control Officials Inc.

**13** Bantawa, K., Rai, K., Limbu, D.S. et al. (2018). Food-borne bacterial pathogens in marketed raw meat of Dharan, Eastern Nepal. *BMC Research Notes* 11: 618. https://doi.org/10.1186/s13104-018-3722-x.

**14** Kananub, S., Pinniam, N., Phothitheerabut, S. et al. (2020). Contamination factors associated with surviving bacteria in Thai commercial raw pet foods. *Veterinary World* 13 (9): 1988–1991. https://doi.org/10.14202/vetworld.2020.1988-1991.

**15** Albracht-Schulte, K., Islam, T., Johnson, P. et al. (2020). Systematic review of beef protein effects on gut microbiota: implications for health. *Advances in Nutrition* 12 (1): 102–114. https://doi.org/10.1093/advances/nmaa085.

**16** Lubbs, D.C., Vester, B.M., Fastinger, N.D. et al. (2009). Dietary protein concentration affects intestinal microbiota of adult cats: a study using DGGE and qPCR to evaluate differences in microbial populations in the feline gastrointestinal tract. *Journal of Animal Physiology and Animal Nutrition* 93 (1): 113–121. https://doi.org/10.1111/j.1439-0396.2007.00788.x.

**17** Kerr, K.R., Vester Boler, B.M., Morris, C.L. et al. (2012). Apparent total tract energy and macronutrient digestibility and fecal fermentative end-product concentrations of domestic cats fed extruded, raw beef-based, and cooked beef-based diets. *Journal of Animal Science* 90 (2): 515–522. https://doi.org/10.2527/jas.2010-3266.

**18** Oberli, M., Lan, A., Khodoroava, N. et al. (2016). Compared with raw bovine meet, boiling but not grilling, barbecuing, or roasting decreases protein digestibility without any major consequences for intestinal mucosa in rats, although the sily ingestion of bovine meet induces histologic modifications in the colon. *The Journal of Nutrition* 146 (8): 1506–1513. https://doi.org/10.3945/jn.116.230839.

**19** Kim, J., An, J.-U., Kim, W. et al. (2017). Differences in the gut microbiota of dogs (Canis lupus familiaris) fed a natural diet or a commercial feed revealed by the Illumina MiSeq platform. *Gut Pathogens* 9 (1): 68. https://doi.org/10.1186/s13099-017-0218-5.

**20** Spears, J.K., Vester Boler, B., Gardner, C., and Li, Q. (2017). Development of the oral microbiome in kittens. In: *Companion Animal Nutrition (CAN) Summit: The Nexus of Pet and Human Nutrition: Focus on Cognition and Microbiome*, 4–7. Helsinki, Finland.

**21** Wedley, A.L., Dawson, S., Maddox, T.W. et al. (2017). Carriage of antimicrobial resistant *Escherichia coli* in dogs: prevalence, associated risk factors and molecular characteristics. *Veterinary Microbiology* 199: 23–30. https://doi.org/10.1016/j.vetmic.2016.11.017. Epub 2016 Nov 23. PMID: 28110781.

**22** Heim, D., Kuster, S., and Willi, B. (2020). Antibiotic-resistant bacteria in dogs and cats: recommendations for owners. *Schweizer Archiv für Tierheilkunde* 132 (3): 141–151. 10.17236/sat00248.

**23** Brejyeh, Z., Jubeh, B., and Karaman, R. (2020). Resistance of gram-negative bacteria to current antibacterial agents and approaches to resolve it. *Molecules* 25 (6): 1340. https://doi.org/10.3390/molecules25061340.

24 Reygaert, W.C. (2018). An overview of the antimicrobial resistance mechanisms of bacteria. *AIMS Microbiology* 4 (3): 482–501. https://doi.org/10.3934/microbiol.2018.3.482.

25 Zhang, G. and Feng, J. (2016). The intrinsic resistance of bacteria. *Yi Chuan* 38 (10): 872–880. https://doi.org/10.16288/j.yczz.16-159.

26 Salyers, A.A. and Amábile-Cuevas, C.F. (1997). Why are antibiotic resistance genes so resistant to elimination? *Antimicrobial Agents and Chemotherapy* 41 (11): 2321–2325.

27 Lorenzo-Díaz, F., Fernández-López, C., Lurz, R. et al. (2017). Crosstalk between vertical and horizontal gene transfer: plasmid replication control by a conjugative relaxase. *Nucleic Acids Research* 45 (13): 7774–7785. https://doi.org/10.1093/nar/gkx450.

28 Johnson, C.M. and Grossman, A.D. (2016). Integrative and conjugative elements (ICEs): what they do and how they work. *Annual Review of Genetics* 49: 577–601. https://doi.org/10.1146/annurev-genet-112414-055018.

29 Verraes, C., Boxstael, S.V., Meervenne, E.V. et al. (2013). Antimicrobial resistance in the food chain: a review. *International Journal of Environmental Research and Public Health* 10 (7): 2643–2669. https://doi.org/10.3390/ijerph10072643.

30 Dimidi, E., Cox, S.R., Rossi, M. et al. (2019). Fermented foods: definitions and characteristics, impact on the gut microbiota and effects on gastrointestinal health and disease. *Nutrients* 11 (8): 1806. https://doi.org/10.3390/nu11081806.

31 Parvez, S., Malik, K.A., Ah Kang, S., and Kim, H.-Y. (2006). Probiotics and their fermented food products are beneficial for health. *Journal of Applied Microbiology* 100 (6): 1171–1185. 10.1111/j.1365-2672.2006.02963.x.

32 Wastyk, H.C., Fragiadakis, G.K., Perelman, D. et al. (2021). Gut-microbiota-targeted diets modulate human immune status. *Cell* 184 (16): 4137–4153. https://doi.org/10.1016/j.cell.2021.06.019.

33 Zhang, C., Derrien, M., Levenez, F. et al. (2016). Ecological robustness of the gut microbiota in response to ingestion of transient food-borne microbes. *The ISME Journal* 10 (9): 2235–2245. https://doi.org/10.1038/ismej.2016.13.

# 19

# Grain and Gluten-Free Diets

Grain-free and gluten-free diets grabbed a share of the human and pet market approximately 15 years ago when there was an increased awareness of celiac and grain intolerance in people. Some of these "grain-free" canine pet diets have been part of ongoing research focused on a possible nutritional-influenced dilated cardiomyopathy in dogs [1]. Research is currently ongoing to determine if there is a correlation between the disease state and these diets, or the ingredients, and how the nutrients they provide are possibly affecting patient health through normal digestion and physiological functions [2].

While grains in general have been thought to be a possible cause of food-borne allergic responses in dogs and cats, in North America, the allergens most likely contributing to cutaneous adverse food reactions in a dog are beef, dairy products, chicken, wheat, and lamb [3]. In cats, the most common allergens causing cutaneous adverse food reactions are beef, fish, and chicken [3].

## 19.1 Grains

Grains ("cereals" or "cereal grains") are the edible seeds of specific grass crops that commonly include but are not limited to wheat, corn, rice, barley, oats, sorghum, soy, and rye [4]. Whole grains are characterized as being high in resistant carbohydrates, meaning they typically

*Small Animal Microbiomes and Nutrition*, First Edition. Robin Saar and Sarah Dodd.
© 2024 John Wiley & Sons, Inc. Published 2024 by John Wiley & Sons, Inc.
Companion website: www.wiley.com/go/saar/1e

contribute fiber (including insoluble non-starch polysaccharides and resistant starch), nutrients (including unsaturated complex lipids), and antioxidants (phenolics), which are important sources of nutrients for the gut microbiota [4, 5]. In general, grains provide three main physiological benefits to the GI microbiome: fiber, lipids, and phenolics [4].

### 19.1.1 Nutrients from Grains

#### 19.1.1.1 Fiber

Even though non-starch polysaccharides are insoluble and poorly fermentable, they have many positive contributions for the host. They create bulk to the feces and reduce intestinal transit times, along with decreasing the pH in the distal colon and increasing fecal butyrate concentrations [4]. Whole grains (oats and barley) that are high in soluble fiber decrease lipoprotein cholesterol and blood pressure, along with improving glucose and insulin responses by binding with bile acids in the small intestine [5, 6]. Grains that provide high amounts of insoluble fiber (wheat) will moderately decrease blood glucose and can be utilized as a prebiotic for GI microbiota. See Chapter 5 for further details on the fiber's effect on the microbiome.

#### 19.1.1.2 Lipids

Currently, it is recognized that higher levels of lipids (particularly saturated fats) can be detrimental to a microbiome, decreasing the diversity of microbiota and proportions of beneficial bacteria [4]. Whole grains are low in fats and the type of fat they provide tends to be unsaturated [4]. Whole grains also provide a good source of plant sterol esters such as α-linolenic acid and linolenic acid. Five α-linolenic acid is found in significant amounts in several seeds, seed oils, and nuts, while linseeds or flaxseeds and their oil generally contain 45–55% of their total fatty acids content in the form of α-linolenic acid [7]. Only 5–10% of fatty acids from soybean oil, rape-seed oil, and walnuts contain are α-linolenic acid. Corn oil, sunflower oil, and safflower oil have significant amounts of linolenic acid and contain only a small amount of α-linolenic acid [7]. See Chapter 5 for further details on lipid's influence on the microbiome.

### 19.1.1.3 Phenolics

Phenolics act as antioxidants in several ways [8]. In whole grains, the antioxidants are bound to the fiber components of the grain which resist enzymatic digestion in the small intestine. These fibers are fermented by favorable microbiota in the large intestine, releasing the phenolic compounds that are rapidly metabolized into usable metabolites. These metabolites may be effective in protecting the intestinal epithelium from free radical damage [4] (Figure 19.1).

### 19.1.2 Obesity's Relationship to Grains

Obesity is inversely related to whole grain intake [5]. Grain processing improves palatability and can have varying effects on nutrition (e.g. the process of milling and grinding flour increases glucose availability and decreases phytochemical content, whereas thermal processing increases available antioxidants). A 4-week crossover study in humans revealed compositional alteration in the GI microbiome and improvements in physiological measures related to metabolic dysfunctions, such as obesity and its correlated comorbidities, when there was a short-term increase in the intake of whole grains [6]. Studies in humans have also shown a bifidogenic effect (increase in Bifidobacterium) and/or an increase in butyrate-producing bacteria with diets high in whole grains [4, 7].

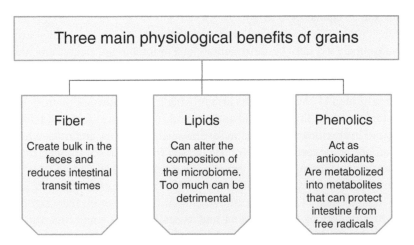

**Figure 19.1** The three main physiological benefits of grains on the GI microbiome.

### 19.1.3   Processing's Effect on Grain Nutrient Profile

Grain processing, while improving palatability, can have varying effects on the nutrition it provides. For example, the milling and grinding process of flour increases glucose availability and decreases phytochemical content. Thermal processing will increase the availability of antioxidants [5].

## 19.2   Gluten

Gluten is the main storage protein (amino acid reserve) of wheat grains. These protein networks consist of a mixture of hundreds of related yet distinct proteins [9]. Gluten mainly consists of proteins gliadin and glutenin, with similar storage proteins like secalin in rye, hordein in barley, and avenins in oats, which are collectively referred to as "gluten" [9]. Gluten is heat stable and acts as a binding and extending agent improving texture, moisture retention, and flavor in extruded diets [9]. Some of these storage proteins like gliadin contain peptide sequences that are highly resistant to gastric, pancreatic, and intestinal proteolytic digestion in the gastrointestinal tract [9]. Grain gluten allergies are extremely rare in dogs, with documented reports in only a couple of dog breeds (Irish Setters and Border Terriers) [10, 11]. Gluten does not cause illness in cats.

## 19.3   Chapter Summary

- Grains have been indicated to be a cause of some diseases such as allergic disease and be non-biologically appropriate sources of nutrients for pets, there is research to show that only wheat in dogs may be the cause of one type of allergic disease [3], and grain gluten allergies are also isolated to only one or two breeds of dogs and never in cats [10].
- In general, whole grains provide three main physiological benefits to the GI microbiome: (i) Fiber, (ii) Lipids, and (iii) Phenolics
- Processing can affect the nutrients provided by whole grains.
- Whole grains have a bifidogenic effect on the GI microbiome, which causes positive shifts and improvements in metabolic conditions.
- Gluten consists of protein reserves that hold multiple amino acids.
- Many storage proteins are resistant to enzymatic digestion by the gastric, pancreatic, and small intestine.

# References

1 Walker, A., DeFrancesco, T., Bonagura, J. et al. (2022). Association of diet with clinical outcomes in dogs with dilated cardiomyopathy and congestive heart failure. *Journal of Veterinary Cardiology* 40: 99–109. https://doi.org/10.1016/j.jvc.2021.02.001.

2 Smith, C.E., Parnell, L.D., Lai, C.Q. et al. (2021). Investigation of diets associated with dilated cardiomyopathy in dogs using foodomics analysis. *Scientific Reports* 11: 15881. https://doi.org/10.1038/s41598-021-94464-2.

3 Mueller, R.S., Olivry, T., and Prélaud, P. (2016). Critically appraised topic on adverse food reactions of companion animals (2): common food allergen sources in dogs and cats. *BMC Veterinary Research* 12: 9. https://doi.org/10.1186/s12917-016-0633-8.

4 Rose, D.J. (2014). Impact of whole grains on the gut microbiota: the next frontier for oats? *British Journal of Nutrition* 112 (S2): S44–S49. 10.1017/S0007114514002244.

5 Harris, K.A. and Kris-Etherton, P.M. (2010). Effects of whole grains on coronary heart disease risk. *Current Atherosclerosis Reports* 12: 368–376. 10.1007/s11883-010-0136-1.

6 Martínez, I., Lattinmer, J.M., Hubach, K.L. et al. (2012). Gut microbiome composition is linked to whole grains-induced immunological improvements. *The ISME Journal* 7: 269–280. 10.1038/ismej.2012.104.

7 Alpha-Linolenic Acid (2016) ScienceDirect. https://www.sciencedirect.com/topics/agricultural-and-biological-sciences/alpha-linolenic-acid (accessed 3 February 2022).

8 Pereira, D.M., Valentão, P., Pereira, J.A. et al. (2009). Phenolics: from chemistry to biology. *Molecules* 14: 2202–2211. 10.3390/molecules14062202.

9 Biesiekierski, J.R. (2017). What is gluten? *Journal of Gastroenterology and Hepatology* 32 (S1): 78–81. https://doi.org/10.1111/jgh.13703.

10 Lowrie, M., Garden, O.A., Hadjivassiliou, M. et al. (2018). Characterization of paroxysmal gluten-sensitive dyskinesia in border terriers using serological markers. *Journal of Veterinary Internal Medicine* 32 (2): 775–781. https://doi.org/10.1111/jvim.15038.

11 Hall, E.J. and Batt, R.M. (1992). Dietary modulation of gluten sensitivity in a naturally occurring enteropathy of Irish setter dogs. *Gut* 33 (2): 198–205. https://doi.org/10.1136/gut.33.2.198. PMID: 1347279; PMCID: PMC1373930.

# 20

# Cannabinoids

Cannabis, *Cannabis sativa,* is a complex plant belonging to the Cannabaceae family [1], with over 540 chemical entities of which more than 60 of them are cannabinoid compounds, some of them with opposing effects [2–4]. Some commonly known chemical entities are cannabinoids, terpenes, and flavonoids. The two main cannabinoid compounds are tetrahydrocannabinol (THC) and cannabidiol (CBD) with over 100 other compounds being identified [3]. When people use the term "marijuana," they are using the part of the plant that contains THC compounds that are associated with an altered mental state [3]. "Hemp" or "industrial hemp" refers to specific strains of the cannabis plant that consistently has no more than 0.3% THC in the flowering heads, branches, and leaves [3]. Hemp has a high content of polyunsaturated fatty acids, phenolic compounds, carbohydrates, vitamins, and minerals [1].

## 20.1   Regulations on Cannabis Products

In the United States, all ingredients that are included in pet food must be generally recognized as safe (GRAS) for the intended species, be an approved food additive, or be a listed ingredient in the Official Publication of the Association of American Feed Controls Officials (AAFCO) as being acceptable for use in animal feed [5]. The US Food and Drug Administration (FDA) regulates the use of cannabis and cannabis-derived products including CBD, including its use in animal feed [6], though individual states may

*Small Animal Microbiomes and Nutrition*, First Edition. Robin Saar and Sarah Dodd.
© 2024 John Wiley & Sons, Inc. Published 2024 by John Wiley & Sons, Inc.
Companion website: www.wiley.com/go/saar/1e

be able to circumvent Federal and state oversight by considering legislation that will allow the use of hemp in animal feed in their respective states. In regard to the 2018 Farm Bill, it does not grant the right to use hemp and hemp products in food for humans or animals [5]. To date the FDA has determined that products containing THC or CBD cannot be sold legally as dietary supplements. Foods that have THC or CBD added cannot be sold legally in interstate commerce, as each state sets laws and regulations about TCH and CBD independently [3]. In February 2022, AAFCO issued an information letter asking for critical scientific research to be completed prior to allowing hemp in animal feed [7].

In Canada, Health Canada, in the Health Products and Food Branch, reviews all drug applications, with the Cannabis Act specifically regulating cannabis products [8]. To date, under the Cannabis Act, pet food would be considered an "edible" product. Initially, the regulations on the production and sale of edibles in Canada will be focused on human consumption, particularly regarding the accessibility of quality-controlled cannabis products [4]. Industrial hemp is regulated under the Industrial Hemp Regulations and while the level of THC is controlled, there is no limit on CBD in industrial hemp [4]. Only limited parts of cannabis or hemp plants may be used as a medicinal ingredient in veterinary health products under the Food and Drug Regulations and can only contain parts of the cannabis or hemp plants that are not considered cannabis under the Cannabis ACT [4]. Examples of this would be hemp-seed derivatives and nonviable seeds, and while mature stalks that do not include any leaves, flowers, seeds or branches, and fiber from such stalks are excluded from the Cannabis Act, they may not be used in veterinary health products [4]. Further information can be found on the Government of Canada website including the cannabis health products guidance page [9].

In the European Union, European countries where cannabis is allowed as a therapy for humans, a veterinarian can prescribe a compound formula based on cannabis derivatives, extemporaneously prepared by a pharmacist [10].

## 20.2 By-products of the Plant as an Ingredient Source

With the legalization of cannabis in many areas of the world, there is an increased human demand for products containing the THC and cannabidiol CBD portions of the plant, along with an increased use in industrial hemp as an alternative. Some identified current and potential uses of hemp are the fiber from stalks can be used in making paper, textiles, rope or twine, and other construction materials, while grain from industrial hemp can be used in food products, cosmetics, plastics, and fuel [11]. In pet food, the potential of hemp being a fiber, fat, and possible plant protein source are all areas where further research is still required [7].

Whole hempseed generally contains about 20–25% proteins including edestin, albumin, and high amounts of amino acid arginine, glutamic acid, methionine, and cystine. Hempseed meal has a major protein content of up to 40% [1]. Carbohydrates make up approximately 25–35% with 10–15% being insoluble fibers [1]. Fat content from hempseed oil is obtained from cold pressing of seeds or by extraction at approximately 25–35% [1]. Hempseed oil contains up to 90% of polyunsaturated fatty acids (PUFAs) and includes both omega-6 fatty acid linoleic acid, and omega-3 fatty acid α-linoleic acid resulting in an omega 6 : omega 3 ratio of 3.5 : 1. Hempseeds and hempseed cakes contain tocopherols. Hempseeds contain 60.85 mg/100 g dry matter of γ-tocopherol, and hempseed cakes contain 33.72 mg/100 g dry matter γ-tocopherol [1].

## 20.3 Concerns About the Health and Safety of Cannabis Products in Animal Feed

While there is potential for some parts of the hemp plant to provide nutrients there are concerns about the performance of animals fed the diets, any alterations in the products these animals provide (meat, eggs, milk), and if any of those changes will affect the end source eating these animal products [7]. Scientific evidence supporting long-term safety for the animals fed cannabis plants, and for the final consumer of these animal influenced products, is still recommended before this product is used for commercial purposes [7].

## 20.4 Cannabidiol Supplementation Effects on the Microbiome

Cannabidiol is currently being supplemented to dogs with possible therapeutic indications for osteoarthritis, anxiety, and phobias, along with epilepsy [12]. While there are a number of studies available looking at the specific therapeutic benefits, there are limited studies looking at the effect on the microbiomes.

In a recent canine study, the metabolites of 16 dogs were analyzed after 3 weeks of treatment with CBD 4.5 mg CBD/kg BW/day. The dogs were all placed on a GI with fiber veterinary line diet (Pro Plan EN with Fibre), 37 days prior to the start of the supplementation and 58 days prior to collection of samples for evaluation. Both the control and CBD supplementation were provided in a treat format, which was made up of chicken, chicken liver, Asian carp, catfish, and in the case of the CBD treats, industrial hemp extract. Results of the addition of the CBD supplementation were an alteration in the canine metabolome, with altered metabolites showing influences on glucose, amino acid, vitamin and nucleotide metabolism, and pathways where CBD may exert beneficial effects as an anti-inflammatory, antioxidant, and antimicrobial [12] (Figure 20.1).

In a study on mice, looking at THC's effect on the GI microbiome and metabolic functions, mice were divided into two groups with both being fed *ad libitum* on either a low fat diet or a high fat diet. THC was then administered daily, with different outcomes observed between diet-induced obese (D/O), and lean mice [13]. Compared to the lean mice, the D/O mice experienced reduced weight, and fat mass gain, a decrease in energy intake, and a decrease in caloric consuming over the 3-week trial period [13]. Locomotion was assessed in this study and

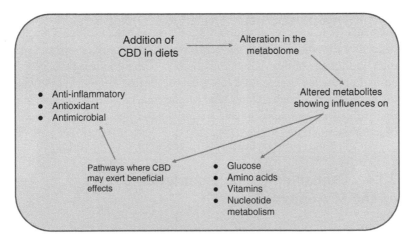

**Figure 20.1** Results of the addition of the CBD supplementation.

found sedation from the TCH not to be the cause of decreased caloric intake [13].

An interesting study in mice looked at the role of GI microbiota in autoimmune encephalomyelitis (EAE) when influenced by THC and CBD [14]. Mice with EAE have high levels of a particular gram-negative bacteria, *Akkermansia muciniphila* (A. muc), which plays a role in higher levels of lipopolysaccharides in the brain resulting in neuroinflammation [14]. When mice were treated with THC and CDB, levels of A. muc and lipopolysaccharides were decreased. These mice also had significantly higher levels of short-chain fatty acids (butyric, isovaleric, and valeric acid) compared to controls. This data suggests that cannabinoids may prevent microbial dysbiosis seen in EAE resulting in suppressed neuroinflammation and attenuating symptoms of the disease [14].

In a study with forty-eight laying hens, one of six diets were offered over a 12-week period [15]. These diets contained hempseed at either a 10, 20, or 30% inclusion or the inclusion of hempseed oil at either 4.5 or 9.0%. The final diet had no additional supplementation as the control diet.

Interestingly, as the intake of alpha-linolenic acid from the hempseed increased, there was a significant increase in the n-3 PUFA contents of yolk total lipid. The values of alpha-linolenic acid increased by 12-fold ($152 \pm 3.56$ and $156 \pm 2.42$ mg/yolk) and docosahexaenoic acid (DHA) by twofold to threefold ($41.3 \pm 1.57$ and $43.6 \pm 1.61$ mg/yolk) over the control [15]. By increasing levels of hemp products in laying hen diets, the level of fatty acid, triacylglycerol (TAG), and total phospholipids were able to be positively manipulated while also enhancing the omega-3 fatty acids [15]. Additionally, within 3 weeks of feeding hens either the hempseed or hemp-oil-containing diets, a reduction in the omega 6 : omega 3 ratio was observed [15].

## 20.5 Antimicrobial Effects of Cannabis

Antimicrobial activity of cannabis derivatives has been identified with oils derived from several cannabinoids showing *in vitro* antimicrobial properties on several bacteria, particularly gram-positive bacteria including methicillin-resistant *Staphylococcus aureus* [1, 16]. Research in this area has not always shown consistent results with the effectiveness of cannabis as an antimicrobial though there is potential for further research in this area [16].

## 20.6 Current Diets on the World Pet Food Market

A diet in Croatia came into the market in 2020 which lists hemp leaves, hemp protein, and, hemp oil as ingredients providing hemp. The diets are canine focused and have an analytical list for each diet with CBD listed at a range of 35–55.5 mg/kg [17].

In North America, there are multiple nutraceuticals and treats on the market, which leads to concerns of dosing, quality, and consistency in the creation and manufacturing process for these products.

## 20.7 Chapter Summary

- Cannabis, *Cannabis sativa,* is a complex plant belonging to the Cannabaceae family.
- The two main cannabinoids compounds are tetrahydrocannabinol (THC) and cannabidiol (CBD) with over 100 other compounds being identified.
- "Hemp" or "industrial hemp" refers to specific strains of the cannabis plant that consistently have no more than 0.3% THC in the flowering heads, branches, and leaves.
- Hemp has a high content of polyunsaturated fatty acids, phenolic compounds, carbohydrates, vitamins, and minerals.
- Each country has different regulations regarding the inclusion of cannabis products in pet food.
- Hempseed has potential to be a good source of protein, fiber, and fat.
- The inclusion of cannabis products in animal feed brings concerns of how it may affect the animal consuming it, the products intended for the food chain, and any effects those products may have on the consumer.
- Cannabis derivatives have shown to have antimicrobial effects.

## References

1 Della, R.G. and Di Salvo, A. (2020). Hemp in veterinary medicine: from feed to drug. *Frontiers in Veterinary Science* 7: 387. https://doi.org/10.3389/fvets.2020.00387.

**2** Atakan, Z. (2012). Cannabis, a complex plant: different compounds and different effects on individuals. *Therapeutic Advances in Psychopharmacology* 2 (6): 241–254. https://doi.org/10.1177/20451253 12457586.

**3** National Academies of Sciences, Engineering, and Medicine (2017). *The Health Effects of Cannabis and Cannabinoids: The Current State of Evidence and Recommendations for Research*. Washington, DC: The National Academies Press https://doi.org/10.17226/24625.

**4** Yakima, R. (2021). Regulating CBD: the pet food industry or the Wild West? *Petfoodindustry.com* - blogs. https://www.petfoodindustry.com/blogs/10-debunking-pet-food-myths-and-misconceptions/post/10075-regulating-cbd-the-pet-food-industry-or-the-wild-west (accessed 16 December 2021).

**5** FDA Regulation of Cannabis and Cannabis-Derived Products, Including Cannabidiol (CBD) (2023). *US Food and Drug Administration*. https://www.fda.gov/news-events/public-health-focus/fda-regulation-cannabis-and-cannabis-derived-products-including-cannabidiol-cbd (accessed 16 December 2021).

**6** Hemp and Hemp Byproducts in Animal Food – AAFCO Position and Call to Action. Association of American Feed Control Officials (2021). www.aafco.org/Portals/0/SiteContent/Announcements/AAFCO_HempUpdate-9-21.pdf (accessed 20 December 2021).

**7** Cannabis Act (2018). Canada; Cannabis Health Products. Government of Canada – Health Canada. www.canada.ca/content/dam/hc-sc/documents/services/drugs-health-products/drug-products/applications-submissions/guidance-documents/cannabis-health-products-guidance-eng(2).pdf (accessed 20 December 2021).

**8** Kirilov, B., Zhelyazkova, M., Petkova-Gueorguieva, E., *et al.* (2020) Regulation and marketing of cannabidiol-containing products in European countries. Pharmacists' knowledge in Bulgaria. *Biotechnology and Biotechnological Equipment*, 34(1): pp. 1158–1165. https://doi.org/10.1080/13102818.2020.1824620

**9** grégorio, C., Lichtfouse, E., Chanet, G., and Crini, N. (2020). Applications of hemp in textiles, paper industry, insulation and building materials, horticulture, animal nutrition, food and beverages, nutraceuticals, cosmetics and hygiene, medicine, agrochemistry, energy production and environment: a review. *Environmental Chemistry Letters* 18: https://doi.org/10.1007/s10311-020-01029-2.

**10** Morris, E.M., Kitts-Morgan, S.E., Spangler, D.M. et al. (2021). Alteration of the canine metabolome after a 3-week supplementation of cannabidiol (CBD) containing treats: An exploratory study of healthy animals. Frontiers in Veterinary Science 8: 685606. https://doi.org/10. 3389/fvets.2021.685606.

**11** Cluny, N.L., Keenan, C.M., Reimer, R.A. et al. (2015). Prevention of diet-induced obesity effects on body weight and gut microbiota in mice treated chronically with Δ9-tetrahydrocannabinol. *PLoS One* 10 (12): e.0144270. https://doi.org/10.1371/journal.pone.0144270.

**12** Al-Ghezi, Z.Z., Busbeem, P.B., Alghetaa, H. et al. (2019). Combination of cannabinoids, Δ9-tetrahydrocannabinol (THC) and cannabidiol (CBD), mitigates experimental autoimmune encephalomyelitis (EAE) by altering the gut microbiome. *Brain, Behavior, and Immunity* 82: 25–35. https://doi.org/10.1016/j.bbi.2019.07.028.

**13** Neijat, M., Suh, M., Neufeld, J. et al. (2016). Hempseed products fed to hens effectively increased n-3 polyunsaturated fatty acids in total lipids, triacylglycerol and phospholipid of egg yolk. *Lipids* 51 (5): 601–614. https://doi.org/10.1007/s11745-015-4088-7.

**14** Karas, J.A., Wong, L.J.M., Paulin, O.K.A. et al. (2020). The antimicrobial activity of cannabinoids. *Antibiotics (Basel).* 9 (7): 406. https://doi.org/ 10.3390/antibiotics9070406.

**15** Products. *Canibis.* www.canibis.eu/ (accessed 16 December 2021)

**16** Della Rocca G, Di Salvo A. Hemp in veterinary medicine: from feed to drug. *Frontiers in Veterinary Science* 2020;7:387. doi:https://doi.org/ 10.3389/fvets.2020.00387.

**17** Karas JA, Wong LJM, Paulin OKA, et al. The antimicrobial activity of cannabinoids. *Antibiotics (Basel).* 2020;9(7):406. doi:https://doi.org/ 10.3390/antibiotics9070406.

# 21

# Insects

Entomophagy or the practice of eating insects has been common for thousands of years [1] though they are considered a more recent emerging ingredient source for commercial pet food diets. Nutritionally insects can provide high amounts of proteins, fats, vitamins, and mineral elements with great economic and environmental advantages [1, 2]. Some of them can transform waste streams into valuable proteins revealing high-feed conversion ratios at low levels of greenhouse gas emission [3]. Historically insects are already a common food for feral cats contributing <0.5% of the total daily energy needs [2, 4]. By 2012 approximately 1900 edible insect species were listed worldwide with desirable species being non-toxigenic and nonpathogenic toward humans and relevant animals [3]. The insect species that have been recognized as promising alternative sources of protein for animal feed are:

- The Black Soldier Fly (BSF) *Hermetia illucens* L. (Diptera: Stratiomyidae)
- The common housefly, *Musca domestica* L. (Diptera: Muscidae)
- The yellow mealworm *Tenebrio molitor* L. (Coleoptera: Tenebrionidae) [5]

## 21.1 Black Soldier Fly Larvae

The Black Soldier Fly Larvae (BSFL) have interesting qualities that make them a contender as a future source of nutrients for pet nutrition.

*Small Animal Microbiomes and Nutrition*, First Edition. Robin Saar and Sarah Dodd.
© 2024 John Wiley & Sons, Inc. Published 2024 by John Wiley & Sons, Inc.
Companion website: www.wiley.com/go/saar/1e

### 21.1.1 Adjustable Nutrient Profile

The amino acid profile can be manipulated by adjusting the feed substrate provided, the environment during growth stages, the age at harvest, and the harvest technique [4, 5].

### 21.1.2 Natural Decomposers

BSFL, along with other insects, can flourish on nutrient-rich organic waste substrates [5, 6]. They can reduce organic waste energy by 50–60% and utilize it as a high-protein energy source [5]. Organic waste examples are animal and human manure, fruits and vegetables residues, general food waste, municipal organic waste, coffee bean pulp, straw, dried distillers' grains with soluble, and fish offal [5]. Microbiota in the midgut of BSFL help digest various substrates with a different nutrient content allowing insects the ability to grow on multi-diet materials [6, 7].

### 21.1.3 Non-Disease Vector Species

During the adult life stage, a BSF has a short life span and does not eat as it has redundant mouthparts, which decrease the risk of disease transmission to other species, unlike the common housefly [6].

### 21.1.4 Reduce Pathogen and Other Vermin on Decaying Matter

BSFL are able to significantly reduce indigenous pathogenic bacteria (examples *Escherichia* sp., *Salmonella* sp.) from organic waste [6]. This is accomplished by reducing bacterial colonies with the high pH conditions of their gut, enzymatic reactions, and competitive gut bacteria that create undesirable growth conditions for the bacteria [4].

### 21.1.5 Production of Antimicrobial Peptides

BSFL has the ability to produce antibacterial peptides (host defense peptides), which are short-chain positively charged peptides against *Helicobacter pylori* [6]. A benefit of peptides in comparison to pharmaceutical antimicrobials is that they are effective in reducing multidrug-resistant bacteria [8] (Figure 21.1).

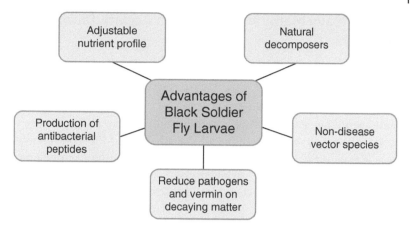

Figure 21.1    Advantages of using Black Soldier Fly Larvae as a protein source.

### 21.1.6    BSFL GI Microbiome

The GI microbiota plays a large role in the digestion and recycling of biomass waste and other nutrients in the BSFL, through the encoding of enzymes in the midgut of BSFL by bacterial genes [6]. These genes (cellulase, protease, and lipase) are able to hydrolyze starch, cellulose, protein, and lipids [6]. A recent study by Ao et al. found *Bacteroidetes*, *Firmicutes*, *Proteobacteria* were dominant in the midgut of BSFL in the bacterial communities of BSFL-fed swine and chicken manure [9]. Klammsteiner et al. found *Actinomyces* spp., *Dysgonomonas* spp., and *Enterococcus* spp. as main members of the BSFL GI microbiome community that provide various functional and metabolic skills that allow the BSFL to thrive in various environments [10]. Rather than diet dictating diversity in BSLF, a stable indigenous collection of bacteria function in the degradation of a broad range of substrates [10].

### 21.1.7    Probiotics for BSFL

The addition of specific live bacteria to food sources is proving to be beneficial for BSFL [6]. In a study by Yu et al., four different strains of *Bacillus subtilis* were added to chicken manure, which resulted in positive changes in growth and development of BSFL [11].

## 21.2 Heavy Metal and Mycotoxin Accumulation in Insects

The accumulation of heavy metals is a concerning contaminant of insects along with exposure to mycotoxins [3]. In BSFL that were highly exposed to heavy metals copper and cadmium the bacterial diversity was significantly reduced [12]. The accumulation of heavy metal ions may vary depending on the type of metal, the species, and the development stage of the insect [3]. For example, BSFs are at risk for the accumulation of cadmium and yellow mealworms for arsenic. The reported species-specific accumulation and metabolism patterns of contaminants emphasize the importance to assess potential safety hazards in a case-by-case approach [3]. For example, the total body burden of these contaminants is mostly found in the gut content of the insects. The risk of species–species contamination could be averted by completing a starving period before harvest [3]. Mycotoxins are low-molecular-weight secondary metabolites produced by fungi found on the food sources for insects (grains, corn, nuts, and some fruit), which are capable of causing adverse effects to insects such as decreased growth [3]. Having considerable thermal resistance, most mycotoxins are not inactivated during cooking. More long-term studies are still required to evaluate the adequacy and safety of insect-based pet foods in dogs and cats, as well as studies that focus on the presence of health-promoting functionalities of insects [2].

## 21.3 Chitin

Chitin is the most abundant aminopolysaccharide polymer and the second most abundant polysaccharide (after cellulose) occurring in nature and is the building material that gives strength to the exoskeletons of crustaceans, insects, and the cell walls of fungi [13]. Chitin has the potential to be a prebiotic for the GI microbiome as it has been shown to improve glucose intolerance, increase insulin secretion, relieve dyslipidemia, and protect intestinal integrity [14]. Additionally, chitin, or its derivative, may have antiviral, anticancer, and antifungal activity, along with antimicrobial properties and a bacteriostatic effect on the gram-negative bacteria *Escherichia coli, Vibrio cholerae,* and *Shigella dysenteriae* [14].

Even though chitin is considered to be an insoluble fiber, humans have digestive enzymes in their GI tract that can partially degrade chitin to chitosan. Chitin is not digestible by dogs, but its derivative chitosan is [15]. Hydrolyzed products of chitosan, such as chitin oligosaccharides, are readily soluble in water because of their shorter chain lengths [14]. In cats, there has been some research on the use of chitosan in combination with calcium carbonate as a phosphate binder for cats with renal dysfunction [16], with some current products on the market utilizing polysaccharide chitosan in renal focused supplement products [17].

## 21.4 The Effects on the Host GI Microbiome

A study in broiler chickens revealed that while a low inclusion of BSFL meal (5%) had a positive influence on the cecal microbiota, a higher inclusion (15%) may result in a partial reduction of microbial diversity, particularly in beneficial bacteria [18] (Figure 21.2).

A 2021 study in piglets looked at BSF as an alternative protein source to a soybean meal-based diet. The BSF diet increased microbial diversity and density, both at phylum and genus level [19]. The results indicated the piglets fed the BSF diet a greater indication of a "healthy gut," which is considered to be an increase in intestinal microbiota diversity, a stable composition of species within the microbiome and a functioning mucosal barrier [19]. A significant increase of *Bifidobacterium* and a decreased abundance of *Streptococcus* was observed in piglets fed the BSF-based diet [19].

A 2021 study by Seo et al. looked at using fermented oat flour, BSFL meal, or a combination of the two as a diet for senior dogs [20]. Twenty female spayed dogs were divided into 4 groups of 5 dogs. One group was the control group, one was fed 10% fermented oat flour, another 5% BSFL meal, with the fourth group a combination of 10% fermented oat flour and 5% BSFL meal for 12 weeks [20]. Compared to the control group, there were no significant differences in food intake, body weight, fecal status, skin condition, or hematological and biochemical parameters [20].

The necessity for alternative protein sources with low environmental impact and their effect on animal and human health. More studies are needed to be able to identify the correct volume for inclusion, with reproducible results among an entire species.

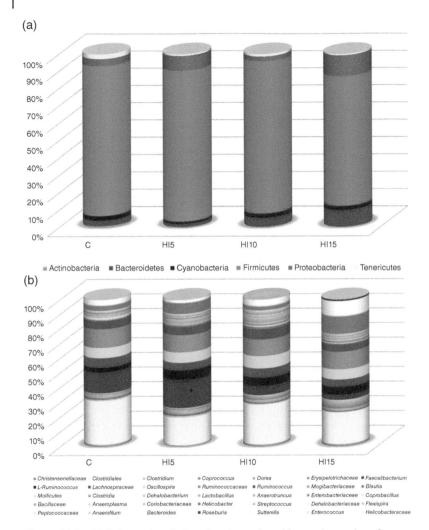

(a)

Actinobacteria    Bacteroidetes    Cyanobacteria    Firmicutes    Proteobacteria    Tenericutes

(b)

| Christensenellaceae | Clostridiales | Clostridium | Coprococcus | Dorea | Erysipelotrichaceae | Faecalibacterium |
| L-Ruminococcus | Lachnospiraceae | Oscillospira | Ruminococcaceae | Ruminococcus | Mogibacteriaceae | Blautia |
| Mollicutes | Clostridia | Dehalobacterium | Lactobacillus | Anaerotruncus | Enterobacteriaceae | Coprobacillus |
| Bacillaceae | Anaeroplasma | Coriobacteriaceae | Helicobacter | Streptococcus | Dehalobacteriaceae | Flexispira |
| Peptococcaceae | Anaerofilum | Bacteroides | Roseburia | Sutterella | Enterococcus | Helicobacteraceae |

**Figure 21.2**  Main bacteria relative abundance found in cecal samples of broiler chickens fed different diets. Figure (a) shows the bacterial phyla while figure (b) shows bacterial genera. C = control; HI5 = 5%; HI10 = 10%; and HI15 = 15% level of inclusion of Black Soldier Fly in meal diets. 18 Creative Commons License: https://creativecommons.org/licenses/by/4.0/.

## 21.5  Chapter Summary

- Insects can provide high amounts of proteins, fats, vitamins, and mineral elements with great economic and environmental advantages.
- The insect species that have been recognized as promising alternative sources of protein for animal feed are:
  - The Black Soldier Fly (BSF) *Hermetia illucens* L. (Diptera: Stratiomyidae)
  - The common housefly *Musca domestica* L. (Diptera: Muscidae)
  - The yellow mealworm *Tenebrio Molitor* L. (Coleoptera: Tenebrionidae)
- BSFL GI microbiome community provides various functional and metabolic skills that allow the BSFL to thrive in various environments [10].
- Rather than diet dictating diversity in BSLF, a stable indigenous collection of bacteria functions in the degradation of a broad range of substrates.
- BSFL that are highly exposed to heavy metals may see detrimental changes to the GI microbiome such as a reduction in bacterial diversity [11].
- The addition of specific probiotics to the feed of BSFL may be beneficial for their growth and development.
- Chitin is an aminopolysaccharide that has the potential to be a prebiotic for the GI microbiome as it has been shown to improve glucose intolerance, increase insulin secretion, relieve dyslipidemia, and protect intestinal integrity [14].
- While chitin is an insoluble fiber source, its derivatives when hydrolyzed may have an increase in water solubility.
- Chitosan combined with calcium carbonate is used in supplements for cats with renal disease as a phosphate blocker.

## References

**1** Tang, C., Yang, D., Liao, H. et al. (2019). Edible insects as a food source: a review. *Food Production, Processing and Nutrition* 1: 8. https://doi.org/10.1186/s43014-019-0008-1.

**2** Bosch, G. and Swanson, K.S. (2021). Effect of using insects as feed on animals: pet dogs and cats. *Journal of Insects as Food and Feed* 7 (5): 795–805. https://doi.org/10.3920/JIFF2020.0084.

**3** Schrögel, P. and Wätjen, W. (2019). Insects for food and feed – safety aspects related to mycotoxins and metals. *Food* 8 (8): 288. https://doi.org/10.3390/foods8080288.

**4** Bessa, L., Pieterse, E., Marais, J. et al. (2020). Why for feed and not for human consumption? The black soldier fly larvae. *Comprehensive Reviews in Food Science and Food Safety* 19: 2747–2763. https://doi.org/10.1111/1541-4337.12609.

**5** Shumo, M., Osuga, I.M., Khamis, F.M. et al. (2019). The nutritive value of black soldier fly larvae reared on common organic waste streams in Kenya. *Scientific Reports* 9: 10110. https://doi.org/10.1038/s41598-019-46603-z.

**6** Siddiqui, S.A., Ristow, B., Rahayu, T. et al. (2022). Black soldier fly larvae (BSFL) and their affinity for organic waste processing. *Waste Management* 140: 1–13. https://doi.org/10.1016/j.wasman.2021.12.044.

**7** Bonelli, M., Bruno, D., Brilli, M. et al. (2020). Black soldier fly larvae adapt to different food substrates through morphological and functional responses of the midgut. *International Journal of Molecular Sciences* 21 (14): 4955. https://doi.org/10.3390/ijms21144955.

**8** Alcarez, D., Wilkinson, K.A., Treihou, M. et al. (2019). Prospecting peptides isolated from black soldier fly (Diptera: Stratiomyidae) with antimicrobial activity against *Helicobacter pylori* (Campylobacterales: Helicobacteraceae). *Journal of Insect Science* 19 (6): 17. https://doi.org/10.1093/jisesa/iez120.

**9** Ao, Y., Yang, C., Wang, S. et al. (2021). Characteristics and nutrient function of intestinal bacterial communities in black soldier fly (Hermetia illucens L.) larvae in livestock manure conversion. *Microbial Biotechnology* 14 (3): 886–896. https://doi.org/10.1111/1751-7915.13595.

**10** Klammsteiner, T., Walter, A., Bogataj, T. et al. (2020). The core gut microbiome of black soldier fly (Hermetia illucens) larvae raised on low-bioburden diets. *Frontiers in Microbiology* 11: 993. https://doi.org/10.3389/fmicb.2020.00993.

**11** Yu, G., Cheng, P., Chen, Y. et al. (2011). Inoculating poultry manure with companion bacteria influences growth and development of black soldier fly (Diptera: Stratiomyidae) larvae. *Environmental Entomology* 40 (1): 30–35. https://doi.org/10.1603/EN10126.

**12** Wu, N., Wang, X., Xu, X. et al. (2020). Effects of heavy metals on the bioaccumulation, excretion and gut microbiome of black soldier fly larvae (Hermetia illucens). *Ecotoxicology and Environmental Safety* 192: 110323. https://doi.org/10.1016/j.ecoenv.2020.110323.

**13** Elieh-ALi-Komi, D. and Hamblin, M.R. (2016). Chitin and chitosan: Production and application of versatile biomedical nanomaterials. *International Journal of Advanced Research (Indore).* 4 (3): 411–427.

**14** Lopez-Santamarina, A., del Carmen Mondragon, A., Lamas, A. et al. (2020). Animal-origin prebiotics based on chitin: an alternative for the future? A critical review. *Food* 9 (6): 782. https://doi.org/10.3390/foods9060782.

**15** Jarett, J., Carlson, A., Serao, M. et al. (2019). Diets with and without edible cricket support a similar level of diversity in the gut microbiome of dogs. *Peer Journal* 7: e7661. https://doi.org/10.7717/peerj.7661.

**16** Wagner, E., Schwendenwein, I., and Zentek, J. (2004). Effects of a dietary chitosan and calcium supplement on Ca and P metabolism in cats. *Berliner und Münchener Tierärztliche Wochenschrift* 117 (7-8): 310–315.

**17** Morin-Crini, N., Lichtfouse, E., Torri, G. et al. (2019). Applications of chitosan in food, pharmaceuticals, medicine, cosmetics, agriculture, textiles, pulp and paper, biotechnology, and environmental chemistry. *Environmental Chemistry Letters* 17: 1667–1692. https://doi.org/10.1007/s10311-019-00904-x.

**18** Biasato, I., Ferrocino, I., Dabbou, S. et al. (2020). Black soldier fly and gut health in broiler chickens: insights into the relationship between cecal microbiota and intestinal mucin composition. *Journal of Animal Science and Biotechnology* 11: 11. https://doi.org/10.1186/s40104-019-0413-y.

**19** Kar, S.K., Schokker, D., Harms, A.C. et al. (2021). Local intestinal microbiota response and systemic effects of feeding black soldier fly larvae to replace soybean meal in growing pigs. *Scientific Reports* 11: 15088. https://doi.org/10.1038/s41598-021-94604-8.

**20** Seo, K., Cho, H.W., Chun, J. et al. (2021). Evaluation of fermented oat and black soldier fly larva as food ingredients in senior dog diets. *Animal (Basel).* 11 (12): 3509. https://doi.org/10.3390/ani11123509.

# Section IV

# Communication and Nutrition Plans for Pet Parents

# 22

# Communicating with Pet Parents

## 22.1 From the Pet Parent Perspective

There are a variety of factors that may preclude pet parents from following your recommendation: Are they able to understand the complexity of the diagnosis or the importance of the diagnostics, particularly in situations where we are discussing new or not completely understood medicine [1]? Can they financially and emotionally afford to follow the recommendations, and do we have alternative routes we can recommend if they are unable to follow the gold standard medical path? These questions become particularly important when we are discussing complexities like the microbiome, where effects of a dysbiosis may have started years prior.

There are multiple concerns for the pet parent during the decision-making process:

1) Concerns for their pet: *Are they in pain? Do they need to stay at the hospital? Are they scared, or being mistreated when they are out of my sight?*
2) Concerns for themselves: *What will this cost? Will I need to be away from my pet? Will this change what I feed my pet? Will I have to medicate my pet? Will my pet be mad at me? How long will this last?*
3) Financial concerns: *What will this cost? Do I have enough money? Do I have support if I don't have enough money? How can I pay for this long term? How expensive are the additional products? What can I do to mitigate my costs now? What can I do to mitigate any future expenses?*

*Small Animal Microbiomes and Nutrition*, First Edition. Robin Saar and Sarah Dodd.
© 2024 John Wiley & Sons, Inc. Published 2024 by John Wiley & Sons, Inc.
Companion website: www.wiley.com/go/saar/1e

4) Concerns about the medical process: *Will I get to research what is happening to my pet before deciding? Are there other options? Can I get a second opinion? What is the timeline?*

Creating trust between pet parents is the main component when developing a veterinarian–client–patient relationship (VCPR). It includes aiding the pet parents in making decisions about their pet's health. Directing pet parents through the clinical decision-making process may be one of the most complex and difficult components of the VCPR relationship [1]. Understanding the expectations of pet parents and collaborating through the process will result in improved overall satisfaction [1]. A recent study by Janke et al. revealed that veterinarians who understand the client's current knowledge level of the topic, tailor the information for each client, and educate the clients about their options can impact pet parents' perceptions of veterinarians' motivations [1].

## 22.2 How the Brain Processes New Information

Understanding the unconscious processes that happen when a person receives information may allow us to be more empathetic to how the pet parent is feeling when we deliver medical information about their pet. This information is not new to the veterinary team; we studied it, experienced multiple cases, and discuss it daily. For pet parents, they may be hearing this information for the first time, or it may contradict information they have believed to be true. They may not understand the language you are using to describe the content or have a lower general understanding of science and pet health than you perceived.

### 22.2.1 The Protection Motivation Theory

This theory was developed by Rogers in 1975 to describe how individuals are motivated to react in a self-protective way toward a perceived threat [2]. This theory has four key elements (Figure 22.1).

#### 22.2.1.1 Receipt of Knowledge
The receipt of information may be perceived as a threat [2]. This perceived threat does not need to be as dramatic as "do this treatment or your pet will die." It can be as simple as the pet parents' perception that

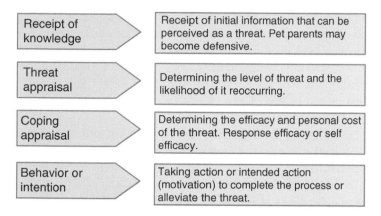

| Receipt of knowledge | Receipt of initial information that can be perceived as a threat. Pet parents may become defensive. |
| Threat appraisal | Determining the level of threat and the likelihood of it reoccurring. |
| Coping appraisal | Determining the efficacy and personal cost of the threat. Response efficacy or self efficacy. |
| Behavior or intention | Taking action or intended action (motivation) to complete the process or alleviate the threat. |

**Figure 22.1** The four elements of the protection motivation theory (PMT).

you think badly of them; maybe the pet's current diet is causing a disease or malnourishment in the pet.

Examples of perceived threats:

1) Feeding table scraps has aided in my pet having diarrhea.
2) My pet still has skin lesions because I did not shampoo him weekly as instructed.
3) My pet is sick, and the vet team won't give him antibiotics.
4) I feed a diet that I thought was the best and now I am being told it is a poor-quality diet, it may be causing my pet to be sick.

Pet parents can become defensive when the initial information is presented. This will stop pet parents from going through the assessment process. Defensiveness can be avoided by using *self-affirmation*. In this theory, people are motivated to maintain a positive self-image [2]. When the threats are perceived to reflect badly on the self-image, the threats are met with resistance. Self-affirmations can restore self-image by allowing individuals to reflect on sources of self-worth. They focus on the positive information and are less likely to become defensive to the perceived threat. For example:

A pet parent has an obese pet that is fed multiple treats per day as a reward for good behavior. When calculated the pet is receiving 35% of its daily energy requirements from treats. If the owner is approached with the information that their pet is overweight and they need to stop giving so many treats or giving treats as often, they may become defensive as they may feel responsible for their pet's poor health condition. This makes them look bad and therefore they do not hear any of the post statement information and will not discuss or consider a weight loss plan for their pet.

In this example, we could instead start by using self-affirmation – "I can tell that you are such loving pet parents and I appreciate your willingness to train and reward your pet for good behavior. To continue to support your pet with his health condition let's look at other forms of treats we could use so you can continue to love him while we work on improving his health."

### 22.2.1.2 Threat Appraisal

Threat appraisal includes determining the level of threat and the likelihood of it reoccurring. Examples of threat appraisals are:

- This is a small change that I can make.
- This is a change that will affect my day-to-day life.
- This is a one-time situation that will be difficult for me to pay for.
- This may repeatedly occur to my pet for the rest of his life.

### 22.2.1.3 Coping Appraisal

By determining the efficacy and personal cost of the threat, the client can decide how to cope with the threat [1]. This may lead to response efficacy where the belief that certain processes will mitigate the threat [1]. Examples of response efficacy are:

- The vet team has a plan that will help my pet.
- Medications and nutrition will benefit my pet's condition.

Alternatively, an individual may experience self-efficacy where an individual's idea of their own ability to implement the required actions to mitigate the threat [1]. Examples of self-efficacy:

- I can stop giving my pet table scraps.
- I can use my savings to pay for my pet's treatment.
- I can change my behaviors to benefit my pet.

#### 22.2.1.4 Behavior or Intention

The behavior includes "taking action" or "intended action" (motivation) to complete the process and alleviate the threat. There can be some difficulties when getting the intended behavior moved into action. Motivation does not equal action and while pet parents may be motivated to help their pets, though they do not follow through with the action plan. This could be the result of multiple barriers such as financial, lifestyle, or a lack of a supporting action plan. "Head in the Sand Phenomenon" or "The Ostrich Effect" is a phenomenon when people choose to ignore the threat as it may be too overwhelming or reflect badly on themselves [3, 4]. There is a conflict between our rational mind knowing that the information is important, and our emotional mind anticipating that the information will be painful [2]. Smoking, for example, has proven to cause a variety of illnesses, diseases, and neoplasia yet despite that information being widely circulated, people continue to smoke and even start smoking despite the information being known.

Behavior can be difficult to change and is driven by cues. Changing behavior can be difficult for pets, pet parents, and the vet team.

- Dogs and cats are highly intelligent and learn how to respond to cues quickly. This can be favorable with a motivated pet parent who is willing to work on a new training plan or it can be detrimental in the case of a persistent pet who continues the unwanted behavior until the pet parent gives a rewarding response.
- Pet parents have the most behavioral changes to make. They need to modify their cues, along with adjusting how they respond to their pets' cues. We are sometimes asking them to sacrifice a perceived positive experience with their pet or change an action they have been repeating for multiple years.
- The vet team has behaviors to modify in this process, with the focus being on how they present the plan to the pet parent. They need to ensure that they don't respond to preconceived ideas and continue to present a plan of action in a nonjudgmental way. For example, if the pet and pet parents are above an ideal body condition, it is important to present an action plan to the pet parent and not assume that the pet parents won't participate in a weight loss plan. Many vet med teams have short pitches for providing pet parents with information. The language in the pitches or how they are presented may require changes and individualism to improve the pet parent's response.

## 22.3   Improving Action Results

Vet teams must improve the consistency and longevity of pet parents following action plans. For example, when you consider approximately 50% of pets in North America are in an obese state [5–7] the multiple health concerns associated with obesity, and how diet management can aid in eliciting a positive shift in GI microbiome health, having a successful action plan becomes vital for improving the longevity and well-being of these pets [8]. To support pet parents in overcoming some of the previously mentioned barriers, we need to provide thorough directions on how to complete the action and how to cope with any foreseeable and unforeseeable barriers.

### 22.3.1   Steps to Create a Successful Action Plan

#### 22.3.1.1   Step 1 Identify the Threat
Identify the threat to the pet parent and utilize self-affirmation in your discussion with the pet parent [3]. Discuss an important or positive aspect about the pet parent before giving the information, which may be perceived as negative, creating defensiveness. Examples of phrases you might use are:

- "I can tell you care about your pet, and he is a big part of the family, . . . (new information)."
- "I can see that you are an amazing pet parent and that you have such a great bond with Fluffy . . . (new information)."
- I appreciate how engaged you are in Fluffy's nutritional health by wanting to feed him a health-conscious diet . . . (new information)."

#### 22.3.1.2   Step 2 Develop a Plan
Develop a plan for the pet parent, including possible cues that may cause temptation and how to avoid or manage behaviors, behavior cues, or other possible barriers. Be as specific as possible in your action plan.

- Create a day-by-day transition plan with exact volumes and times for meals to be fed.
- List any housekeeping tips such as food storage or feeding equipment cleaning.
- List known behaviors and alternative ways to react to the cue behaviors.

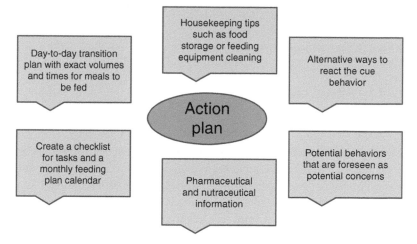

**Figure 22.2** Elements of an efficient action plan.

- List possible behaviors that have not been discussed but are foreseen as potential concerns (what happens when family comes to visit – how do we change their actions?).
- List the exact name, dose, and frequency of any supplements or medications along with possible side effects or interactions that should be avoided.
- Create a checklist for the pet parents to acknowledge when tasks have been completed to allow for accountability.
- Create monthly feeding plan calendars. Have words of encouragement throughout the month (Figure 22.2).

## 22.4 Supporting Pet Parents Through the Decision-Making Process

### 22.4.1 Dr. Google

Most pet parents will complete some form of research and interpretation of provided information post-diagnosis [1]. While many pet parents recognize that information found on the internet may not be a reliable source, it can provide the veterinary team an opportunity to start a discussion [1]. Providing clients with reputable sites is the ideal way to support pet parents who have a desire to research and validate information from validated sites [1].

### 22.4.2 Provide Learning Tools

Diagnostics and treatment options should be provided to pet parents in a step-by-step plan, which discloses the value of each step, with an allowance of input from the pet parent. A variety of learning tools or resources should be provided to help pet parents who learn in different ways. Providing visual aids, written handouts, or website addresses to approved internet platforms may decrease the risk of pet parents conducting their research from less accurate or reliable platforms. Pet parents want to understand; language utilized in the tool should be expressed at a level of comprehension for the individual pet parent [1] (Figure 22.3).

### 22.4.3 Understanding Financial Constraints

Finances must be considered when we consider the pet parent. A pet parent may be willing to complete all courses of action to help their pet, while their finances do not allow for this action. Other pet parents may have preconceived levels of value on the veterinary services or on the pet itself. They may be able to afford treatment for their pet but have a conflict with the value to cost ratio. Behavioral economics refers to the science of understanding why humans may not make logical decisions and how to utilize these subconscious irrationalities to help them make better choices [9]. The concept of "the nudge" is an intervention to help the pet parent do the right thing, allowing them to have free will with no incentive or punishment, by simply making it slightly easier for them to make the right choice [9]. Hospitals can utilize principles to affect human behavior to help pet parents decide to follow our recommendation. Some examples are:

- Decoys – Provide pet parents with options. When provided with a lower, middle, and higher cost option, most buyers will reach for the middle option. If the ideal option is listed as the middle option, we may be able to direct the pet parent to take the desired recommendation [9].

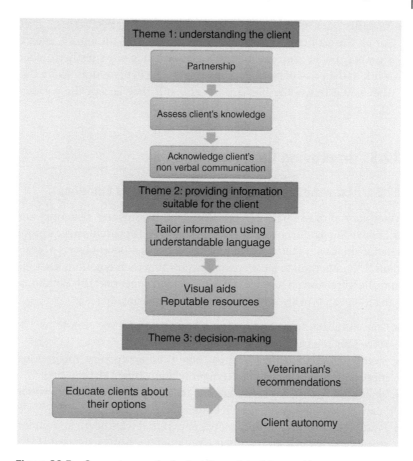

**Figure 22.3** Concept map of a logical flow of decision-making expectations and information exchange between a veterinary professional and pet owners. *Source:* Janke et al. [1] / PLOS / Public Domain CC BY 4.0.

- Reciprocity – People like the idea of returning a feeling or action. By creating a nutrition plan for "their pet" you have provided them with something that is special for them [9]. In return they may be more likely to follow your dietary recommendation.
- Social Norms – Utilizing social media to share stories [9] about pets in the hospital can be a way to increase trust with other pet parents. This outside influence may aid in pet parents' ability to agree to your recommendations.

- Defaults – Set up pricing or packages in a way that expresses a need for all the services. Most people will choose a default option even if they may not be required to [9]. You may include pre-anesthetic blood work in the price of sterilization surgery. The pet parent is aware that they could refuse the blood work and still they accept the package as it is.

## 22.5 Improving Conversations

### 22.5.1 Lose the Judgment – Validate Pet Parents Emotions

Veterinary professionals can validate pet parents by listening and acknowledging their concerns and emotions [1]. Pet parents have unique relationships with their pets, which may result in different levels of emotions. It is important to let pet parents know that their emotions are valid and offer direction on how we can support their concerns [10]. Emotional validation can provide some benefits to the relationship [11]:

- Communicate acceptance – by acknowledging their emotions you show that you care for and accept them [11].
- Strengthen relationships – when there is an acceptance you can feel more connected and build a stronger relationship [11].
- Show value – the pet parent will feel that they are important to you as you have acknowledged their feelings [11].
- Better emotional regulation – a pet parent that feels heard and understood may have the level of their emotional intensity decreased [11].

In a study examining how validation or invalidation of emotional experiences moderates personality characteristics and aggression, it was observed that people with a tendency to be more aggressive had increased aggressive behavior when invalidated versus when their emotions were validated [12]. Examples of validation phrases are [11]:

- "I can see how you would feel that way."
- "That must be very difficult."
- "I feel the same way."
- "How frustrating!"
- "I bet you're frustrated."
- "I'm here for you" (Figure 22.4).

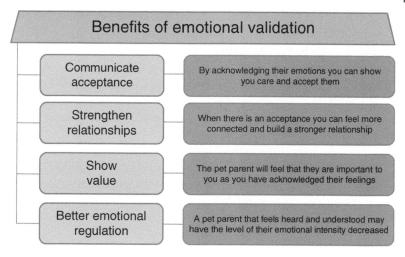

**Figure 22.4** Benefits of providing emotional validation to the pet parents.

## 22.6 Providing Continuing Support to Pet Parents

Post-consultation support for the pet parent is extremely important in ensuring that the continuation and success of the nutrition or treatment plan. Changing behaviors can be difficult, along with identifying the behavior cues that initiate the unwanted behavior [3]. By completing frequent and consistent touchpoints with the pet parents, we can help support them to stay on track and follow the action plan appropriately.

### 22.6.1 Staying in Touch

Technology has provided veterinary teams with multiple ways to stay in contact with pet parents. The pet parent's preferred method should be investigated as this may affect the outcome of the sessions. For example, a pet parent who does not like to speak on the phone may not respond to your calls, whereas if you had sent a text, they may be more engaging about following up with their pet's health. Some options you can present to the pet parent are:

- Phone calls – this can be a more personal way to reach out to pet parents. By hearing and speaking to a pet parent you have the added addition of hearing their tone while individualizing your tone and language to better communicate with them.

- Texting – this form of communication is a nice way to reach out to pet parents that are busy or more difficult to engage in longer conversations. Caution must be taken in the language used in texts and ensure that there is a true understanding in the exchange of information. Alternate tools for communicating may be required if more in-depth conversations or directions are required.
- Email/messaging – this type of communication can be a great way to send specific instructions or provide information where you can take the time to ensure you have created a positive letter in a language the pet parent can understand. When a client may have multiple cross-questions, this form of communication can be very time-consuming and ineffective.
- Teleconsultation (virtual) – As a growing tool for communication, virtual consultations are becoming a more sought out way to communicate with pet parents. For pets who have a stable health condition, and do not require diagnostics, this form of communication may be the ideal way to perform routine touchpoints. There may be a greater form of trust developed through the use of visual and auditory connections between the veterinary team member and the pet parent. This connection is similar to an in-person visit and has become a more normalized way of staying in touch, with many families using these types of platforms to stay connected in recent years when social distancing has become a more common way of life.
  - a) Forms – utilizing questionnaire-type forms (Google Forms) is a way to receive information from pet parents on how they are doing with the action plan. This is a unilateral form of communication and will require a response utilizing one of the other communication tools.
  - b) Group supports – the creation of positive support groups may help pet parents relate to others experiencing the same stressors with their pets. This could include in-person groups where pet parents of weight loss management pets meet at a park to go for monthly walks with their pets and virtual support groups where pet parents can post photos of their pets and add memories to a blog. Creating this type of community within the veterinary hospital is a wonderful way to support pet parents along with creating long-lasting trust.

### 22.6.2 How Often to Request Contact

The frequency of the touchpoints will depend on the support required by the pet parent. Questions to consider when determining the frequency are:

- How stable is the pet's health condition?
- How many barriers are there for the pet parents?
- How are the pet parents managing the action plan?
- What is the health condition?
- How soon could the symptoms return and cause increased health risks?
- How often do the pet parents want to have support?

Giving the pet parents contact options and allowing them to have some say in the frequency will aid in the success of repeat consultations.

## 22.7 Chapter Summary

- Pet parents want to be included in the decision-making process concerning their pet's health and treatment plan [1], though a variety of factors may preclude them from being able to follow your recommendation.
- Creating trust between pet parents is the main component when developing a veterinarian–client–patient relationship (VCPR). It includes aiding the pet parents in making decisions about their pet's health, and it may be one of the most complex and difficult components of the VCPR relationship.
- The protection motivation theory (PMT) describes how individuals are motivated to react in a self-protective way toward a perceived threat [2]. This theory has four key elements:
  - Receipt of Knowledge
  - Threat Appraisal
  - Coping Appraisal
  - Behavior or Intention
- Changing behavior can be difficult and requires on-going support to ensure the illicit of new behaviors.
- Self-affirmation is identifying and communicating an important or positive aspect about the pet parent before giving information, which may be perceived as negative. This action will aid in preventing defensiveness.

- Action plans should include:
  - Day-by-day transition plan with exact volumes, and times for meals to be fed.
  - Housekeeping tips such as food storage or feeding equipment cleaning.
  - Alternative ways to react to the cue behaviors.
  - Potential behaviors that are foreseen as potential concerns.
  - Pharmaceutical and nutraceutical information.
  - Create a checklist for tasks and a monthly feeding plan calendar.
- Providing visual aids, written handouts, or website addresses to approved internet platforms may decrease the risk of pet parents conducting their research from less accurate or reliable platforms.
- Behavioral economics refers to the science of understanding why humans may not make logical decisions, and how to utilize these subconscious irrationalities to help them make better choices [9].
- Emotional validation can provide some benefits to the relationship [11]:
- Post-consultation support for the pet parent is extremely important in ensuring that the continuation and success of the nutrition or treatment plan. We can keep in touch with pet parents via a wide range of communication tools with the frequency depending on the individual case and pet parent requirement for support.

## References

1 Janke, N., Coe, J.B., Bernardo, T.M. et al. (2021). Pet owners' and veterinarians' perceptions of information exchange and clinical decision-making in companion animal practice. *PLoS One* 16 (2): e0245632. https://doi.org/10.1371/journal.pone.0245632.

2 Westcott, R., Ronan, K., Bambrick, H. et al. (2017). Expanding protection motivation theory: investigating an application to animal owners and emergency responders in bushfire emergencies. *BMC Psychology* 5: 13. 10.1186/s40359-017-0182-3.

3 Webb, T.L. and Sheeran, P. (2006). Does changing behavioral intentions engender behavior change? A meta-analysis of the experimental evidence. *Psychological Bulletin* 132 (2): 249–268. https://doi.org/10.1037/0033-2909.132.2.249.

**4** Webb, T.L., Chang, B.P.I., and Benn, Y. (2013). 'The ostrich problem': motivated avoidance or rejection of information about goal progress. *Social and Personality Psychology Compass* 7: 794–807. https://doi. org/10.1111/spc3.12071.

**5** Banfield Pet Hospital (2017). State of pet health. https://www.banfield. com/pet-health/state-of-pet-health (accessed 4 January 2022).

**6** Association for Pet Obesity Prevention (2018). Pet obesity survey results. https://petobesityprevention.org/2018 (accessed 4 January 2022).

**7** Pet Food Alberta (2012). Trending – obesity in pets. https://www1.agric. gov.ab.ca/$department/deptdocs. nsf/all/bdv14368/$file/Obesity FactsheetFinalized%282%29kk.pdf?OpenElement (accessed 4 January 2022).

**8** Kieler, I.N., Kamal, S.S., Vitger, A.D. et al. (2017). Gut microbiota composition may relate to weight loss rate in obese pet dogs. *Veterinary Medicine and Science* 3 (4): 252–262. https://doi.org/10.1002/vms3.80.

**9** Moore-Jones, J. (2019). Principal, unleashed coaching and consulting. Beyond the shelter. *8th Annual G2Z Summit and Workshops.* https:// www.g2z.org.au/assets/pdf/Jessica%20Moore%20Jones%20paper% 20Behavioural%20economics.pdf (accessed 3 January 2022).

**10** Thomas, V. (2012). A comprehensive guide to effective communication between veterinarian and client: from a terminal diagnosis to an end-of-life discussion. Honors College thesis. Oregon State University. https://ir.library.oregonstate.edu/concern/honors_college_theses/ x633f2851 (accessed 8 January 2022).

**11** Clinical Nutrition Service (2019). How do I switch my pet's food? https://vetnutrition.tufts.edu/2019/11/how-do-i-switch-my-pets-food/ (accessed 8 January 2022).

**12** Herr, N.R., Meier, E.P., Weber, D.M. et al. (2017). Validation of emotional experience moderates the relation between personality and aggression. *Journal of Experimental Psychopathology* 8 (2): 126–139. https://doi.org/10.5127/jep.057216.

# 23

## Documenting a Nutrition History

Nutrition is now considered to be a fifth vital assessment – temperature, pulse, respiration, pain, and nutritional assessment. When we consider how an imbalance in the gut microbiome can cause poor health outcome later in life, obtaining a historical and current nutrition history is a vital part of completing a physical examination and intake.

## 23.1 How to Ask the Right Questions

To obtain a thorough nutrition history, we must allow the clients to engage and recall their daily routines ensuring they provide us with a complete view of what the pet is eating daily.

There are different ways we can ask questions that will set the pet parent to answer in a certain way. These techniques can help control the volume or the type of information. Some commonly used questioning techniques are:

### 23.1.1 Closed-Ended Questions

Using these types of questions will limit answers to a single word or few words in response [1]. Information will be direct (yes/no) and may not provide detailed information.

*Small Animal Microbiomes and Nutrition*, First Edition. Robin Saar and Sarah Dodd.
© 2024 John Wiley & Sons, Inc. Published 2024 by John Wiley & Sons, Inc.
Companion website: www.wiley.com/go/saar/1e

Some example questions could be

- Do you feed your pet treats?
- Do you feed your pet kibble, canned, raw, or homemade food?
- How often do you feed your pet?
- Do you give your pet any human food?

These questions could lead to defensiveness if stated in the wrong tone or if perceived by the client to have a positively and negatively viewed answer.

For example, if the pet is experiencing gastrointestinal illness, and the pet parent is asked, "did you give him any food other than his dog food?". The pet parent may wonder if you might accuse them of causing the problem, as they give their pet a drive-thru hamburger every day. They may answer "no" to deflect any possible chance this threat could be their fault. As discussed in Chapter 22, this could lead to defensiveness and barriers early on in the conversation.

### 23.1.2 Open-Ended Questions

These questions prompt pet parents to answer with sentences, lists, and stories, giving deeper and new insights [1]. These types of questions will encourage pet parents to share which will allow for a better exchange of information.

Some open-ended question examples are:

- Tell me all the food that goes into your pet's mouth from when you wake up until bedtime.
- Describe what your pet does behaviorally, to earn a treat reward.
- Explain in detail how your pet acts when you offer him the new diet

### 23.1.3 Probing Questions

These questions will prompt pet parents to respond in more detail. It is a way to ensure you have received all the information. These questions may be utilized after an open or closed-ended question to retrieve more details.

- Example questions
  - What are the things you like about feeding this diet?
  - Can you describe exactly what your pet does before he vomits?
  - Tell me more about why you chose that type of diet for your pet (Figure 23.1).

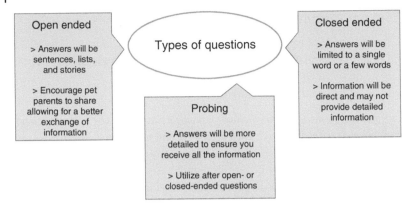

Figure 23.1  Types of questions and responses.

### 23.1.4  Using Appropriate Tone

The use of a proper tone should be in conjunction with your question. Our tone communicates our emotions behind our words [2]. A study on humans where the tone on certain words was provided in either neutral, sad, or happy tones. Words that were given with a sad tone were later perceived as negative, while words given in a happy tone were rated to be more positive [2].

### 23.1.5  Timing Is Everything

When we require a pet parent to recall a nutrition history, we are asking them to recall memories. The concern is what memories about their pet's nutrition can they recall? "It's the green bag with a dog on the front," "I think it's called True Werewolf, or something like that" or "It has triangle kibble." A pet parent may not find it a priority to store the details of the pet food we are looking to obtain.

## 23.2  Nutrition Questionnaire

One solution to the incomplete nutrition history is to provide the pet parent with a Nutrition Questionnaire days before a nutrition consultation. This technique will allow the pet parent time to recall and retrieve all the information you are requiring. There are benefits to completing a nutrition history:

- More efficient use of time. Having the pet parent complete the nutrition questionnaire before the examination allows for the veterinarian or vet nurse (tech) to focus on probing questions if needed and decrease the history-taking process.
- More accurate, and thorough history. By allowing pet parents time to recall their pet's previous diets, in greater detail.
- Time to contemplate the previous nutrition provided. This is particularly important for practitioners who are not as comfortable or experienced in making nutrition recommendations. Giving a deadline to the pet parent to submit the form 24 hours before the appointment can allow the practitioner adequate time to assess the information and create a plan of how they would like to proceed during the consultation.

### 23.2.1 What to Include in a Nutrition History

As part of the fifth vital assessment, the current diet including the volume and frequency should be recorded in the patient's file. In conjunction with taking a current weight, the percentage of weight loss should be recorded if applicable. A noninitiated weight loss of 10% has been associated with disease cachexia, with a 5% loss being a sign of possible pre-cachexia [3]. In a small pet, 5% can equate to a 0.2 kg loss.

A more in-depth history should include a timeline of diets including the volume and frequency of meals. How far back nutrition history is required may depend on the health status of the pet and the depth that the consultation is required to investigate. Ideally, a gold standard nutrition history would include nutrition back to the dam at the time of pregnancy through to the current diet, along with any pharmaceutical treatments during that same time frame. Knowing the large shift that some pharmaceuticals (antibiotics, antifungals) can have on the microbiome [4], it is important to have a good medical history when compiling previous nutrition information. The World Small Animal Veterinary Association (WSAVA) "Nutrition Toolkit" has in it a "Short Diet History Form" which can be used or modified to suit your team's particular assessment requirements [5].

### 23.2.1.1 A More In-Depth History Form Should Inquire about

1) Current Diet – including treats, other food, and supplements. (name brand, volume, and frequency). Homemade diets should include the recipe with the volume of ingredients and feeding plan.

2) Historical Diet – including treats or supplements given in the past (name brand, volume, frequency, and the time frame of when this diet/treat/supplement was provided). Homemade diets should include the recipe with the volume of ingredients and feeding plan.

3) Pet's relationship with food – How does the pet behave when fed – eats right away, grazes, needs to be hand-fed. Is there any food competition in the house (children, other pets)?

4) Exercise – Type of exercise including the intensity and frequency of the activity.

5) How the meals, water, and supplements are provided – dish type or administration tool, who provides the meal? Where is the meal fed? Who administers supplements? How often is the water changed? What type of water is provided? Where is the food, water dishes located?

6) Other pets in the home – if so, name the species and breed. Discuss the pet's relationship, and how the pets are fed (together, separate room, etc.).

7) How is the pet housed? (Indoor, outdoor). Where is the litter box or pee pads located?

8) People in the family – How many people live in the home? How many are teenagers? Elementary age? Toddlers or younger?

9) Medical concerns – Any medications that the pet has been prescribed – previous and current. With dosage and frequency for current medications. Does your pet have any medical problems (previous and current)? Has your pet lost or gained weight? Does your pet have allergies?

10) Food Storage – How is your pet's food stored? How long do you leave your pet access to meals? Does your pet have access or get access to other food – garbage, counters, steal food? How long of a supply of food is purchased at a time?

11) What is important to the pet parent when choosing pet food? Location of purchase, quality, perceived quality, convenience, cost, features (organic, natural, health condition focused), dental care, food sensitivity, skin and coat condition, palatability, stool quality.

12) Who does the pet parent use as a source for nutrition information for their pet? Internet searches, specific internet site, podcast, veterinarian, breeder, family/friends, pet store, books [6].

## 23.3 Chapter Summary

- Nutrition is now considered to be a fifth vital assessment – temperature, pulse, respiration, pain, and nutritional assessment.
- Questioning techniques can help control the volume or the type of information
  - Closed-ended questions – using these types of questions will limit answers to a single word or few words in response [1].
  - Open-ended questions – prompt pet parents to answer with sentences, lists, and stories, giving deeper and new insights [1].
  - Probing questions – will prompt pet parents to respond in more detail. It is a way to ensure you have received all the information.
- The use of a proper tone should be in conjunction with your question. Our tone communicates our emotions behind our words [2].
- Providing pet parents with a nutrition history questionnaire, days prior to the consultation can benefit the consultation process.
  - More efficient use of time.
  - More accurate, and thorough history.
  - Time to contemplate the previous nutrition provided.
- The extent of the nutrition history required is case dependant and may include:
  - Current diet
  - Historical diet
  - Pet's relationship with food
  - Exercise
  - How the meals, water, and supplements are provided
  - Other pets in the home
  - How is the pet housed? (Indoor, outdoor).
  - People in the family
  - Medical concerns
  - Food storage
  - What is important to the pet parent when choosing pet food?
  - Who does the pet parent used as a source for nutrition information for their pet?

# References

1 Coe, J.B., Adams, C.L., and Bonnett, B.N. (2007). A focus group study of veterinarians' and pet owners' perceptions of the monetary aspects of veterinary care. *Journal of the American Veterinary Medical Association* 231 (10): 1510–1518. https://doi.org/10.2460/javma.231.10.1510. PMID: 18020992.

2 Schirmer, A. (2010). Mark my words: tone of voice changes affective word representations in memory. *PLoS One* 5 (2): e9080. 10.1371/journal. pone.0009080.

3 Blum, D., Stene, G.B., Solheim, T.S. et al. (2014). Validation of the consensus – definition for cancer cachexia and evaluation of a classification model – a study based on data from an international multicentre project (EPCRC-CSA). *Annals of Oncology* 25 (8): 1635–1642. 10.1093/annonc/mdu086.

4 Langdon, A., Crook, N., and Dantas, G. (2016). The effects of antibiotics on the microbiome throughout development and alternative approaches for therapeutic modulation. *Genome Medicine* 8: 39. https://doi.org/ 10.1186/s13073-016-0294-z.

5 WSAVA (2020). Short diet history form. https://wsava.org/wp-content/ uploads/2020/01/Diet-History-Form.pdf (accessed 4 March 2022).

6 Clinical Nutrition Service: University of Guelph (2018). Diet history form for pet owners. https://www.ovchsc.ca/files/2018/10/451244-Sep2018-Clinical-Nutrition-Diet-History-Form.pdf (accessed 4 March 2022).

# 24

# Dietary Treatment Plans

As nutrition is the fifth vital assessment pillar, veterinary professionals should include a nutrition recommendation with every consultation [1]. Nutrients are vital to provide energy and aid in the completion of multiple physiological processes. Since nutrition is required by a pet throughout life, veterinary teams should appreciate the value of making a dietary recommendation and creating a nutrition plan for patients at every visit.

## 24.1 Pet Parents Want Veterinary Nutrition Recommendations

Surveys completed in the United States by Packaged Facts (APPA National Pet Owners Survey, 2021–2022) and AnimalBiome (State of the Gut Report, September 2022) revealed that pet parents trust their veterinarians and are looking to them to provide information and recommendations. A study by Janke and Coe et al. [2] that survey both pet parents and veterinarians identified that a "team" approach with pet parents can result in better recommendation compliance [2].

## 24.2 Increasing the Value of Nutrition Plans

Knowing the value of nutrients in pet health, providing a balanced diet, and including balanced energy should be addressed at every veterinary appointment. Consider feeding dosages like drug dosages; an excess of

*Small Animal Microbiomes and Nutrition*, First Edition. Robin Saar and Sarah Dodd.
© 2024 John Wiley & Sons, Inc. Published 2024 by John Wiley & Sons, Inc.
Companion website: www.wiley.com/go/saar/1e

nutrients may create a state of malnutrition, or gut dysbiosis, possibly instigating or influencing a metabolic or inflammatory disease state like obesity. Conversely, supplying insufficient nutrients may not obtain the desired result and may lead to a malnourished or nutritional deficiency. Veterinary professionals should create specific diet recommendations and feeding plans for their patients including calculating the specific volume based on the energy requirements. Much like calculating drug dosages, nutritional math can provide us with more specific information about how to properly dose the patient. By utilizing dietary plans, we can offer our clients specialized nutritional calculations leaving an increased feeling of trust with the client and more accurate treatment for the patient.

## 24.3  Components of a Nutrition Plan

Pet Nutrition Alliance is an organization that consists of individuals from national and international veterinary and veterinary nutrition focused organizations. According to Pet Nutrition Alliance, "a nutrition plan includes providing a complete and balanced diet for patients, establishing nutrient goals, selecting an appropriate food, and determining how much to feed." [3] An extensive nutrition plan could also include details as part of the action plan for overcoming barriers and information regarding how the nutrients in the diet will be beneficial to the pet. Any special instructions on diet preparation, storage, and possible health risks should also be noted in the plan (Figure 24.1).

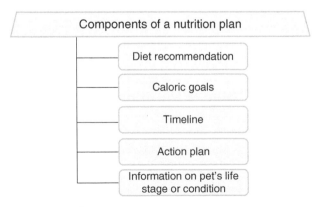

**Figure 24.1**  Components of a nutritional plan.

### 24.3.1 Diet Recommendation

The diet, regardless of the type, should provide complete and balanced nutrition with a few exceptions for short-term recommendations. The length of time to feed these diets depends on the diet, and the health condition. The timeline will depend on the type and volume of nutrient imbalance. The diet recommendation should be appropriate for the life stage and provide appropriate nutrient levels for comorbidities [3, 4]. The diet recommendation needs to also be appropriate for the pet parent, taking into consideration any barriers that may prevent them from purchasing or feeding your recommendation, along with ensuring it meets the pet parents' nutritional expectations for their pet.

### 24.3.2 Caloric Goals

Daily caloric calculations should be made based on the pet's weight, body, and muscle condition score [4].

#### 24.3.2.1 Main Meal(s)
Daily caloric goals will then need to be divided into meals and the volume of the diet(s) should be calculated [4].

#### 24.3.2.2 Treat Goals
The daily caloric goal of treats should be no more than 10% of the daily energy requirements. Treats include any food that is not considered to be complete and balanced nutrition. Treat caloric goals once removed from the daily requirements should be calculated into the number of treats that can be provided to the pet each day [4]. Further details on nutrition calculations can be found in Chapter 25.

### 24.3.3 Timeline

Provide the pet parent with a transition feeding plan along with a timeline of when to have the pet's weight, body, and muscle condition reassessed. The daily calories can be recalculated if required to meet the caloric goals. Giving pet parents short- and long-term goals can aid in the success of the plan. For example, successful weight loss plans can take a year for a pet to reach its ideal weight. It can be difficult for a pet parent to change necessary behaviors to help their pet meet these goals initially and continue the new behaviors over an extended time [5].

### 24.3.3.1 Action Plan

Address here any foreseeable barriers that may hinder the success of the nutrition plan. This may include how to administer pharmaceuticals or nutraceuticals, how to continue to reward a pet that is on a weight loss plan, how to entice a hyporexic pet to eat, and possibly reiterating something in the timeline to help the pet parent continue with the plan [5].

### 24.3.3.2 Information About the Pet's Condition or Life Stage

This section of a plan can be beneficial for the pet parent. This information should focus on why the recommendation and caloric calculation relate to the pet in its current health state. Pet parents are likely to complete research. It is important to provide them with factual information and links to trusted sites where they will see and read similar information that supports your recommendation [2]. This area could also discuss how the recommendation is supporting the pet parents' expectations in a diet for their pet. For example, if the pet parent only wants to purchase a diet from a grocery store, we can address that to meet the pet parents needs by recommending diet A, and while we hope that this diet will be able to meet the pet's needs, we can recommend diet B from the pet store or diet C from the vet clinic if we find diet A is not providing sufficient nutritional support. There can be a brief discussion of how diet C includes additional supplements that will benefit the pet's condition along with having increased digestibility.

## 24.4 Chapter Summary

- Components of nutrition are required daily by the patient to ensure energy needs along with a proper balance of vitamins and minerals, which is why veterinary teams need to first understand the value of making a dietary recommendation and creating a nutrition plan for their patients.
- Pet parents want our nutrition recommendations
- Comparing nutrition plans with medical treatment plans

- Veterinary professionals should create specific diet recommendations and feeding plans for their patients including calculating the specific volume based on the energy requirements. Feeding dosages should be compared to drug dosages; an excess of nutrients may create a dysbiotic state, possibly influencing an illness or disease, while supplying insufficient nutrients may not obtain the desired result or create a nutritional deficiency.
- "A nutrition plan includes providing a complete and balanced diet for patients, establishing nutrient goals, selecting an appropriate food, and determining how much to feed." [3] Components of a plan are:
  - Diet recommendation
  - Caloric goals
  - Timeline
  - Action plan
  - Information for the pet parent about their pet's life stage or condition

# References

1 Blees, N. R., Vandendriessche, V. L., Corbee, R. J., Picavet, P., & Hesta, M. (2022). Nutritional consulting in regular veterinary practices in Belgium and the Netherlands. *Veterinary Medicine and Science*, 8(1), 52–68. https://doi.org/10.1002/vms3.679

2 Janke, N., Coe, J.B., Bernardo, T.M. et al. (2021). Pet owners' and veterinarians' perceptions of information exchange and clinical decision-making in companion animal practice. *PLoS One* 16 (2): e0245632. https://doi.org/10.1371/journal.pone.0245632.

3 Pet Nutrition Alliance Creating a nutritional plan. https://petnutrition-alliance.org/site/pnatool/creating-nutrition-plan (accessed 28 February 2022).

4 Hand et al. (2010). Small Animal *Clinical Nutrition* 5th Edition. MMI, 1,3–18

5 Webb, T.L. and Sheeran, P. (2006 Mar). Does changing behavioral intentions engender behavior change? A meta-analysis of the experimental evidence. *Psychological Bulletin* 132 (2): 249–268. https://doi.org/10.1037/0033-2909.132.2.249. PMID: 16536643.

# 25

# Calculations for the Nutrition Consultation

## 25.1 Energy Requirements

Energy requirements should be calculated for every patient in every consultation [1]. Calculations should include resting energy requirements (RERs) and maintenance energy requirements (MERs). Much like calculating drug dosages, calculating daily energy requirements is necessary:

1) To ensure that adequate energy is being provided
2) To ensure an abundance of energy is not being provided
3) Providing one of the options above may result in deficiencies or excess of vitamins and minerals in commercial diets (Table 25.1).

### 25.1.1 Resting Energy Requirements

RER is the energy required when a patient is awake and at rest. This would be the state of most hospitalized patients. There are two basic equations that most practitioners utilize, a surface area and linear formula, with weight restrictions on the linear calculation [2]. The linear calculation $((BW_{(kg)} \times 30) + 70)$ is less accurate when completed on weights that are less than 2 kg or over 30 kg. Utilizing the surface area calculation will result in more accurate results for all weights [2]. Bodyweight should be calculated in kg (Figure 25.1).

$$RER = BW(kg)^{0.75} \times 70 \text{ (Surface area formula) [2]}$$

*Small Animal Microbiomes and Nutrition*, First Edition. Robin Saar and Sarah Dodd.
© 2024 John Wiley & Sons, Inc. Published 2024 by John Wiley & Sons, Inc.
Companion website: www.wiley.com/go/saar/1e

**Table 25.1** Legend conversion chart.

| Acronyms | Conversions |
|---|---|
| BW=body weight in kg | 1 kg = 2.2 lbs |
| BWC = current body weight in kg | 16 oz = 1 lb = 0.45 kg<br>Conversion: lbs/2.2 = kg or kg × 2.2 = lbs |
| BW$_e$ = expected adult body weight in kg | 250 ml per cup = 8 fluid oz per cup = ½ pint = 1 cup |
| ME = metabolizable energy | 15 ml = 1 tbsp 5 ml = 1 tsp 1 oz = 30 ml = 3 tbsp<br>1000 ml = 1 l 1 kg = 1 l |

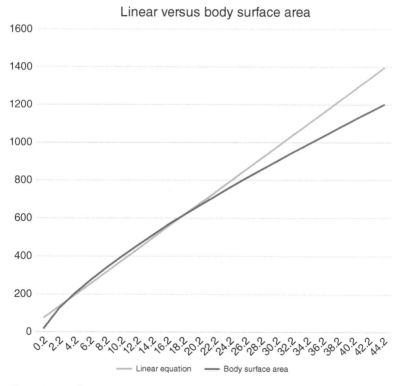

**Figure 25.1** Graph depicting differences between linear and body surface area RER calculations. *X*-axis is the body weight in kg. *Y*-axis is the number of calories.

## 25.1.2 Maintenance Energy Requirements

This is the energy the patient requires to meet basic physiologic needs along with any additional energy requirements related to growth, gestation, lactation, activity, or disease energy expenditures [2]. The RER is multiplied by a factor depending on the energy needs of the pet.

MER = RER × Maintenance Energy Factor [2]

Maintenance energy factors [3]:

| Dogs | Cats |
|---|---|
| Intact adult × 1.8 | Intact adult × 1.4 |
| Neutered adult × 1.6 | Neutered adult × 1.2 |
| Inactive or obese prone × 1.2–1.4 | Inactive or obese prone × 1.0 |
| Weight loss × 1.0 | Weight loss × 0.8 |
| Active light to moderate work × 1.6–5.0 | Active × 1.4–1.6 |
| Weight gain 1.2–1.4 × RER at the ideal weight | Weight gain 1.2–1.4 × RER at the ideal weight |
| Growth ≤16 weeks × 3 | Growth ≤16 weeks × 3 |
| Growth ≥17 weeks × 2 | Growth ≥17 weeks × 2 |
| Moderate to high activity × 5–10 | Moderate to high activity × 2–3 |

## 25.1.3 Calculation for Growth

There is an increased demand for energy during growth as energy is required for tissue energy and development. Growing puppies require two times as much energy per gram body weight as adult dogs [4].

1) Simple – RER × 3.0 (for puppies up to 16 weeks/4 months)
    i) RER × 2.0 (for puppies ≥17 weeks/4 months)
2) Calculation based on estimated adult weight [4]
    i) (Dogs) $130 \times BWc^{0.75} \times 3.2 \, (2.71828^{-0.87(BWc \div BWe)} - 0.1)$
    ii) (Cats) $100 \times BWc^{0.67} \times 6.7 \, (2.71828^{-0.189(BWc \div BWe)} - 0.66)$

## 25.1.4 Calculating for Pregnancy

Energy requirements for pregnancy do not increase until approximately 5 weeks post-breeding. Energy needs can increase from 25 to 60%

depending on the size of the bitch, with larger dogs having greater energy requirements. Queens generally gain 40–50% during pregnancy [4].

Bitches: ME kcal/day $= 130 \times BW^{0.75} + (26 \times BW)$

Queens: ME kcal/day $= 140 \times BW^{0.67}$

### 25.1.5 Calculating for Lactation

Lactation represents the greatest energy demand on an animal. It can be difficult for a lactating animal to ingest sufficient calories to meet all requirements, which can vary depending on the number of offspring. Energy requirements usually reach 2–4 times maintenance requirements during lactation in queens and bitches [4].

| Nursing bitches ME (kcal/day) [3] Puppies (#) | MER | Nursing queens ME (kcal/day) [3] Week of lactation | MER |
|---|---|---|---|
| 1 | $3.0 \times$ RER | Week 1–2 | RER + 30% per kitten |
| 2 | $3.5 \times$ RER | Week 3 | RER + 45% per kitten |
| 3–4 | $4.0 \times$ RER | Week 4 | RER + 55% per kitten |
| 5–6 | $5.0 \times$ RER | Week 5 | RER + 65% per kitten |
| 7–8 | $5.5 \times$ RER | Week 6 | RER + 90% per kitten |
| $\geq 9$ | $\geq 6.0 \times$ RER | | |

## 25.2 Calculating kcal/cup or kcal/can from Energy Requirement

By taking the energy requirements and dividing them by the kcal per cup (or can), we can calculate the daily volume of food required [4]. If the daily energy requirements are divided between two separate diets, for example kibble and canned diets, total calories from one type of diet are subtracted from the daily energy requirements with the balance then divided by the second diet's calories.

Feeding 1 diet – MER ÷ kcal per cup(can) = volume to be fed per day

Feeding 2 diets – Calculate the desired volume of diet 1(1 can[cup], ½ can. ¼ can) = kcal to be fed diet 1, then MER – diet 1 kcal = partial MER, partial MER ÷ diet 2 kcal = volume of diet 2 to be fed.

## 25.2.1 Formulations

### 25.2.1.1 Calculating Diet 1 kcal where a Set Percentage of the can/cup or Multiple cans(cups) Volumes are Predetermined

1) kcal/can(cup) ÷ (# of times the can or cup of diet will be divided)
2) kcal/can(cup)×(# of times the can or cup of the diet will be added)
3) kcal/can(cup)×(percentage of the diet to be fed)
   i) Example 1: MER of 1200 kcal/day with 397 kcal/can feeding ¼ can per day, and 265 kcal/cup kibble
   397 kcal/can ÷ 4 = 99.25 kcal can per day
   ii) Example 2: MER 342 kcal/day with 67 kcal/can feeding 2 cans per day, and 501 kcal/cup kibble
   o 67 kcal/can×2 = 134 kcal can per day
4) MER − kcal diet 1 = Remaining MER kcals
   i) Example 1: MER of 1200 kcal/day with 397 kcal/can feeding ¼ can per day, and 265 kcal/cup kibble
   1200 kcal/day − 99.25 kcal can = 1100.75 kcal Remaining MER kcal
   ii) Example 2: MER 342 kcal/day with 67 kcal/can feeding 2 cans per day, and 501 kcal/cup kibble
   342 kcal/day − 134 kcal can = 208 Remaining MER kcal
5) Remaining MER kcal ÷ kcal per cup (can) diet 2 = kcal to be fed diet 2
   i) Example 1: MER of 1200 kcal/day with 397 kcal/can feeding ¼ can per day, and 265 kcal/cup kibble
   1100.75 kcal/day ÷ 265 = 4.15 cup kibble per day
   ii) Example 2: MER 342 kcal/day with 67 kcal/can feeding 2 cans per day, and 501 kcal/cup kibble
   208 kcal/day ÷ 501 kcal/cup = 0.42 cup kibble per day

## 25.3 Calculating kcal per day by Weight (grams)

When weighing portions for diet control, you will need to calculate the grams to be fed per day or per meal. For this calculation, you will use metabolizable energy (ME) [4].

kcal required/day ÷ kcal/kg×1000 = gram/day

# 25.4 Calculating Calories from Nutrients and Metabolizable Energy

The guaranteed analysis can help us calculate how many calories are coming from proteins, fats, or carbohydrates otherwise known as nitrogen-free extract (NFE) [4]. This may be a beneficial calculation when pet parents want to compare diets when product guides are unavailable. Each nutrient (protein, fat, and carbohydrate) provides a set amount of kcal/g with protein = 3.5 kcal/g, carbohydrates providing 3.5 kcal/g, and fat providing the most energy-dense calories per gram at 8.5 kcal/g [4].

## 25.4.1 Calculating NFE

The guaranteed analysis does not include simple carbohydrates or NFE. To calculate this amount, you will start at 100% (the total volume of nutrients in the diet) and subtract the percentages of protein, fat, fiber, moisture, and ash. The ash content is not routinely noted and can be estimated to be 2.5% for canned diets and 8% for kibble [4].

NFE = 100 – % crude protein – % crude fat – % crude fiber – % moisture – % ash
(ash = 2.5% for canned diets and 8% for kibble) [2]

## 25.4.2 Calculating % of kcals from the Macronutrients

To calculate the kcals provided from the main nutrients, you will multiply the percentage of nutrient content from the guaranteed analysis by the energy factor for the nutrient [4].

Protein = 3.5 kcal/g × % crude protein
Fat = 8.5 kcal/g × % crude fat
Carbohydrate (NFE) = 3.5 kcal/g × % crude NFE

## 25.4.3 Calculating Metabolizable Energy

Metabolizable energy (ME) is the amount of energy that is available to the tissue for use. It is represented in kcal/kg and is the value most often used to express the energy content in pet foods [2] Some diets do not list the kcal/kg or kcal/cup on the bag of food, which leaves the guaranteed analysis, and a few simple calculations to determine calorie content in the diet [2].

ME kcal/kg = 10[(8.5 kcal/g×% crude fat)+(3.5 kcal/g×% crude protein)+(3.5 kcal/g×% crude NFE)

## 25.5 Calculating Percentage of Body Weight Loss

A patient that loses more than 5% body weight in a short time should indicate to the veterinary staff a possible early indicator of a health concern with a 10% unanticipated body weight loss indicating cachexia where general guidelines for initiating nutritional support [2, 3]. Calculating the percentage of weight loss change, especially in a cat or small breed dog, can be a diagnostic tool. For example, a cat that weighed 4.5 kg (9.9 lbs) 1 month ago has a current weight of 4.2 kg (9.24 lbs), which equals a 6.7% weight loss. Had this calculation not been completed, it may not be obvious that the pet is losing a possibly significant amount of weight, which may indicate the necessity for further diagnostics or at minimum to monitor this pet's weight [4].

%BW Δ = (Previous BW − current BW) ÷ previous BW × 100

## 25.6 Calculating Energy Requirements for a Critical Care Patient

When a patient has been hyporexic or anorexic for an extended time (3 days or longer), it is beneficial to start energy requirements at 25–50% RER to ensure we do not instigate a metabolic derangement such as refeeding syndrome [2]. Refeeding syndrome refers to the metabolic alterations that occur after nutritional support is started in a severely malnourished, underweight, and/or starved patient [2]. Starting with a reduced amount of the required RER and increasing slowly over 3–7 days, we decrease the risk of inducing metabolic, glucose, and electrolyte imbalances in the patient [2]. A critical care patient can then be maintained on its RER during its stay in the critical care department. Once the patient is no longer critical, the energy requirements can be calculated based on energy factors and weight management.

## 25.7 Calculating Water Requirements

Water requirements are related to maintaining water balance. Body water lost by urination, defecation, evaporation, and perspiration are replaced by one of two sources:

1) water derived from the metabolism of nutrients
2) water that is consumed as a liquid or as a portion of the food [3].

## 25.8 Calculating Metabolic Water

Metabolic water can account for 5–10% of the total water requirement with an average of 13 ml produce per 100 kcal of ME ingested [4]. Oxidation of macronutrients will result in varying amounts of water. One gram of oxidized fat will result in 1.071 g of metabolic water, 1 g of glucose results in 0.556 g of metabolic water, and 1 g of protein results in 0.396 g of metabolic water [2]. We can calculate the daily water requirements by multiplying RER × 1.6 for dogs and RER × 1.2 for cats [2].

## 25.9 Feeding and Transition Plan Formulations

Once you have determined the volume of food to be fed each day, you can calculate the volume to be fed per meal. The number of meals per day may be determined by:

1) The life stage of the pet.
2) The health status of the pet.
3) The type of disease processes the pet may be experiencing.
4) The volume of food required – increased number of meals for larger daily volume requirements.
5) Preference of the pet parent.

### 25.9.1 Calculating Meals by kcal per Meal [2]

- kcal/day ÷ # of meals per day = kcal per meal

### 25.9.2 Calculating Meals by Volume per Meal [2]

- The volume of food per day (g) ÷ # of meals per day = volume (g) per meal

## 25.10   Creating a Feeding Plan

Creating a feeding plan for a pet may include general guidelines for a transition plan from the previous diet to the current diet, or an immediate transition. An immediate transition plan is ideal if the previous diet is no longer appropriate, the pet is in a hyporexic or anorexic state for more than 3 days, or the previous diet is unavailable to complete a general transition [2, 3]. An immediate transition plan should start at a lower energy requirement provided in multiple small meals. This format provides a reduced risk of GI upset or dysbiosis, which can occur when there is an immediate diet transition without caloric restriction. Dysbiosis and GI upset can occur due to a lack of digestive enzymes in the small intestine to fully complete nutrient absorption, resulting in an excess of undigested nutrients being fermented and altering growth, and metabolite production by the GI microbiome.

### 25.10.1   General Guidelines for Diet Transitions [4]

|  | DAY 1 | DAY 2 | DAY 3 | DAY 4 | DAY 5 | DAY 6 | DAY 7 |
| --- | --- | --- | --- | --- | --- | --- | --- |
| Previous diet | 90% | 75% | 50% | 50% | 25% | 10% | — |
| New diet | 10% | 25% | 50% | 50% | 75% | 90% | 100% |

### 25.10.2   Immediate Diet Transition (For Critical Care and Initial Calorie Restricted Diet Changes) [4]

- Day 1 – feed 50% RER divided into 4–6 meals
- Day 2 – feed 75% RER divided into 4–6 meals
- Day 3 – feed RER divided into 4 meals
- Days 4 and 5 – feed 25% (MER-RER) + RER divided into 3–4 meals
- Days 6 and 7 – feed 50% (MER–RER) + RER divided into 3–4 meals
- Days 8 and 9 – feed 75% (MER–RER) + RER divided into 2–3 meals
- Days 10–14 – feed MER divided into 2–3 meals

## 25.11   Chapter Summary

- Resting energy requirements (RER) – RER = $BW^{0.75} \times 70$
  Example: A dog weighs 18.6 kg RER = $18.6^{0.75} \times 70 = 626.94977$
  (627 kcal/day)

- Maintenance energy requirements (MER) – RER × Energy Factor
  The factor used depends on the energy requirements for the pet (0.8–2 or greater).
- Growth
  - (*Simple*) – RER × 3.0 (up to 16 weeks of age) or RER × 2.0 (>14 weeks of age)
  - (Calculation based on estimated adult weight [2])
    - Dogs 130 × BWc0.75 × 3.2 (2.71828 − 0.87 (BWc ÷ BWe) − 0.1)
    - Cats 100 × BWc 0.67 × 6.7 (2.71828 − 0.189 [BWc ÷ BWe] − 0.66)
- Calculation for pregnancy
  - Bitches: $130 \times BW^{0.75} + (26 \times BW)$
  - Queens: $140 \times BW^{0.67}$
- Calculation for lactation
  - Depends on the number and age of neonates in the litter
- Calculating kcal/cup or can from energy requirement
  - MER ÷ kcal per cup (can) = volume to be fed per day.
- Calculating kcal per day by weight
  - kcal required/day ÷ kcal/kg × 1000 = gram/day
- Calculating metabolizable energy
  - Calculate carbohydrates (nitrogen-free extracts – NFE)
    - NFE = 100 – % crude protein – % crude fat – % crude fiber – % moisture – % ash (Ash = 2.5% for canned diets and 8% for kibble) [2]
    - ME kcal/kg = 10[(8.5 kcal/g × % crude fat) + (3.5 kcal/g × % crude protein) + (3.5 kcal/g × % crude NFE)]
- Calculating percentage of body weight change
  - %BW Δ = (Previous BW – current BW) ÷ previous BW × 100
- Calculate for critical care patient
  - Day 1 – feed 50% RER divided into 4–6 meals
  - Day 2 – feed 75% RER divided into 4–6 meals
  - Day 3 – feed RER divided into 4 meals
  - Days 4 and 5 – feed 25% (MER-RER) + RER divided into 3–4 meals
  - Days 6 and 7 – feed 50% (MER-RER) + RER divided into 3–4 meals
  - Days 8 and 9 – feed 75% (MER–RER) + RER divided into 2–3 meals
  - Days 10–14 – feed MER divided into 2–3 meals
- Calculate water requirements
  - Dogs – RER × 1.6
  - Cats – RER × 1.2

- Moisture in the diet
  - % moisture × gram in can
- Metabolic water – One gram of oxidized fat will result is 1.071 g of metabolic water, 1 g of glucose results in 0.556 g metabolic water, and 1 g of protein results in 0.396 g of metabolic water

## References

**1** WSAVA Global nutrition guidelines. https://wsava.org/global-guidelines/global-nutrition-guidelines (accessed 14 April 2022).

**2** Wortinger, A. and Burns, K.M. (2015). Energy balance; nutrition calculations; assisted feeding in dogs and cats; cancer. In: *Nutrition and Disease Management for Veterinary Technicians and Nurses*, 2e (ed. A. Wortinger and K.M. Burns), 42–54. Wiley.

**3** Hand, M.S., Thatcher, C.D., Remillard, R.L. et al. (2010). Macronutrients. In: *Small Animal Clinical Nutrition*, 5e (ed. M.S. Hand et al.), 52. Mark Morris Institute.

**4** Delaney, S.J. and Fascetti, A.J. (2012). Basic nutrition overview. In: *Applied Veterinary Clinical Nutrition* (ed. A.J. Fascetti and S.J. Delaney), 9–22. Wiley.

# Index

*Small Animal Microbiomes and Nutrition*, First Edition. Robin Saar and Sarah Dodd.
© 2024 John Wiley & Sons, Inc. Published 2024 by John Wiley & Sons, Inc.
Companion website: www.wiley.com/go/saar/1e